Straight A's
in
Psychiatric &
Mental Health
Nursing

Straight A's
in
Psychiatric & Mental Health Nursing

LIPPINCOTT WILLIAMS & WILKINS
A **Wolters Kluwer** Company

Philadelphia • Baltimore • New York • London
Buenos Aires • Hong Kong • Sydney • Tokyo

STAFF

Executive Publisher
Judith A. Schilling McCann, RN, MSN

Senior Acquisitions Editor
Elizabeth Nieginski

Editorial Director
David Moreau

Clinical Director
Joan M. Robinson, RN, MSN

Senior Art Director
Arlene Putterman

Editorial Project Manager
Tracy S. Diehl

Clinical Project Manager
Beverly Ann Tscheschlog, RN, BS

Editors
Dave Beverage, Laura Bruck,
Karen C. Comerford, Diane Labus,
Brenna H. Mayer

Clinical Editor
Maryann Foley, RN, BSN

Copy Editors
Kimberly Bilotta (supervisor),
Heather Ditch, Shana Harrington,
Danielle Michaely, Kelly Pavlovsky,
Pamela Wingrod

Designers
Jan Greenberg (project manager),
Lynn Foulk

Digital Composition Services
Diane Paluba (manager),
Joyce Rossi Biletz, Donna S. Morris

Manufacturing
Patricia K. Dorshaw (director),
Beth J. Welsh

Editorial Assistants
Megan L. Aldinger, Karen J. Kirk,
Linda K. Ruhf

Indexer
Karen C. Comerford

STRPMH011105—020907

**Library of Congress
Cataloging-in-Publication Data**

Straight A's in psychiatric and mental health nursing.
    p. ; cm.
    Includes bibliographical references and index.
    1. Psychiatric nursing—Outlines, syllabi, etc. 2. Psychiatric nursing—Examinations, questions, etc. I. Lippincott Williams & Wilkins.
    [DNLM: 1. Psychiatric Nursing—Examination Questions. WY 18.2 S8966 2006]
RC440.S772 2006
616.89'0231'076—dc22
ISBN13: 978-1-58255-448-8
ISBN10: 1-58255-448-X (alk. paper)   2005022019

Contents

Advisory board   vi

Contributors and consultants   vii

How to use this book   ix

Foreword   x

1   Introduction to psychiatric nursing   1

2   Disorders of children and adolescents   39

3   Disorders of elderly people   65

4   Schizophrenic disorders   92

5   Mood disorders   117

6   Anxiety disorders   142

7   Somatoform disorders   173

8   Dissociative disorders   203

9   Personality disorders   219

10   Eating disorders   257

11   Substance abuse disorders   272

12   Sexual disorders   323

NANDA nursing diagnoses   350

Glossary   353

Selected references   357

Index   359

Advisory board

Ivy Alexander, PhD, CANP
Assistant Professor, Yale University
New Haven, Conn.

Susan E. Appling, RN, MS, CRNP
Assistant Professor, Johns Hopkins University School of Nursing
Baltimore

Paul M. Arnstein, PhD, APRN-BC, FNP-C
Assistant Professor, Boston College

Bobbie Berkowitz, PhD, CNAA, FAAN
Chair & Professor, Psychosocial & Community Health; University
    of Washington
Seattle

Karla Jones, RN, MSN
Nursing Faculty, Treasure Valley Community College
Ontario, Ore.

Manon Lemonde, RN, PhD
Associate Professor, University of Ontario (Oshawa) Institute of Technology

Sheila Sparks Ralph, DNSC, RN, FAAN
Director & Professor, Division of Nursing & Respiratory Care; Shenandoah
    University
Winchester, Va.

Kristine Anne Scordo, PhD, RN, CS, ACNP
Director, Acute Care Nurse Practitioner Program; Wright State University
Dayton, Ohio

Robin Wilkerson, PhD, RN,BC
Associate Professor, University of Mississippi
Jackson

Contributors and consultants

Noreen R. Brady, RN, PhD, CNS, LPCC
Assistant Professor of Nursing
Director, Sarah Cole Institute for Best Nursing Practices Based on Evidence
Frances Payne Bolton School of Nursing
Case Western Reserve University
Cleveland

Wendy Tagan Conroy, RN, MSN, FNP, BC
Nurse Practitioner
City of Portland (Maine) Public Health Department

Linda Carman Copel, RN, PhD, CS, DAPA
Associate Professor
Villanova (Pa.) University College of Nursing

Anne H. Fishel, APRN, BC, PhD
Professor
University of North Carolina
Chapel Hill

James Johnson, RN, BSN
Nurse Manager
University of Pennsylvania Health System
Presbyterian Medical System
Philadelphia

David C. Keller, APRN, MS
Assistant Professor
Utah Valley State College
Orem

Cheryl Laskowski, APRN, DNS, CS
Assistant Professor of Nursing
University of Vermont
Burlington

Marilyn Little, APRN,BC, MS
Professor
Salt Lake Community College
Salt Lake City

Barbara Maxwell, RNC, MSN
Assistant Professor of Nursing
State University of New York–Ulster
Stone Ridge

Barbara Scheirer, RN, BS, MSN
Assistant Professor
Grambling (La.) State University

Kathleen R. Tusaie, APRN-BC, PhD
Assistant Professor
The University of Akron (Ohio) College of Nursing

Mary E. Weyer, RN, EdD, APN, CS
Associate Professor
Deicke Center for Nursing Education
Elmhurst (Ill.) College

Nancy Wood, RN, MSN
Instructor of Nursing
Maysville (Ky.) Community and Technical College

Rick Zoucha, APRN,BC, DNS, CTN
Associate Professor
Duquesne University School of Nursing
Pittsburgh

How to use this book

Straight A's is a multivolume study guide series developed especially for nursing students. Each volume provides essential course material in a unique two-column design. The easy-to-read interior outline format offers a succinct review of key facts as presented in leading textbooks on the subject. The bulleted exterior columns provide only the most crucial information, allowing for quick, efficient review right before an important quiz or test.

Special features appear in every chapter to make information accessible and easy to remember. **Learning objectives** encourage the student to evaluate knowledge before and after study. **Chapter overview** highlights the chapter's major concepts. Within the outlined text, color is used to highlight critical information and key points. Key points may include cardinal signs and symptoms, current theories, important steps in a nursing procedure, critical assessment findings, crucial nursing interventions, or successful therapies and treatments. **NCLEX® checks** at the end of each chapter offer additional opportunities to review material and assess knowledge gained before moving on to new information.

Other features appear throughout the book to facilitate learning. **Time-out for teaching** highlights key areas to address when teaching patients. **Clinical alerts**, which appear in color throughout the book, point out essential information on how to provide safe, effective care. Lastly, a brand-new Windows-based software program (see CD-ROM on inside back cover) poses more than 250 multiple-choice and alternate-format NCLEX-style questions in random or sequential order to assess your knowledge.

The *Straight A's* volumes are designed as learning tools, not as primary information sources. When read conscientiously as a supplement to class attendance and textbook reading, *Straight A's* can enhance understanding and help improve test scores and final grades.

Foreword

I met James in the hospital after his third near-fatal suicide attempt. Although he was young and in the midst of his third year of medical school, he was deeply hopeless and felt he had nothing to live for. I was a new graduate nurse and felt I had everything to live for. Consequently, his surrender to bipolar disorder puzzled me.

Several years of working with a dedicated team of providers helped James develop a life that included a successful medical practice, a partner, a home, and children. Later, as an advanced practice nurse with a private psychotherapy practice, I provided family therapy for James. I learned that in James' complex world of chronic symptoms and lifelong treatment, the notion of hope was an essential intervention that helped him choose life instead of death.

Hope is a powerful emotion. In today's psychiatric and mental health nursing world, we know so much more about the complex factors that affect behavior, motivation, perception, thinking, and emotion. We can integrate knowledge of physiological, genetic, hormonal, neurobiological, and environmental factors into our existing interventions to help our patients cope with their mental health challenges and achieve full lives.

However, with all we now know about psychiatric disorders, it's crucial to stay up-to-date on current facts. *Straight A's in Psychiatric & Mental Health Nursing* provides quick and direct access to the most recent information about major mental disorders. Organized by the categories of the *Diagnostic and Statistical Manual for Mental Disorders,* Fourth Edition, Text Revision, each chapter begins with an overview of the major features of each disorder, theories of origin, and challenges to overcome.

The book provides highlighted points that summarize such topics as major disorders, defining characteristics, signs and symptoms, and diagnostic testing.

In addition to the simple outline format in the main text, this book offers students the option of going straight to the most critical facts or doing a more thorough review. Students will find the book's text useful because each section summarizes key information, including nursing interventions and treatments.

The outer columns of *Straight A's in Psychiatric & Mental Health Nursing* feature main points every psych student should use to brush up on key topics or study right before a quiz or exam. In addition, students can prepare for their licensing examination by testing themselves with the NCLEX® questions at the end of each chapter or with the CD-ROM in the back of the book, which contains more than 250 traditional and alternate-format questions.

In addition to student nurses, practicing nurses in any clinical setting will find this text useful as a ready-reference. Increasingly, patients with depression, anxiety, dementias, and somatoform and eating disorders seek help in primary care and general medical settings. This text will assist in making a correct diagnosis and referrals for patients with primary mental health challenges.

It's an exciting time for psychiatric and mental health nursing. As our understanding of the issues creates accessible therapies, nurses will continue to be the ones who help patients integrate these therapies into their lives. *Straight A's in Psychiatric & Mental Health Nursing* can provide you with the knowledge you need to help treat psychiatric patients — even those with the most severe and persistent mental disorders. Then, maybe these patients can learn to live full, successful, hopeful lives.

Linda S. Beeber, APRN,BC, PhD
Professor
The University of North Carolina
at Chapel Hill
School of Nursing

1

Introduction to psychiatric nursing

LEARNING OBJECTIVES

After studying this chapter, you should be able to:

- Identify the nurse's role in psychiatric care.
- Describe the phases of the therapeutic relationship.
- Discuss ways to enhance communication with patients.
- Identify therapies used to treat psychiatric disorders.
- Explain the components of the psychiatric nursing assessment.
- List the members of the multidisciplinary care team.
- Discuss the ethical and legal issues in psychiatric care.

CHAPTER OVERVIEW

Patients with mental illness and emotional problems can be found in any clinical setting. It isn't surprising that, at some point in their career, nurses will find themselves caring for someone with depression, anxiety, a thought disorder, dementia, or some other commonly encountered psychiatric problem.

Providing effective, therapeutic nursing care requires careful consideration of the psychological and physiologic aspects of health, as many medical conditions are linked to—or lead to—emotional and mental distress. Recognizing emotional problems and how they affect the patient's overall health is crucial to psychiatric nursing.

Advances in mental health field

- Neurobiological
- Research and technology
- Increased number and diversity of programs available
- Increased media attention
- Increased focus on holistic health
- Consumer involvement
- Sociologic studies

CHANGING THE MENTAL HEALTH PERSPECTIVE

● **Dramatic changes in mental health field**
- Health care professionals' knowledge about mental health and its link to physical health has grown tremendously, mainly due to scientific research and technological advances
  - Neurobiological advances: revolutionized our understanding of the physiologic factors affecting mental functioning and emotional states
  - Research and technology: provided improved diagnosis and treatment of psychiatric disorders (especially in the realm of drug therapy for acute disorders)
- The increased number and diversity of mental health programs available to individuals has lead to better awareness of mental illness and more opportunities to seek and obtain help
  - Community mental health programs: include family advocacy programs, substance abuse rehabilitation programs, stress-management workshops, bereavement groups, victim assistance programs, and domestic violence shelters
  - Public education systems: offer classes and disperse information on mental health issues
- Increased media attention has provided an open forum for discussion of mental health issues
  - Numerous publications on self-help and coping
  - Television's standardized coverage of mental health topics
- Increased focus on holistic health has resulted in closer ties between psychiatry and medicine
- Consumer involvement in mental health programs has paved the way for increases in psychiatric consultation and hospitalization coverage
- Sociologic studies and other research have identified significant changes contributing to the increased incidence of mental and emotional disorders
  - Alteration in the traditional family structure: contributes to the loss of extended family and greater numbers of single parents, dysfunctional families, troubled children, and homeless people
  - Loss of effective support systems: contributes to strained ability to cope with problems (see *Links between stress and disease*)
- Identification of ongoing social problems and trends in mental illness has helped target high-risk populations and has helped illustrate the need for better prevention and effective interventions
  - Teenage depression and suicide: rate has more than tripled in the past 20 years
  - Alcohol and substance abuse: continues to rise and includes an alarming number of children and young adults
  - Depression among elderly persons: commonly suffer from isolation, loneliness, and fear of violent crime

Links between stress and disease

Hans Selye, a pioneer in stress research, found a link between the environment and biological response. He noted that emotional and physical stress cause a pattern of responses that, unless treated, lead to infection, illness, disease and, eventually, even death. Selye called this set of responses the *general adaptation syndrome* and identified three stages – alarm reaction, resistance, and exhaustion.

ALARM REACTION
During this stage, any type of physical or mental trauma triggers immediate biological responses designed to counter the stress. These responses depress the immune system, which lowers resistance and makes the person more susceptible to infection and disease. Unless the stress is severe or prolonged, though, the person recovers rapidly.

RESISTANCE
This stage begins when the body starts to adapt to prolonged stress. The immune system shifts into high gear to meet increased demands. At this point, the person becomes more resistant to illness.

However, the perception of a threat lingers, so the body never reaches complete physiologic equilibrium. Instead, it stays aroused, which places stress on body organs and systems.

Because adaptation appears to work initially, a person in the resistance stage may become complacent and assume he's immune to the effects of stress – and thus fail to take steps to relieve it.

EXHAUSTION
With chronic stress, adaptive mechanisms eventually wear down, and the body can no longer meet its increased demands. Immunity and resistance decline dramatically, and illness is likely to set in. The point at which exhaustion occurs differs among individuals.

INTERRUPTING THE STRESS RESPONSE
Selye laid the groundwork for the use of relaxation techniques in interrupting the stress response, thereby reducing susceptibility to illness and disease.

3 stages of general adaptation syndrome
- Alarm reaction
- Resistance
- Exhaustion

Classification of mental disorders
- The current classification of psychiatric and mental disorders used by health providers and insurance carriers was developed by the American Psychiatric Association (APA); its widespread use has lead to better patient diagnosis and communication among the health care community
- The APA published the *Diagnostic and Statistical Manual of Mental Disorders, Fourth Edition, Text Revision* (*DSM-IV-TR*) in 2000 (see *Understanding the DSM-IV-TR*, page 4)

Mental disorder classification
- APA's *DSM-IV-TR*; developed in 2000
- Used by health providers and insurance carriers

- Axis I: Clinical disorders
- Axis II: Personality disorders and mental retardation
- Axis III: General medical conditions
- Axis IV: Psychosocial and environmental problems
- Axis V: GAF

Understanding the *DSM-IV-TR*

The American Psychiatric Association's *Diagnostic and Statistical Manual of Mental Disorders,* Fourth Edition, Text Revision *(DSM-IV-TR)* defines a mental disorder as a clinically significant behavioral or psychological syndrome or pattern associated with at least one of these criteria:
- current distress (a painful symptom)
- disability (an impairment in one or more important areas of functioning)
- a significantly greater risk of suffering, death, pain, and disability
- an important loss of freedom.

The syndrome or pattern must not be merely an expected, culturally sanctioned response – such as grief over the death of a loved one. Whatever its original cause, it must currently be considered a sign of behavioral, psychological, or biological dysfunction.

FIVE AXES
For greater diagnostic detail, the *DSM-IV-TR* uses a multiaxial approach, which specifies that every patient be evaluated on each of five axes.
- *Axis I: Clinical disorders* – mental disorders comparable to general medical illnesses

- *Axis II: Personality disorders and mental retardation* – personality disorders and traits as well as mental retardation
- *Axis III: General medical conditions* – general medical illnesses or injuries
- *Axis IV: Psychosocial and environmental problems* – life events or problems that may affect diagnosis, treatment, and prognosis of the mental disorder
- *Axis V: Global assessment of functioning (GAF)* – level of functioning, reported as a number from 0 to 100 based on the patient's overall psychological, social, and occupational function.

MULTIAXIAL DIAGNOSIS
After being evaluated on these five axes, a patient's diagnosis may look like this example:
- Axis I: adjustment disorder with anxious mood
- Axis II: obsessive-compulsive personality
- Axis III: Crohn's disease, acute bleeding episodes
- Axis IV: recent remarriage, death of father
- Axis V: GAF = 83.

ROLE OF PSYCHIATRIC NURSES

● **Overview**
- The American Nurses Association (ANA) considers psychiatric nursing a specialized area of nursing practice — one that's based on theories of human behavior as its science and the "therapeutic use of self" as its art
- The National Institute of Mental Health recognizes psychiatric nursing as a core mental health discipline
- The nurse's role in helping emotionally troubled patients has grown considerably; she has many new roles
  - Carries out the traditional task of administering prescribed drugs and monitoring drug effects
  - Acts as the primary therapist or directs behavior therapies in some cases
  - Uses an interpersonal approach to promote, maintain, restore, and rehabilitate individual, family, and community mental health and functioning

– Draws on the psychosocial and biophysical sciences as well as theories of personality and human behavior when providing care
- The nurse's clients may include individuals, families, groups, or communities, depending on the setting and type of practice
    – Common settings: psychiatric hospitals, community mental health centers, general hospitals, community health agencies, outpatient clinics, homes, schools, and prisons
    – Types of practice: health maintenance organizations, primary care practices, private practices, crisis units, and industrial centers
- The nurse may assume one or more roles in a practice setting
    – Staff nurse
    – Liaison between patient and other health care team members
    – Administrator
    – Consultant
    – In-service educator
    – Clinical practitioner
    – Researcher
    – Program evaluator
- To provide effective, therapeutic care, psychiatric nurses must possess and demonstrate necessary skills
    – Practical, orderly way of dealing with people who have diverse and complex problems
    – Ability to plan, implement, and evaluate care
    – Ability to establish a meaningful therapeutic relationship with patients
    – Self-awareness of attitudes and feelings

Scope of practice
- The level at which psychiatric nurses practice is determined by various factors, including nurse practice acts, professional boards and standards, and the nurse's self-motivation
- Nurse practice acts regulate entry into the profession and define the legal limits of nursing practice; the nurse is responsible for knowing her state's regulations
    – Advanced practice: requirements usually addressed by state nurse practice act; may need second licensure at advanced level
    – Authority to write prescriptions: may be granted to advanced-degree nurses; varies from state to state
- Professional practice standards define nursing practice and performance; first developed by the ANA in 1973, they were most recently revised in 2000 (see *ANA standards of care for psychiatric and mental health nursing,* pages 6 and 7)
- Psychiatric nurses may practice as either generalists or specialists, depending on their education and experience
- Psychiatric nurses may be certified by professional organizations
    – ANA certification: requires a formal review, including a written test
    – Certification credentials: include psychiatric nurse generalist, psychiatric clinical nurse specialist, and psychiatric nurse practitioner
- A health care organization's philosophy of mental health and mental illness — and its approach toward treatment — help shape the expectations of both the nurse and patient
- The psychiatric nurse's level of performance is greatly influenced by many factors

(Text continues on page 10.)

Key facts about the role of the psychiatric nurse

Common settings
- Psychiatric hospitals
- Community mental health centers
- General hospitals
- Community health agencies
- Outpatient clinics
- Homes
- Schools
- Prisons

Types of practice
- Health maintenance organizations
- Primary care practices
- Private practices
- Crisis units
- Industrial centers

Scope of practice for psychiatric nurses

- Nurse practice acts regulate entry into profession and define legal limits.
- Nurse must know her state's regulations.
- Professional practice standards define nursing practice and performance.
- Nurse may practice as generalist or specialist.
- Nurse may be certified by professional organizations.

ANA standards of care for psychiatric and mental health nursing

In 1973, the American Nurses Association (ANA) issued standards designed to improve the quality of care provided by psychiatric and mental health nurses. Last revised in 2000, these standards apply to generalists and specialists working in any setting in which psychiatric and mental health nursing is practiced.

Listed below are these standards of care and standards of professional performance, along with rationales. *Note:* Standards Vh through Vj apply only to the advanced practice registered nurse in psychiatric and mental health (APRN-PMH) specialist.

ANA standards of care for psychiatric and mental health nursing

- Standard I: Assessment
- Standard II: Diagnosis
- Standard III: Outcome identification
- Standard IV: Planning
- Standard V: Implementation
- Standard VI: Evaluation

STANDARDS OF CARE

Standards of care pertain to professional nursing activities demonstrated through the nursing process. These standards encompass assessment, diagnosis, outcome identification, planning, implementation, and evaluation.

The nursing process is the foundation of clinical decision making and encompasses all significant action taken by nurses in providing psychiatric and mental health care to all patients.

Standard I: Assessment

The nurse collects patient health data.

Rationale: The assessment interview — which requires linguistically and culturally effective communication skills, interviewing, behavioral observation, database record review, and comprehensive assessment of the patient and relevant systems — enables the psychiatric and mental health nurse to make sound clinical judgments and plan appropriate interventions.

Standard II: Diagnosis

The nurse analyzes assessment data to determine applicable diagnoses.

Rationale: The basis for providing psychiatric and mental health nursing care is recognizing and identifying patterns of response to actual or potential psychiatric illnesses, mental health problems, and potential comorbid physical illnesses.

Standard III: Outcome identification

The nurse identifies expected outcomes individualized for the patient.

Rationale: Within the context of providing nursing care, the ultimate goal is to influence health outcomes and improve the patient's health status.

Standard IV: Planning

The nurse develops a care plan that's negotiated among the patient, nurse, family and significant others, and health care team. The plan prescribes evidence-based interventions to attain expected outcomes.

Rationale: A care plan is used to guide therapeutic intervention, systematically document progress, and achieve expected patient outcomes.

Standard V: Implementation

The nurse implements the interventions identified in the care plan.

Rationale: Nurses use a wide range of interventions designed to prevent mental and physical illness and to promote, maintain, and restore mental and physical health. They select interventions according to their practice level. At the basic level, nurses may select counseling, milieu therapy, self-care activities, psychobiological interventions, health teaching, case management, health promotion and maintenance, crisis intervention, community-based care, psychiatric home health care, telehealth, and various other approaches to meet the patient's mental health needs.

ANA standards of care for psychiatric and mental health nursing (continued)

In addition to the interventions available to the basic-level psychiatric and mental health nurse, the APRN-PMH may provide consultation, engage in psychotherapy, and prescribe pharmacologic agents where permitted by state statutes or regulations.

STANDARD Va: COUNSELING

The nurse uses counseling interventions to assist patients in improving or regaining their previous coping abilities, fostering mental health, and preventing mental illness and disability.

STANDARD Vb: MILIEU THERAPY

The nurse provides, structures, and maintains a therapeutic environment in collaboration with the patient and other health care providers.

STANDARD Vc: PROMOTION OF SELF-CARE ACTIVITIES

The nurse structures interventions around the patient's activities of daily living to foster self-care and mental and physical well-being.

STANDARD Vd: PSYCHOBIOLOGICAL INTERVENTIONS

The nurse uses knowledge of psychobiological interventions and applies clinical skills to restore the patient's health and prevent further disability.

STANDARD Ve: HEALTH TEACHING

Through health teaching, the nurse assists patients in achieving satisfying, productive, and healthy patterns of living.

STANDARD Vf: CASE MANAGEMENT

The nurse provides case management to coordinate comprehensive health services and ensure continuity of care.

STANDARD Vg: HEALTH PROMOTION AND HEALTH MAINTENANCE

The nurse uses strategies and interventions to promote and maintain mental health and prevent mental illness.

Standard VI: Evaluation

The nurse evaluates the patient's progress in attaining expected outcomes.

Rationale: Nursing care is a dynamic process involving change in the patient's health status over time, giving rise to the need for new data, different diagnoses, and modifications in the care plan. Therefore, evaluation is a continuous process of appraising the effect of nursing and treatment regimens on the patient's health status and expected outcomes.

ADVANCED PRACTICE INTERVENTIONS

The following interventions may be performed only by the APRN-PMH.

Standard Vh: Psychotherapy

The APRN-PMH uses individual, group, and family psychotherapy and other treatments to assist patients in preventing mental illness and disability, treating mental health disorders, and improving mental health status and functional abilities.

Standard Vi: Prescriptive authority and treatment

The APRN-PMH uses prescriptive authority, procedures, and treatments in accordance with state and federal laws and regulations to treat symptoms of psychiatric illness and improve functional health status.

Standard Vj: Consultation

The APRN-PMH provides consultation to enhance the abilities of other clinicians, provide services for patients, and effect change in the system.

ANA standards of care for psychiatric and mental health nursing

Standard V interventions
- Standard Va: Counseling
- Standard Vb: Milieu therapy
- Standard Vc: Promotion of self-care activities
- Standard Vd: Psychobiological interventions
- Standard Ve: Health teaching
- Standard Vf: Case management
- Standard Vg: Health promotion and health maintenance

ANA advanced practice interventions

- Standard Vh: Psychotherapy
- Standard Vi: Prescriptive authority and treatment
- Standard Vj: Consultation

Theoretical models of behavior

- Attempt to explain how human behavior and other factors affect mental health
- Psychoanalytic model (Freud)
- Interpersonal model (Sullivan, Peplau)
- Social model (Caplan, Szasz)
- Existential model (Frankl, Perls, May)
- Nursing model (Rogers, Orem, Sister Roy, Peplau)
- Medical model
- Communication models (Berne, Bandler, Grindler)
- Behavioral model (Skinner, Wolpe, Eysenck)
- Humanistic model (Maslow)

Theoretical models of behavior

Learning about the various models of human behavior gives you a better understanding of psychiatric disorders. These models are summarized below.

Remember, though, that human behavior isn't fully understood, so no model or theory is considered right or wrong or better or worse than any other. Commonly, psychiatric and mental health nurses use an eclectic approach, drawing on several theoretical models.

PSYCHOANALYTIC MODEL (FREUD)

According to the psychoanalytic model, the personality consists of the:
- *id,* encompassing the primitive instincts and energies underlying all psychic activity
- *ego,* the conscious part of the personality, and the part that most immediately controls thought and behavior
- *superego,* the conscience.

During childhood, development occurs in five psychosexual stages — oral, anal, phallic, latency, and genital. Deviations in behavior result from unsuccessful task accomplishment during earlier developmental stages. Freud also proposed that behavior is motivated by anxiety, the cornerstone of psychopathology.

Understanding the psychosexual stages of childhood provides a framework for the nurse to understand adult behaviors. Also, the nurse can promote effective parenting by teaching parents about the child's needs during each psychosexual stage.

INTERPERSONAL MODEL (SULLIVAN, PEPLAU)

The interpersonal model holds that human development results from interpersonal relationships, and that behavior is motivated by avoidance of anxiety and attainment of satisfaction.

Peplau drew on Sullivan's original theory to propose an interpersonal nursing theory, which advanced the practice of psychiatric nursing by defining it as an interpersonal process. She proposed that:
- nurses must promote the nurse-patient relationship to build trust and foster healthy behavior
- therapeutic use of self promotes healing
- the therapeutic relationship is directed toward meeting the patient's needs.

SOCIAL MODEL (CAPLAN, SZASZ)

The social model proposes that the entire sociocultural environment influences mental health. Deviant behavior is defined by the culture in which a person lives. Undesirable or abnormal behavior in one society may be considered normal in another. In addition, social conditions and interactions predispose people to mental illness.

EXISTENTIAL MODEL (FRANKL, PERLS, MAY)

The existential model centers on a person's present experiences rather than his past ones. It holds that alienation from the self causes deviant behavior, and that people can make free choices about which behaviors to display.

Based on the existential model of behavior, nursing developed the concept that the nurse works to restore the patient to a state of "full life" from a state of "self-alienation."

NURSING MODEL (ROGERS, OREM, SISTER ROY, PEPLAU)

The nursing model emphasizes the person as a biopsychosocial being. This holistic approach focuses on caring rather than curing, and promotes collaboration between the nurse and patient. It establishes the nursing process as the basis for providing care.

According to the nursing model, the patient's needs direct the therapeutic relationship and the patient's reactions to nursing interventions guide future interventions.

MEDICAL MODEL

The medical model holds that disease is the cause of deviant behavior. It focuses on diagnosis and treatment of the disease. Application of the medical model to mental illness has led to identification of neurochemicals as possible causes of deviant behavior. The medical model also accepts socioenvironmental influences as potential causes of deviant behavior.

COMMUNICATION MODELS (BERNE, BANDLER, GRINDLER)

Communication theory proposes that all human behavior is a form of communication and that the meaning of behavior depends on the clarity of communication between the sender and receiver. Unclear communication produces anxiety, which results in behavior deviations.

The communication pattern used with individuals, families, and social and work groups identifies the causes of the behavioral deviation. When communication improves, so does behavior.

Nurses draw on the communication model when they teach patients effective communication techniques.

BEHAVIORAL MODEL (SKINNER, WOLPE, EYSENCK)

According to the behavioral model, all behavior — including mental illness — is learned. Unlike other models, which focus on the patient's emotions, behavioral theory focuses on the patient's actions.

Behaviorists believe that behavior that's rewarded will persist. Desired behaviors can be learned through rewards, and negative behaviors can be eliminated through punishment. Thus, people can learn to behave in socially desirable ways.

HUMANISTIC MODEL (MASLOW)

In the humanistic model, understanding human behavior requires familiarity with a hierarchy that has six levels of need.
- Level 1: physiologic survival (food, oxygen, and rest)
- Level 2: safety, security, and self-preservation
- Level 3: love and belonging (developing fulfilling relationships)
- Level 4: esteem and recognition (feeling like a worthwhile, contributing member of society, appreciating one's own uniqueness)
- Level 5: self-actualization (self-fulfillment)
- Level 6: truth, harmony, beauty, and spirituality

Nursing draws from the humanistic model by striving to meet patients' lower-level needs before higher-level ones. By performing a needs assessment, the nurse determines appropriate intervention strategies to help patients meet their needs.

- Willingness to act as an agent of change
- Thorough knowledge of personal strengths and weaknesses
- Realization of clinical competence

● **Theoretical frameworks of psychiatric nursing**
- Psychiatric nursing is historically based on theoretical concepts that attempt to explain how human behavior and other factors affect mental health (see *Theoretical models of behavior,* pages 8 and 9)
- Nurses may incorporate the principles and techniques of one or more conceptual frameworks when providing patient care

NURSE-PATIENT RELATIONSHIP

● **Overview**
- The first step is to establish a therapeutic relationship—one based on caring, sensitivity, genuineness, and empathy
- The nurse's words and actions should convey respect for the patient and acknowledge the importance of his feelings, thoughts, and needs
- The relationship should be goal-oriented, purposeful, time-limited, and focused on the patient's needs and growth
- An effective nurse-patient relationship empowers the patient
- Establishment of an effective relationship requires gaining the patient's trust

● **Phases of the nurse-patient relationship**
- Preinteraction phase occurs before any direct patient contact
    - May last a few seconds or several weeks
    - Involves the nurse reflecting on her beliefs and attitudes
    - Involves reviewing appropriate records in preparation for working with the patient
- Orientation (introductory) phase, also called the getting-to-know-you phase, sets the tone for the relationship
    - Involves making introductions, defining each person's role in the relationship, and beginning of trust development
    - Usually initiated by the nurse, who sets limits for the professional relationship and establishes the focus for conversation based on assessment data
    - May include the patient and nurse making an agreement, writing a contract, or discussing and establishing goals
    - May involve the patient's resistance to treatment, testing the nurse's true intent, or denial that a problem exists
- Working (exploration) phase involves intensely focusing on and evaluating the patient's problems and working toward achieving established goals
    - Characterized by the nurse assuming role of counselor and facilitator, with the patient actively participating
    - Enables the patient to freely examine problems, attempt to gain insight, or find solutions to problems
- Termination (resolution) phase is marked by reviewing and summarizing the patient's progress
    - Involves the nurse and patient, who together determine whether goals have been met and, if not, why
    - Considered the formal ending of relationship, in which the nurse acknowledges the patient's feelings about termination

---

Phases of nurse-patient relationship

- Preinteraction phase: occurs before direct patient contact
- Orientation (getting-to-know-you) phase: sets tone for relationship
- Working (exploration) phase: focuses on and evaluates patient's problems; works toward achieving established goals
- Termination (resolution) phase: marked by reviewing and summarizing patient's progress

– May involve the patient feeling hurt or angry at the nurse's abandonment; the nurse anticipates these feelings and discusses them with the patient before termination

COMMUNICATING WITH PATIENTS

● **General information**
  - Effective communication is key to psychiatric nursing
  - Communication involves both sending and receiving messages; it can be verbal or nonverbal
  - Usually, people send verbal and nonverbal messages simultaneously

● **Verbal communication**
  - In psychiatric nursing, verbal communication usually takes place as the spoken word
  - Sometimes verbal communication involves the written word (as when providing written instructions on taking self-administered medications)
  - Various factors can influence verbal communication, including the patient's and nurse's past experiences, background, and feelings; other factors affecting the patient are especially important to consider
    – Native language
    – Culture or nationality
    – Sexual orientation or gender
    – Age and developmental considerations
    – Roles and responsibilities
    – Social background or status
    – Space and territoriality
    – Physical, mental, and emotional state
    – Values
    – Environment
  - Overcoming potential obstacles to communication requires self-awareness on the nurse's part as well as knowledge of and sensitivity to the patient's experiences, beliefs, and background
    – Can be especially challenging if the underlying disorder involves delusions, paranoia, hallucinations, dementia, or thought disorders (see *Reducing communication barriers,* pages 12 and 13)
    – May be helpful to use an interpreter if the patient doesn't speak English well
    – May require use of a communication aid (a pad and felt-tipped pen, a dry-erase board, sign language, or flash cards with common words or phrases) if the patient is speech-impaired
  - The psychiatric nurse practices intent listening (listening attentively to content and meaning) to hear and analyze what the patient is saying and to interpret his communication pattern

● **Nonverbal communication**
  - Also known as *body language;* includes eye contact, facial expression, posture, gait, gestures, touch, physical appearance or attributes, dress or grooming, affect, and even silence
  - Most communication is nonverbal
  - The nurse must be aware of her own body language in addition to analyzing the patient's body language; gestures, expressions, and posture must convey the proper messages — friendliness, openness, and acceptance of the patient

Verbal communication

Influences
● Patient's and nurse's past experiences, background, and feelings
● Native language
● Culture or nationality
● Sexual orientation or gender
● Age and developmental considerations
● Roles and responsibilities
● Social background or status
● Space and territoriality
● Physical, mental, and emotional state
● Values
● Environment

Obstacles
● Requires nurse self-awareness and knowledge of and sensitivity to patient's experiences, beliefs, and background
● Can be especially challenging
● May be helpful to use interpreter or communication aids

Nonverbal communication

● Also known as *body language*

Types
● Eye contact
● Facial expression
● Posture
● Gait
● Gestures
● Touch
● Physical appearance or attributes
● Dress or grooming
● Affect
● Silence

Types of communication barriers

- Language difficulties or differences
- Impaired hearing
- Inappropriate responses
- Thought disorders
- Paranoid thinking
- Hallucinations
- Delusions
- Delirium
- Dementia

Reducing communication barriers

Acknowledging and reducing communication barriers can promote a more effective relationship with psychiatric patients.

LANGUAGE DIFFICULTIES OR DIFFERENCES

Use words appropriate for the patient's educational level. Avoid medical terms that he's unlikely to understand.

Be aware of words that may have more than one meaning. To some patients, for instance, the word "bad" may also be slang for "good."

If the patient speaks a foreign language or uses an ethnic dialect, obtain an interpreter to help you communicate. However, remember that a third person's presence may make the patient less willing to share his feelings.

IMPAIRED HEARING

If the patient can't hear you clearly, he may misinterpret your questions or responses. Check whether he's wearing a hearing aid. If so, is it turned on? If not, can he read lips? If possible, face him and speak clearly and slowly, using common words. Keep your questions short, simple, and direct.

If the patient has a severe hearing impairment, he may have to communicate in writing, or you may need to collect information from his family or friends.

If the patient is elderly, speak in low-pitched tones. With aging, the ability to hear high-pitched tones deteriorates first.

INAPPROPRIATE RESPONSES

Avoid appearing as if you're discounting the patient's feelings, as by changing the subject abruptly. Otherwise, the patient may get the impression that you're uninterested, anxious, or annoyed — or that you're judging him.

THOUGHT DISORDERS

If the patient's thought patterns are incoherent or irrelevant, he may be unable to interpret messages correctly, fo-

- Silence is a strategic communication tool
  - Can be used to give the patient time to talk, think, and gain insight into problems
  - Requires practice and timing; using it too much or at the wrong times could give the impression of lack of interest or judgment
- Attentive listening is always essential
  - Face the patient
  - Acknowledge him and maintain eye contact
  - Stay relaxed, with legs and arms uncrossed, possibly leaning forward slightly
  - Convey acceptance when the patient speaks
  - Don't interrupt or argue, but provide verbal feedback as appropriate
- Ideally, the patient's nonverbal and verbal messages should be congruent (matching)

Therapeutic communication

- Primary intervention in psychiatric nursing; serves as the foundation for an effective nurse-patient relationship
  - When approached correctly, helps to reduce stress, encourage insight, and support problem solving

cus on the interview, or provide appropriate responses. When assessing him, ask simple questions about concrete topics, and clarify his responses. Encourage him to express himself clearly.

PARANOID THINKING

Approach a paranoid patient in a nonthreatening way. Avoid touching him, which he may misinterpret as an attempt to harm him. Also, keep in mind that a paranoid patient may not mean the things he says.

HALLUCINATIONS

A hallucinating patient can't hear or respond appropriately. Show concern but don't reinforce his hallucinatory perceptions.

Be as specific as possible when giving commands. For instance, if he says he's hearing voices, tell him to stop listening to the voices and listen to you instead.

DELUSIONS

A deluded patient defends irrational beliefs or ideas despite factual evidence to the contrary. Some delusions may be so bizarre that you'll recognize them immediately. Others may be hard to identify.

Neither condemn nor agree with delusional beliefs; also avoid dismissing a statement because you think it's delusional. Instead, gently emphasize reality without arguing.

DELIRIUM

A delirious patient experiences disorientation, hallucinations, and confusion. Misinterpretation and inappropriate responses commonly result. Talk to him directly, ask simple questions, and offer frequent reassurances.

DEMENTIA

The patient with dementia (irreversible deterioration of mental capacity) may experience changes in memory and thought patterns. His language may become distorted or slurred.

When interviewing him, minimize distractions. Use simple, concise language. Avoid making statements that could be easily misinterpreted.

- When done incorrectly or nontherapeutically, can create stumbling blocks in the relationship (see *Nontherapeutic ways of communicating*, page 14)
- Techniques include asking open-ended questions, validating, clarifying, sharing impressions, restating, focusing, suggestive collaboration, and offering information
- Open-ended or general questions are used to initiate a conversation
  - Open-ended: encourages the patient to talk about any subject that comes to mind ("What would you like to talk about today?")
  - Closed-ended: limits the range of responses, eliciting merely a "Yes" or "No" response ("Would you like to talk about anything today?")
- Validating — reviewing and rephrasing key patient statements — helps ensure that the nurse has correctly understood what the patient has said; it also encourages the patient to elaborate
- Asking the patient to clarify a confusing or vague message shows a desire to understand what he's saying
  - May also elicit precise information crucial to his treatment or recovery
  - Can be used to better understand the patient's expression of time, reality, or sequence

Therapeutic communication

- Open-ended questions: initiate conversation and encourage patient to talk; closed-ended questions: limit range of responses
- Validating: reviews and rephrases key patient statements
- Clarifying: shows desire to understand patient's statements
- Sharing impressions: describes patient's feelings, and then seeks corrective feedback from him
- Restating: summarizes patient's message in nurse's own words and allows patient to respond
- Focusing: lets nurse redirect patient's attention toward something specific
- Suggestive collaboration: gives patient chance to explore pros and cons of suggested approach
- Offering information: explains components or purpose of activity or procedure

Nontherapeutic ways of communicating

- Attacking or defending
- Casting judgment
- Interrogating
- Minimizing
- Playing Ann Landers
- Pressuring
- Running off at the mouth
- Rushing
- Taking sides

Nontherapeutic ways of communicating

Nontherapeutic techniques work against establishing an effective nurse-patient relationship. Avoid these pitfalls when interacting with patients.

ATTACKING OR DEFENDING
- Getting angry with the patient
- Arguing with him
- Challenging him or his beliefs
- Being defensive

CASTING JUDGMENT
- Judging the patient
- Criticizing him
- Showing approval or disapproval

INTERROGATING
- Asking him why
- Asking excessive, inappropriate, or leading questions
- Inquiring excessively about sensitive areas or making the patient feel uncomfortable

MINIMIZING
- Stereotyping the patient
- Not listening to him
- Not perceiving him as human
- Not taking his beliefs seriously
- Failing to maintain eye contact
- Changing the subject inappropriately
- Working on a task while he's talking to you

- Letting your mind wander during a conversation
- Using clichés

PLAYING ANN LANDERS
- Giving advice
- Offering false reassurance

PRESSURING
- Trying to talk the patient into accepting treatment

RUNNING OFF AT THE MOUTH
- Talking on and on
- Not letting the patient respond
- Repeating a point you just made
- Interpreting or speculating on the dynamics of patient problems
- Making inappropriate comments

RUSHING
- Responding to the patient before he finishes speaking
- Finishing his sentences for him

TAKING SIDES
- Joining attacks led by the patient
- Participating in criticism of staff members

- Sharing impressions involves describing the patient's feelings, then seeking corrective feedback from him
    - Lets the patient clarify misperceptions or misunderstanding and gives a better understanding of his true feelings
    - Shouldn't be challenging or confrontational
- Restating involves summarizing the patient's message in the nurse's own words and then allowing him to respond
    - Shows that the nurse is paying attention and wants to hear more
    - Encourages the patient to expand on what he has said
- Focusing lets the nurse redirect the patient's attention toward something specific — especially if he's vague or rambling
- Suggestive collaboration gives the patient a chance to explore the pros and cons of a suggested approach
- Offering information involves explaining the components or purpose of an activity or procedure; it's integral to patient teaching

PSYCHIATRIC NURSING ASSESSMENT

● **General information**
  - Psychiatric assessment is the scientific process of identifying a patient's psychosocial problems, strengths, and concerns
  - It serves as the basis for treating patients with psychiatric disorders
  - The information gathered permits caregivers to analyze the patient's mental, emotional, and behavioral status
  - During the assessment, mental status tests may also be administered

● **Psychiatric nursing interview**
  - A systematic psychiatric interview helps the nurse to gather broad information
    - Assesses the patient's psychological functioning
    - Identifies the underlying or precipitating cause of his current problem
    - Identifies the patient's coping methods and their effect on his psychosocial growth
    - Formulates a care plan
    - Assesses patient progress and the effectiveness of treatments
  - The patient may not understand the purpose of the interview; the nurse may need to explain why the information is necessary and help him recognize the benefits of dealing with problems openly
  - There are general guidelines for conducting a patient interview
    - Ensuring the patient's privacy, including asking the patient who should be present during the interview (for instance, an adolescent may refuse to discuss sexual activity in front of a parent)
    - Choosing a quiet, calm, private setting, as interruptions and distractions threaten confidentiality and may interfere with effective listening
    - Reassuring the patient that he's safe (if necessary)
    - Showing support and sensitivity
    - Listening carefully and objectively to make the patient feel comfortable enough to discuss his problems, and responding with sensitivity (see *Interview do's and don'ts*, page 16)
    - Using reliable information sources (for example, if a mentally ill patient seems unreliable or can't provide answers to important questions, ask for permission to interview family members or friends; if he can answer questions but his responses are questionable, verify the information through family members, friends, or other health care personnel)
    - Checking hospital records from previous admissions, if possible, and comparing the patient's past behavior, symptoms, and circumstances with the current situation
    - Considering the patient's culture (be aware that some cultures frown on discussing intimate details with strangers, even nurses); gather cultural information early in the interview, and tailor questions accordingly
  - When meeting a patient for the first time, the nurse should follow certain steps
    - Introducing herself and explaining the purpose of the interview
    - Asking the patient how he would like to be addressed
    - Sitting at a comfortable distance from the patient and giving him undivided attention, while maintaining a professional but friendly attitude; if

---

Psychiatric nursing assessment

- Scientific process of identifying patient's psychosocial problems, strengths, and concerns

Key facts about nursing interview

- Assesses patient's psychological functioning
- Identifies underlying or precipitating cause
- Identifies patient's coping methods
- Formulates care plan
- Assesses patient progress

Guidelines for patient interview

- Ensure patient's privacy.
- Choose quiet, calm, private setting.
- Reassure patient.
- Show support and sensitivity.
- Listen carefully and objectively.
- Use reliable information sources.
- Check hospital records.
- Consider patient's culture.

Guidelines for first encounter

- Introduce yourself and give reason for interview.
- Ask patient how he'd like to be addressed.
- Sit a comfortable distance from patient.
- Speak calmly.

Interview do's and don'ts

- Do set clear goals.
- Do heed unspoken signals.
- Do check yourself.
- Don't rush.
- Don't make assumptions.
- Don't judge patient.

Interview do's and don'ts

When interviewing psychiatric patients, follow these guidelines.

DO SET CLEAR GOALS

The assessment interview isn't meant to be a random discussion. Make sure you have set clear goals, such as obtaining information, screening for abnormalities, or investigating for an identified psychiatric condition (depression, paranoia, or suicidal thoughts, for instance).

DO HEED UNSPOKEN SIGNALS

Listen carefully for indications of anxiety or distress. What topics does the patient ignore or pass over vaguely? You may find important clues in his method of self-expression and in the subjects he avoids.

DO CHECK YOURSELF

Monitor your own reactions. The psychiatric patient may provoke an emotional response strong enough to interfere with your professional judgment. For instance, a depressed patient may make you depressed, a hostile one may provoke your anger, an anxious one may cause you to feel anxiety, and a violent, psychotic patient who has lost touch with reality may induce fear.

DON'T RUSH

Don't rush through the interview. Remember—building a trusting therapeutic relationship takes time.

DON'T MAKE ASSUMPTIONS

Don't make assumptions about how past events affected the patient emotionally. Try to discover what each event meant to him.

If, for instance, he says one of his parents died, don't assume that the death provoked sadness. A death by itself doesn't cause sadness, guilt, or anger. What matters is how the patient perceives the loss.

DON'T JUDGE THE PATIENT

Don't let personal values cloud your professional judgment. For example, when assessing the patient's appearance, judge attire on its appropriateness and cleanliness, not on whether it suits your taste.

the patient has the potential for violence, sitting close to the door rather than in a corner of the room
- Speaking in a calm, nonthreatening tone to encourage the patient to be candid
- Determining the patient's age, sex, ethnic origin, primary language, birthplace, religion, and marital status (use this information to validate his medical record)
- Gathering information about the patient's educational level, housing conditions, income, current employment status, and family — all of which may provide clues to his current problem
- Assessing his economic and personal situation to aid in determining their impact on his current psychological status (keep in mind that a patient experiencing economic or personal hardships is more likely to show symptoms of distress during an illness)
• It's important to find out about the patient's cultural beliefs because they can affect his response to illness, his adaptation to hospital care, and his behavior during the interview
- Behaviors considered appropriate in mainstream American culture: may be frowned on in other cultures

– Many cultures view mental illness as a stigma: the family of a mentally ill person may keep that person hidden and refuse to answer questions about him

– Cultural beliefs: may affect the patient's or family's treatment decisions

• When possible, note specific details to fully explore the patient's chief complaint

– When the patient's symptoms began, whether they had an abrupt or gradual onset, how severe they are, how long they last, and how they affect his level of functioning

– For a recurring problem, what prompted him to seek help at this time

– Patient's description of the problem (use direct quotes when documenting); be aware that some patients don't have overriding concerns; others may insist that nothing is wrong

– Overt signs of mental illness (patients enmeshed in a medical problem may fail to recognize their own depression or anxiety and require careful observation)

– Nonverbal clues indicating the problem

– Information provided by the patient's family or friends (especially helpful when patient's unaware of the problem)

– Patient's expectations about treatment (such as improved self-image or cessation of hallucinations)

• If the patient is capable of holding an in-depth conversation, obtain a detailed personality profile

– Ego functioning (usual coping mechanisms, especially his ability to handle stress; use of violence, withdrawal, or denial; impulse control; and degree of insight and judgment)

– Sense of identity (look for indications of the patient's talents, accomplishments, adaptability, and capacity to find emotional support)

– Developmental level (note any stumbling blocks to maturation process)

• Explore previous psychiatric or psychological disturbances the patient may have had (such as episodes of delusions, violence, attempted suicide, drug or alcohol abuse, or depression) and previous psychiatric treatment he may have received

• Obtain a detailed psychosocial history

– Relationships, lifestyle, coping skills, sexual habits, diet, sleep pattern, and use of alcohol, tobacco, or drugs

– Work, school, religious practices, community life, and hobbies or interests

– Social network and support systems

– Significant life changes (recent marriage, divorce, illness, job loss, or death of a loved one), including how he felt when these changes occurred

• Obtain a detailed family history

– Family customs, child-rearing practices, and emotional support received during childhood (observe how the patient reacts when disclosing family history)

– Emotional health of relatives (including any family history of substance abuse, alcoholism, suicide, psychological disorders, psychiatric hospitalization, child abuse, or violence)

– Physical disorders affecting family members

• Review the patient's medical history, noting any kidney or liver failure, infection, thyroid or metabolic disorders, or increased intracranial pressure; these

Key facts about patient's cultural beliefs

● Can affect response to illness, adaptation to care, and behavior during interview
● Acceptable American behaviors may be frowned on in other cultures
● Many cultures view mental illness as stigma
● May affect treatment decisions

Interview to-do list

● Explore patient's chief complaint.
● Obtain detailed personality profile, including ego functioning, sense of identity, and developmental level.
● Obtain detailed psychosocial history.
● Obtain detailed family history.
● Review patient's medical record.
● Take detailed medical history.

could cause disorientation, distorted thought processes, depression, or other signs or symptoms of mental illness
- Take a detailed medication history, keeping in mind that certain drugs may cause or contribute to signs or symptoms of mental illness
  - All medications the patient takes, including over-the-counter drugs and nutritional and herbal supplements (note any potential drug interactions)
  - Compliance with use of prescribed medications (especially antipsychotic, antidepressant, anxiolytic, or antimanic drugs)
  - Improvement in symptoms since starting drug therapy
  - Adverse reactions to medications

Mental status evaluation

- The mental status examination (MSE), commonly included as part of the psychiatric interview, is a tool for assessing psychological dysfunction and identifying causes of psychopathology; the nurse may be responsible for conducting all or a portion of the MSE
  - Examines the patient's level of consciousness (LOC), general appearance, behavior, speech, mood and affect, intellectual performance, judgment, insight, perception, and thought content
  - Aids in accurate interpretation of the psychiatrist's findings and assists in planning appropriate nursing interventions
- Assess the patient's LOC—an indication of basic brain function
  - Identifies the intensity of stimulation needed to arouse the patient (such as speaking in a normal conversational tone, using a loud voice, light touch, vigorous shaking, or painful stimulation)
  - Assesses response to stimulation, including the degree and quality of movement, speech content and coherence, and level of eye opening and eye contact
  - Notes and documents the patient's actions after the stimulus is removed
  - Determines if LOC is impaired (could indicate a brain tumor or abscess, hematoma, hydrocephalus, electrolyte or acid-base imbalance, or toxicity caused by liver or kidney failure, alcohol, or drugs)
  - Refers any patient with an altered LOC for a more complete medical examination
- Evaluate the patient's general appearance (may reflect his emotional and mental state)
  - Dressing and grooming, and whether they're appropriate for the patient's age and gender
  - Excessive cosmetics use, piercing, or tattoos
  - Cleanliness of skin, hair, nails, and teeth; note any abnormalities (for example, a disheveled appearance may indicate self-neglect or a preoccupation with other activities)
  - Weight and height
  - Skin coloring, skin condition, and body build; note abnormalities (for instance, a pale, emaciated, sad appearance may signal depression)
  - Obvious physical impairments or unpleasant odors
  - Posture, head position, and gait; identify deviations (a slumped posture may mean depression, fatigue, or suspiciousness; an uneven or unsteady gait, physical abnormalities or the influence of drugs or alcohol)
  - Facial expression, including gaze, grimacing, and eye contact
  - Patient's perceptions about his health; note any discrepancies with nurse's observations

- Evaluate the patient's behavior
  - Appropriateness of gestures (disconnected gestures may indicate hallucinations; for example, a patient who experiences auditory hallucinations may speak to someone who isn't there and tilt his head to listen)
  - Mannerisms, including tics or tremors, nail biting, fidgeting, and pacing; note any unusual mannerisms (such as gazing and speaking to someone who isn't present)
  - Attitude (note whether the patient is cooperative, mistrustful, hostile, or embarrassed)
- Evaluate the patient's activity level (whether he's restless, calm, tense, rigid, or unable to sit still)
- Evaluate the patient's speech for content and quality (content includes words used; quality, the pattern, use of repetition, rate, or amount of speech)
  - Illogical choice of topics; irrelevant or illogical replies to questions; speech defects (stuttering; excessively fast or slow speech); sudden interruptions; excessive volume or barely audible speech; altered vocal tone and modulation; slurring; excessive number of words (overproductive speech); or minimal, monosyllabic responses (underproductive speech)
  - If the patient communicates only with gestures, whether this is an isolated behavior or part of a pattern of diminished responsiveness
  - How much time elapses before the patient reacts to questions (taking excessive time to respond is considered *latency* of speech)
  - Speech characteristics that may indicate altered thought processes (such as illogical or irrelevant replies to questions; minimal or monosyllabic responses; convoluted or excessively detailed speech; repetitious speech patterns; flight of ideas; sudden silence for no obvious reason)
- Assess the patient's mood (pervasive feeling or state of mind) and affect (expression of mood)
  - Current feelings (ask him to describe these feelings in concrete terms, and have him suggest possible reasons for these feelings)
  - Manifestations of mood and affect (such as excitement or depression, crying, sweating, heavy breathing, or trembling)
  - Mood swings and ability to keep mood changes under control
  - Indications of mood in facial expression and posture, noting inconsistencies between body language and mood
  - Indications of mood disorder, such as lability of affect (rapid, dramatic fluctuation in the range of emotions), flat affect (unresponsive range of emotion, which may signify schizophrenia or Parkinson's disease), or inappropriate affect (inconsistency between affect and mood such as the patient smiling when discussing an anger-provoking situation)
- Assess the patient's abstract reasoning, judgment, and problem-solving abilities
- Evaluate the patient's orientation to time, place, and person; ask him to state his name and the time, date, place, and present circumstance
- Check for signs of confusion or disorientation (patient may be experiencing delusions, hallucinations, obsessions, compulsions, fantasies, or daydreams)
- Assess the patient's recent and remote memory; keep in mind that a patient may make up plausible answers to mask memory deficits (confabulation)
  - Immediate recall: telling the patient, "I want you to remember three words: apple, house, and umbrella." Then asking, "What are the three words I want you to remember?"

Evaluating patient's speech

- Illogical choice of topics
- Communicating with gestures only
- How soon patient reacts to a question
- Illogical thought patterns

Evaluating patient's mood

- Current feelings
- How mood is manifested (crying, depressed, sweating, trembling)
- Facial expressions and posture
- Affect (flat, inappropriate)

Types of memory

- Immediate recall
- Delayed recall
- Recent memory
- Distant past

Final steps in MSE

- Assess patient's attention span and ability to concentrate.
- Assess patient's ability to understand material.
- Test patient's ability to think abstractly.
- Determine patient's store of common knowledge.
- Assess patient's ability to evaluate choices.
- Assess patient's insight.
- Test patient's sensory perception and coordination.
- Examine patient's thought content and pattern for clarity, including abnormal beliefs, morbid thoughts, and delusions.
- Assess for changes in patient's sex drive.
- Evaluate patient's competence.
- Assess patient's defense mechanisms.
- Assess for evidence of self-destructive behavior or suicidal tendencies.

– Delayed recall: asking the patient to repeat the same words after an interval of 5 to 10 minutes
– Recent memory: asking about an event that happened within the past few hours or days (such as, "When were you admitted to the hospital?"); the nurse should already know the correct response or be able to validate it with a family member
– Distant past: asking the patient where he was born or where he attended high school; keeping in mind that recent memory loss with intact remote memory may indicate an organic mental disorder
- Assess the patient's attention span and ability to concentrate on a task for an appropriate length of time; if the patient has a short attention span, remember to provide simple, written health care instructions
- Assess the patient's ability to understand material, and retain and repeat the content (for example, ask the patient to read part of a news article and explain it; if the patient can't read, use alternative methods to assess his ability to understand)
- Test the patient's ability to think abstractly by asking him the meaning of a common proverb such as, "People in glass houses shouldn't throw stones"
- Determine the patient's store of common knowledge by asking questions appropriate to his age and learning level such as, "Who's the vice president?"
- Assess his ability to evaluate choices and draw appropriate conclusions by asking questions that emerge naturally during conversation (such as, "What would you do if….")
- Assess the patient's insight by asking, "What do you think is causing your anxiety?" or "Have you noticed a recent change in yourself?"
- Test the patient's sensory perception and coordination by having him copy a simple drawing; also note any evidence of hallucinations or illusions (both involve perceptual distortions)
- Examine the patient's thought content and pattern for clarity, connection to reality, and logical progression
  – Abnormal beliefs and morbid thoughts or preoccupations (such as suicidal, self-destructive, violent, or superstitious thoughts; recurring dreams; distorted perceptions of reality; or feelings of worthlessness)
  – Delusions (false beliefs with no firm basis in reality), ideas of reference (misinterpreting others' acts in a highly personal way), and obsessions (preoccupations or recurring thoughts that interfere with daily living)
- Assess for changes in the patient's sex drive
  – Should recognize many may be uncomfortable discussing sexuality
  – Should introduce the subject of sex tactfully but directly
  – Should avoid language that assumes a heterosexual orientation
- Evaluate the patient's competence, understanding of reality, and the consequences of his actions (helps determine if the patient understands the implications of his illness, its treatment, and the consequences of avoiding treatment)
  – Use extreme caution when assessing for changes in competence; unless the patient's behavior strongly indicates otherwise, assume he's competent
  – Legally, only a judge has the authority to declare a person incompetent to make decisions regarding personal health and safety or financial matters
- Assess the patient's use of defense mechanisms—behaviors that operate on an unconscious level to protect the ego and reduce stress—noting excessive reliance on any particular mechanisms (see *Defining defense mechanisms*)
- Assess for evidence of self-destructive behavior or suicidal tendencies

Defining defense mechanisms

People use defense, or coping, mechanisms to relieve anxiety. The definitions below will help you determine whether your patient is using one or more of these mechanisms.

ACTING OUT

Acting out refers to repeating certain actions to ward off anxiety without weighing the possible consequences of those actions. For example, a husband gets angry with his wife and starts staying at work later.

COMPENSATION

Also called *substitution,* compensation involves trying to make up for feelings of inadequacy or frustration in one area by excelling or overindulging in another. For example, an adolescent takes up jogging because he failed to make the swim team.

DENIAL

A person in denial protects himself from reality — especially the unpleasant aspects of life — by refusing to perceive, acknowledge, or face it. For example, a woman newly diagnosed with end-stage cancer says, "It'll be okay. It's not a big deal."

DISPLACEMENT

In displacement, the person redirects his impulses (commonly anger) from the real target (because that target is too dangerous) to a safer but innocent person. For example, a patient yells at a nurse after becoming angry at his mother for not calling him.

FANTASY

Fantasy refers to creation of unrealistic or improbable images as a way of escaping from daily pressures and responsibilities or to relieve boredom. For example, a person may daydream excessively, watch TV for hours on end, or imagine being highly successful when he feels unsuccessful. Engaging in such activities makes him feel better for a brief period.

IDENTIFICATION

In identification, the person unconsciously adopts the personality characteristics, attitudes, values, and behavior of someone else (such as a hero he emulates and admires) as a way to allay anxiety. He may identify with a group to be more accepted by them. For example, an adolescent girl begins to dress and act like her favorite pop singer.

INTELLECTUALIZATION

Also called *isolation,* intellectualization refers to hiding one's emotional responses or problems under a façade of big words and pretending there's no problem. For example, after failing to obtain a job promotion, a worker explains that the position failed to meet his expectations for climbing the corporate ladder.

INTROJECTION

A person introjects when he adopts someone else's values and standards without exploring whether they fit him. For example, an individual begins to follow a strict vegetarian diet for no apparent reason.

PROJECTION

In projection, the person attributes to others his own unacceptable thoughts, feelings, and impulses. For example, a student who fails a test blames his parents for having the television on too loud when he was trying to study.

(continued)

Defense mechanisms

- Acting out
- Compensation
- Denial
- Displacement
- Fantasy
- Identification
- Intellectualization
- Introjection
- Projection
- Rationalization
- Reaction formation
- Regression
- Repression
- Sublimation
- Undoing

Defining defense mechanisms *(continued)*

RATIONALIZATION

Rationalization occurs when a person substitutes acceptable reasons for the real or actual reasons that are motivating his behavior. The rationalizing patient makes excuses for shortcomings and avoids self-condemnation, disappointments, and criticism. For example, an individual states that she didn't win the race because she hadn't gotten a good night's sleep.

REACTION FORMATION

In reaction formation, the person behaves the opposite of the way he feels. For example, love turns into hate and hate into love.

REGRESSION

Under stress, a person may regress by returning to the behaviors he used in an earlier, more comfortable time in his life. For example, a previously toilet-trained preschool child begins to wet his bed every night after his baby brother is born.

REPRESSION

Repression refers to unconsciously blocking out painful or unacceptable thoughts and feelings, leaving them to operate in the subconscious. For example, a woman who was sexually abused as a young child can't remember the abuse but experiences uneasy feelings when she goes near the place where the abuse occurred.

SUBLIMATION

In sublimation, a person transforms unacceptable needs into acceptable ambitions and actions. For example, he may channel his sex drive into sports and hobbies.

UNDOING

In undoing, the person tries to undo the harm he feels he has done to others. For example, a patient who says something bad about a friend may try to undo the harm by saying nice things about her or by being nice to her and apologizing.

– A mentally healthy person: may intentionally take death-defying risks (such as engaging in dangerous sports); a self-destructive person: takes risks that are death-seeking, not death-defying
– Not all self-destructive behavior is suicidal in intent: some patients engage in such behavior because it helps them feel alive (for example, patients who have lost touch with reality may cut or mutilate body parts to focus on physical pain, which may be less overwhelming than emotional distress; called *self-injury*)
– Depression signs and symptoms: could mean suicidal tendencies; patients considered high risk when they begin to feel more energy (typically after starting antidepressant therapy)
– Statements or evidence of hopelessness: assess the patient for suicide risk (see *Recognizing and responding to suicidal patients*)
– Suicidal crisis: requires immediate steps to protect the patient from harm

● **Personality and projective tests**
  • These tests provide insight into the patient's personality, mood, and psychopathology
  • Tests include Beck Depression Inventory, Draw-a-Person Test, Minnesota Multiphasic Personality Inventory (MMPI), Sentence Completion Test, and Thematic Apperception Test

Personality and projective tests

● Beck Depression Inventory
● Draw-a-Person Test
● MMPI
● Sentence Completion Test
● Thematic Apperception Test

Recognizing and responding to suicidal patients

Assess your patient for these indications of suicidal ideation (thoughts of suicide):

- withdrawal from others (social isolation)
- signs and symptoms of depression — crying, sadness, fatigue, helplessness, poor concentration, reduced interest in sex and other pleasurable activities, constipation, and weight loss
- overwhelming anxiety (the most common trigger for a suicide attempt)
- saying farewell to friends and family
- putting affairs in order
- giving away possessions
- conveying covert suicide messages and death wishes
- making obvious suicidal statements such as, "I'd be better off dead."

RESPONDING TO A SUICIDE THREAT

If you believe the patient intends to attempt suicide, assess the seriousness of his intent and the immediacy of the risk. Consider a patient with a chosen method who plans to commit suicide in the next 48 to 72 hours at high risk.

Tell the patient you're concerned, and urge him to avoid self-destructive behavior until the staff has an opportunity to help him. Then consult with the treatment team about arranging for psychiatric hospitalization or a safe equivalent such as having someone watch him at home.

SAFETY PRECAUTIONS

If you believe the patient is at high risk for suicide, initiate these safety precautions:

- Provide a safe environment. Check for and correct any conditions that pose a danger. Look for exposed pipes, windows without safety glass, and access to the roof or an open balcony.
- Remove dangerous objects — belts, razors, suspenders, light cords, glass, knives, scissors, nail files, and clippers.
- Be alert when the patient shaves, takes medication, or uses the bathroom.
- Make the patient's specific restrictions clear to staff members.
- Plan for one-on-one observation of the patient.
- Clarify day staff and night staff responsibilities.

STAY CLOSE

Helping the patient build emotional ties to others is the ultimate means of preventing suicide. Besides observing the patient, maintain personal contact with him. Encourage continuity of care and consistency of primary nurses.

WHEN TO KEEP SECRETS

A patient may ask you to keep his suicidal thoughts confidential. Remember that such requests are ambivalent — a suicidal patient typically wants to escape the pain of life, but he also wants to live. A part of him wants you to tell other staff members about his suicidal thoughts so he can be kept alive.

Tell the patient you can't keep secrets that endanger his life or conflict with his treatment. You have a duty to keep him safe and ensure the best care.

Indications of suicidal ideation

- Withdrawal from others
- Signs and symptoms of depression (crying, sadness, fatigue, helplessness, poor concentration)
- Overwhelming anxiety
- Saying farewell
- Putting affairs in order
- Giving away possessions
- Conveying covert suicide messages
- Making obvious suicidal statements

Responding to suicide threat

- Provide safe environment.
- Remove dangerous objects.
- Be alert when patient shaves, takes medication, or uses bathroom.
- Make patient's specific restrictions clear to staff.
- Plan for one-on-one observation of patient.
- Clarify day staff and night staff responsibilities.
- Maintain personal contact with patient.
- Don't keep secrets that endanger patient's life.

- Other assessment tests may be given to aid diagnosis (see *Psychiatric assessment tests*, page 24)
- The Beck Depression Inventory helps diagnose depression and determine its severity
  - Provides objective evidence of the need for treatment
  - Can be used to monitor the patient's response during treatment

Psychiatric assessment tests

- Mini–Mental Status Examination
- Cognitive capacity screening examination
- Cognitive assessment scale
- Global deterioration assessment scale
- Functional dementia scale
- Eating attitudes test
- Michigan alcoholism screening test
- CAGE questionnaire
- Cocaine addiction severity test and cocaine assessment profile

Beck Depression Inventory

- Helps diagnose depression and determine its severity
- Provides objective evidence of need for treatment
- Self-administered and self-scored
- Focuses on both cognitive and physical symptoms

Draw-a-Person Test

- Patient draws human figure of each sex
- Psychologist correlates interpretation with diagnosis
- Can be used to estimate child's developmental level

MMPI

- Structured paper-and-pencil test
- Assesses personality traits and ego function
- Consists of 566 items
- Translated by psychologist
- Provides information about patient's coping strategies, defenses, strengths, gender identification, and self-esteem

---

Psychiatric assessment tests

In addition to the Beck Depression Inventory, the Minnesota Multiphasic Personality Inventory, and other widely used tests, some patients may undergo the tests listed below.

- Mini–Mental Status Examination: measures orientation, registration, recall, calculation, language, and graphomotor function
- Cognitive capacity screening examination: measures orientation, memory, calculation, and language
- Cognitive assessment scale: measures orientation, general knowledge, mental ability, and psychomotor function
- Global deterioration scale: assesses and stages primary degenerative dementia based on orientation, memory, and neurologic function
- Functional dementia scale: measures orientation, affect, and ability to perform activities of daily living
- Eating attitudes test: detects patterns that suggest an eating disorder
- Michigan alcoholism screening test: 24-item, timed test in which a score of 5 or higher classifies the patient as an alcoholic
- CAGE questionnaire: four-question tool in which two or three positive responses indicate alcoholism
- Cocaine addiction severity test and cocaine assessment profile: used when cocaine use is suspected

---

- Self-administered and self-scored; asks patients how often they experience symptoms of depression (poor concentration, suicidal thoughts, guilt feelings, and crying)
- Focuses on both cognitive symptoms (impaired decision making) and physical symptoms (appetite loss)
- High scores on physical symptoms common among elderly and physically ill patients (possibly due to effects of aging or physical illness as well as depression)
- In the Draw-a-Person Test, the patient draws a human figure of each sex
  - Interpreted by psychologist, who systematically correlates interpretation with diagnosis
  - Can also be used to estimate child's developmental level
- The MMPI is a structured paper-and-pencil test that assesses personality traits and ego function in adolescents and adults
  - Consists of 566 items; usually can be completed with little or no help (particularly if patient can read English)
  - Translated by psychologist (develops a patient psychological profile and combines the profile with data gathered from the interview)
  - Provides information about the patient's coping strategies, defenses, strengths, gender identification, and self-esteem
  - May strongly suggest a diagnostic category, point to a suicide risk, or indicate potential for violence (risk of suicide or violence requires patient monitoring)
  - May indicate a need for further physical and psychological evaluation if results show frequent physical complaints (possible hypochondria)

- In the Sentence Completion Test, the patient completes a series of sentences ("When I get angry, I…"); the patient's response may reveal his fantasies, fears, aspirations, or anxieties
- In the Thematic Apperception Test, the patient is shown a series of pictures depicting ambiguous situations and is asked to tell a story describing each picture; the psychologist evaluates the stories systematically to gain insight into the patient's personality, especially regarding interpersonal relationships and conflicts

● **Physical examination**
- It's usually ordered because some psychiatric problems may stem from organic causes or medical treatment
- Examination is accomplished via inspection, palpation, percussion, and auscultation

DIAGNOSIS AND PLANNING

● **General information**
- Appropriate nursing diagnoses are developed after completion of a thorough patient assessment, based on subjective and objective assessment findings
- Planning involves setting and prioritizing goals, formulating nursing interventions, and developing a care plan in conjunction with the patient based on the nursing diagnoses chosen
- Effective planning involves various areas
  - Specific patient needs
  - Consideration of the patient's strengths and weaknesses
  - Encouragement of the patient to help set achievable goals and participate in his own care
  - Feasible interventions
  - Activities that fall within the scope of applicable nursing practice acts

● **Care plan**
- It serves as a written guide for — and documentation of — the patient's care
- It also helps ensure continuity of care delivered by all health care team members
- It should be revised and updated as needed

● **Goal setting**
- Formulation of the plan involves the development of one or more goals for each applicable nursing diagnosis
- Appropriate goals help guide the selection of nursing interventions and serve as criteria for evaluating care
- Goals may be short- or long-term, with short-term goals taking priority over long-term ones
- Each goal must follow certain criteria
  - Relate directly to the nursing diagnosis
  - Be measurable and realistic
  - Be stated as a desired patient outcome of nursing care
  - Reflect the desires of the patient and his family
  - Be stated in a way that the patient and his family can understand

Key facts about implementation

- Begins when care plan is completed, and ends when established goals are achieved
- For effective implementation, members of multidisciplinary team must collaborate closely
- Regular reassessment necessary to ensure that planned interventions continue to be appropriate
- Periodic reassessment helps ensure flexible, individualized, and effective care plan

Treatment options for psychiatric disorders

- Drug therapy
- Psychotherapy
- Behavior therapy
- Milieu therapy
- Detoxification programs
- ECT

IMPLEMENTATION

- **General information**
  - Implementation begins when the care plan is completed, and ends when established goals are achieved
  - During the implementation step, the nurse works with the patient and his family to accomplish the interventions and move toward the outcomes specified in the plan
  - For implementation to be effective, members of the multidisciplinary team must collaborate closely
  - Regular reassessment is necessary to ensure that planned interventions continue to be appropriate
  - Periodic reassessment helps ensure a flexible, individualized, and effective care plan

- **Treatments**
  - A wide range of treatments are available and include drug therapy, counseling, detoxification programs, and electroconvulsive therapy (ECT)
  - Drug therapy may include the use of antidepressants, antianxiety agents, or antipsychotics, which often require dosage adjustments and careful monitoring
  - Types of counseling include psychotherapy, behavior therapy, and milieu therapy
  - Psychotherapy (psychological treatment of mental and emotional disorders) involves a range of approaches—from in-depth psychoanalysis to one-day crisis counseling
    - Usually involves two or more forms of therapy to ensure success
    - Regardless of approach, aims to change the patient's attitudes, feelings, or behavior (see *Types of psychotherapy*)
  - Behavior therapy assumes that problematic behaviors are learned and, through special training, can be unlearned and replaced by acceptable behaviors
    - Unlike psychotherapy, doesn't try to uncover the reasons for these behaviors
    - Tends to de-emphasize the patient's thoughts and feelings about them (see *Behavior therapy*, pages 28 and 29)
  - Milieu therapy uses the patient's environment as a tool for overcoming mental and emotional disorders; the patient's surroundings become a therapeutic community
    - May take place in a hospital or a community setting; units are typically unlocked and activities are carried out in a community room, which serves as the center for meetings, recreation, and meals
    - Involves the patient's active participation in planning, implementing, and evaluating care; patient shares responsibility for establishing group rules and policies along with staff and other patients
    - Includes individual, group, and occupational therapy provided by staff (who are usually dressed in street clothes)
  - Detoxification programs are designed to help patients achieve abstinence
    - Offer a relatively safe alternative to self-withdrawal after prolonged dependence on alcohol or drugs

Types of psychotherapy

The therapist may act as a neutral observer or active participant. The success of therapy depends largely on patient-therapist compatibility, treatment goals, and the patient's commitment to therapy.

INDIVIDUAL THERAPY

Individual therapy involves a series of counseling sessions, which may be short- or long-term. After working with the patient to establish appropriate goals, the therapist mediates the patient's disturbed behavior patterns to promote personality growth and development.

GROUP THERAPY

Guided by a psychotherapist, a group of people (ideally four to ten) experiencing similar emotional problems meets to discuss their concerns. The duration of group therapy may vary from a few weeks for acute conditions requiring hospitalization to several years for chronic conditions. Group therapy can be especially useful in treating addictions.

COGNITIVE THERAPY

According to cognitive theory, depression stems from low self-esteem and a belief that the future is bleak and hopeless. The goal of cognitive therapy is to identify and change the patient's negative generalizations and expectations — and thereby reduce depression, distress, and other emotional problems.

The therapist assigns homework, such as making lists of pleasurable activities and reducing automatic negative thoughts and conclusions.

FAMILY THERAPY

Family therapy aims to alter relationships within the family and change the problematic behavior of one or more members. Useful in treating childhood or adolescent adjustment disorders, marital discord, and abusive situations, family therapy may be short- or long-term.

CRISIS INTERVENTION

Crisis intervention seeks to help patients develop adequate coping skills to resolve an immediate problem. The crisis may be developmental (such as a marriage or the death of a family member) or situational (such as a natural disaster or an illness).

Therapy focuses on helping the patient resume the precrisis functional level. It usually involves just the patient and therapist but sometimes includes family members. It may consist of one session or multiple sessions over several months.

Types of psychotherapy

- Individual therapy
- Group therapy
- Cognitive therapy
- Family therapy
- Crisis intervention

- – Held in outpatient centers or special units, which provide symptomatic treatment as well as counseling or psychotherapy on an individual, group, or family basis
- – Require skill, compassion, and commitment on part of the nurse and other staff
- – Require the nurse to be in control of her own feelings of anger and frustration because people who abuse substances typically have low self-esteem and subsequently may try to manipulate others
- ECT, one of the most controversial treatments in psychiatry, is sometimes used to treat severe depression; according to APA guidelines, it should be used only in treating severe, debilitating mental disorders

Behavior therapy

Suitable for adults or children, behavior therapy can be used either with an individual or with groups of patients who have similar problems.

The behavioral approach relies on therapies designed to change behavioral patterns. Commonly used therapies include assertiveness training, aversion therapy, desensitization, flooding, positive conditioning, response prevention, thought stopping, thought switching, and token economy.

ASSERTIVENESS TRAINING

Assertiveness training uses positive reinforcement, shaping, and modeling to reduce anxiety. It teaches the patient ways to express feelings, ideas, and wishes without feeling guilty or demeaning others.

You can help the patient by providing examples of appropriate behavior and suggesting situations in which he can be more assertive.

AVERSION THERAPY

In aversion therapy, a painful stimulus is applied to create an aversion to the obsession underlying the patient's undesirable behavior.

DESENSITIZATION

The treatment of choice for phobias, desensitization slowly exposes the patient to something he fears. Because phobias reflect unresolved conflicts, desensitization works best if used with other treatments. The patient learns to use deep breathing or another relaxation technique when confronted with a staged series of anxiety-producing situations.

During desensitization, provide the patient with reassurance and review relaxation techniques. Monitor his response to each anxiety-producing situation, and emphasize that he need not proceed to the next one until he feels ready.

FLOODING

Also called *implosion therapy*, flooding can bring rapid relief from phobias such as travel phobias. Like desensitization, it involves direct exposure to an anxiety-producing situation. However, instead of using relaxation techniques, it assumes that anxiety and panic can't persist and that confrontation helps the patient overcome fear.

Types of behavior therapy

- Assertiveness training
- Aversion therapy
- Desensitization
- Flooding
- Positive conditioning
- Response prevention
- Thought stopping
- Thought switching
- Token economy

– Requires written and informed consent in most states
– Potential candidates: severely depressed patients for whom psychotherapy and medication have proven ineffective; patients at immediate risk for suicide (because ECT produces much faster results than antidepressants); patients with certain psychotic syndromes
– Probably works by temporarily altering some of the brain's electrochemical processes, although exact mechanism is unclear
– Involves injection of short-acting general anesthetic along with succinylcholine (to temporarily paralyze muscles) and passage of a small electric current to brain for 1 second or less through electrodes placed above the temples (patient's brain waves and heart rhythm are monitored), producing a seizure, which lasts 30 seconds to 1 minute or slightly longer
– May be followed by brief period of confusion, headache, or muscle stiffness upon awakening (usually within 15 minutes after procedure); symptoms typically ease within 20 to 60 minutes

During flooding, monitor the patient for signs of excitation. If he faints or has another extreme reaction, remove him from the anxiety-producing situation and assess for signs and symptoms of psychological trauma.

POSITIVE CONDITIONING

Building on the principle of desensitization, positive conditioning attempts to gradually instill a positive or neutral attitude toward a phobia. This technique introduces a pleasurable stimulus such as music. The therapist encourages the patient to heighten the pleasurable stimulus by associating it with other pleasurable experiences. Next, the therapist introduces the phobic stimulus along with the pleasurable one. Gradually, the patient develops a positive response to the phobia.

If your patient is undergoing positive conditioning, reinforce relaxation techniques and provide encouragement.

RESPONSE PREVENTION

Response prevention seeks to prevent compulsive behavior through distraction, persuasion, or redirection of activity. To be effective, it may require that the patient enter a hospital and his family get involved in treatment.

THOUGHT STOPPING

Thought stopping helps the patient break the habit of fear-inducing anticipatory thoughts. He's taught to stop such thoughts by saying "stop" and then focusing his attention on achieving calmness and muscle relaxation.

THOUGHT SWITCHING

In thought switching, the patient learns to replace fear-inducing self-instructions with competent self-instructions. The therapist teaches the patient to substitute positive thoughts for fear-inducing ones until the positive thought is strong enough to overcome the fear-inducing one.

TOKEN ECONOMY

Using token economy, the therapist rewards acceptable behavior by giving out tokens, which the patient uses to "buy" a privilege or object. The therapist also may withhold or rescind tokens as punishment or to avert undesirable behavior.

During this treatment, monitor the patient's behavior and provide or withhold rewards consistently and promptly.

Key facts about ECT

- Used only in treating severe, debilitating mental disorders
- Requires written informed consent in most states
- Probably works by temporarily altering some of brain's electro-chemical processes, although exact mechanism is unclear
- May be followed by brief period of confusion, headache, or muscle stiffness upon awakening (usually within 15 minutes after procedure); symptoms typically ease within 20 to 60 minutes

– Usually involves a total of six to twelve treatments, with two or three treatments given weekly

EVALUATION

● **General information**
  - During evaluation, the nurse assesses the patient's progress in terms of how closely the patient has met goals included in the care plan
  - Although technically considered the final step in the nursing process, evaluation occurs throughout the entire nurse-patient relationship

● **Meeting goals**
  - The nurse looks at each of the outcome criteria (goals) stipulated in the care plan and collects additional data, as necessary, to determine whether treatment has been successful
  - Goals that remain partially met or totally unmet may require additional patient treatment or modification of the care plan

Legal importance of documentation

- Must be complete, consistent, accurate, and timely
- Provides legal proof of nature and quality of patient care
- Can be used as defense against allegations of negligence, improper treatment, and omissions in care

Key facts about psychiatric care trends and concerns

- Steady decline in federal funding has reduced mental health services and limited training of new mental health professionals.
- Funding cuts have placed future control of mental health services at state and local community levels.
- Collaboration between community psychiatric facilities and long-term inpatient state facilities has increased.
- Deinstitutionalization has increased number of both homeless and incarcerated persons with mental illness.
- Number of patients with dual diagnosis of chronic mental illness and substance abuse or dependence has been rising.

● Documentation

- Complete, accurate, and timely documentation is crucial to the continuity of patient care and has many legal implications
- The medical record is a legal and business record with many uses
  - Provides legal proof of the nature and quality of care that the patient received
  - Must be factual, consistent, timely, and complete
  - Can be used as a defense against allegations of negligence, improper treatment, and omissions in care
- Health care professionals have a legal duty to maintain the medical record in sufficient detail; inadequate documentation of care may result in liability or denial of reimbursement by third-party payers
- Documentation of care has become synonymous with care itself, and failure to document implies failure to provide care

MULTIDISCIPLINARY CARE

● Multidisciplinary team

- It typically includes many professionals of varying backgrounds and expertise
- Each member has specific responsibilities related to patient care

● Focus of care

- All team members focus on promoting the patient's psychological well-being
- Collaboration and coordination among members are essential

TRENDS AND CONCERNS IN PSYCHIATRIC CARE

● General information

- The steady decline in federal funding for mental health programs has markedly reduced mental health services and limited the training of new mental health professionals
- Funding cuts have placed the future control of mental health services at the state and local community levels
- Collaboration between community psychiatric facilities (short-term inpatient, outpatient, and auxiliary services) and long-term inpatient state facilities has increased

● Deinstitutionalization

- The push to deinstitutionalize mentally ill patients began several decades ago, with a shift toward providing mental health services for patients in the community
- Deinstitutionalization has increased the number of both homeless and incarcerated persons with mental illness
- Despite more public education programs and greater awareness of mental illness, the mentally ill continue to suffer stigmatization and prejudice

● Drugs and dual diagnoses

- The proliferation of street drugs poses a challenge to psychiatric treatment; some illicit drugs can cause permanent brain damage or lead to addiction with just one or two uses

- The number of patients with a dual diagnosis of chronic mental illness and substance abuse or dependence has been rising
- Patients with dual diagnoses require long-term treatment; many don't respond to conventional treatment protocols

LEGAL AND ETHICAL ISSUES

● **General information**
- Legal and ethical issues help shape the role of the psychiatric nurse
- Psychiatric nurses are held to the same standards of reasonable and prudent behavior expected of other professionals with the same education in similar circumstances
  - Must provide care that meets professional standards established by the ANA
  - Must know and abide by statutory provisions concerning patient admissions into psychiatric care
- Nurses and other health care providers must never violate the rights of mentally ill or developmentally disabled patients who, although dependent, have all of the same basic rights as other members of society. Any breach of these rights can have serious legal consequences
- Mentally ill and developmentally disabled persons are further protected by laws to ensure their right to fair and ethical treatment

● **Right to treatment**
- The courts have generally interpreted the U.S. Constitution to mean that mentally ill and developmentally disabled persons have a right to fair and humane treatment, including during hospitalization
- The Americans with Disabilities Act of 1990 ensures a disabled citizen's rights by providing a "national mandate for the elimination of discrimination against individuals with disabilities"
- In 1980, Congress passed the Mental Health Systems Act, which established a universal bill of rights for mental health patients
- The bill of rights specifies that treatment given meets certain criteria
  - By adequate staff
  - In the least restrictive setting
  - In privacy
  - In a facility that provides a comfortable bed, an adequate diet, and recreational facilities
  - With the patient's informed consent before unusual treatment
  - With payment for work done in the facility, outside of program activities
  - According to an individual treatment plan
- Nurses have a duty to ensure that the patient knows what treatment he needs and how he'll get it, to help prepare him for eventual discharge
  - Identifying the patient's major problems
  - Determining what the patient can do for himself and what others must do for him
  - When possible, allowing the patient to participate in formulating his treatment plan (unless there's a documented reason why he can't or shouldn't be involved)

How treatment must be given
- By adequate staff
- In least restrictive setting
- In privacy
- In facility that provides comfortable bed, adequate diet, and recreational facilities
- With patient's informed consent before unusual treatment
- With payment for work done in facility, outside of program activities
- According to individual treatment plan

Rights of mentally ill patients
- Right to treatment
- Right to refuse treatment
- Rights of minors
- Right to informed consent
- Right to privacy
- Reproductive and sexual rights

Criteria for court-ordered treatment

- Need has been clearly established
- Patient poses danger to himself or others
- Physician and treatment team demonstrate need for continued inpatient treatment

Evaluating informed consent

- Can consent for treatment or special procedure be obtained the same way it is from another patient?
- Does patient fully understand procedure he's to undergo, including risks and alternatives?
- Does patient have authority to give his own consent, or must someone else give it?

Consent to medical research

- Guidelines are complicated and raise unresolved questions.
- Potential risks must be weighed against potential benefits.
- Federal regulations guide methods for treatment.

● Right to refuse treatment
- Under most circumstances, a patient can't be kept in a hospital against his will, nor can he be denied the right to refuse treatment
- Despite the patient's wishes, treatment may be ordered by the court under special circumstances—only after need has been clearly established
  - When the patient poses a danger to himself or others
  - When the physician and treatment team demonstrate a need for continued inpatient treatment
- Nurses are expected to be familiar with the relevant laws of their practicing state

● Rights of minors
- When a mentally ill or developmentally disabled minor is admitted to the hospital, legal responsibility must be established immediately
- Usually, a parent accompanying the minor is legally responsible
- If the minor has been institutionalized before entering the hospital, the hospital may be responsible if the parents have waived responsibility and the institution has written evidence to prove it

● Right to informed consent
- Informed consent is the admitting provider's responsibility
- Each situation requires careful analysis to determine if the patient needs help in making health care decisions
- When consent is required from a mentally ill or developmentally disabled patient, three questions can be used to evaluate the situation
  - Can consent for treatment or a special procedure be obtained the same way it is from another patient?
  - Does the patient fully understand the procedure he's to undergo, including the risks and alternatives?
  - Does the patient have the authority to give his own consent, or must someone else give it?
- If the patient can't provide informed consent (isn't of sound mind or can't understand the nature, purpose, alternatives, and risks of the proposed treatment), consent must be obtained from his legal guardian; if the legal guardian is unavailable, the court is authorized to handle such matters and may authorize treatment
- The nurse can best protect the patient's right to informed consent by making sure the physician has provided him (or his guardian) with the required information and by documenting that consent was valid
- The nurse should refuse to participate in procedures for which informed consent hasn't been obtained, unless her absence would place the patient in danger; liability issues may apply
  - If the nurse participates: she could be held liable, along with the physician and the facility
  - If the patient is a minor: double liability is possible; parents could sue now, and the patient could sue when he comes of age

● Consent to medical research
- Guidelines for consent to medical experimentation and drastic, questionable, or extreme forms of treatment are complicated and raise many unresolved questions

- Institutional Review Boards should review research proposals before they are implemented, to weigh potential risks against potential benefits
- Strict federal regulations guide how experimental treatments can be carried out; such treatments must be used with extreme caution in mentally ill patients, who are considered a vulnerable group

Right to privacy

- The law tries to protect all citizens from unwarranted intrusion into their private lives
- Nurses have a professional and ethical responsibility to protect a patient's privacy including those of mentally ill patients
  - Requires more than just keeping patient information confidential
  - May involve teaching the patient about his privacy rights (he may not know what the right to privacy means or that he has such a right)
  - Includes following ANA Code of Ethics and the American Hospital Association's Patient Bill of Rights
- The law requires disclosure of confidential information only in certain circumstances
  - Suspected child abuse
  - Criminal cases
  - Government requests
  - When the public has a right to know
  - If the patient is an imminent risk to himself or others, safety takes precedence over confidentiality; in such cases, the nurse is legally bound to disclose the danger (known as *duty to inform*)

Reproductive and sexual rights

- The U.S. Supreme Court has upheld the reproductive and sexual rights of mentally ill patients
  - Right to marry
  - Right to have children
  - Right to use contraception, abortion, or sterilization, if desired
  - Right to follow a lifestyle of their own choosing

Advocacy options

- Guardianship issues may be a concern
  - If a patient is a minor, may be the parents, a legal or court-appointed guardian, or the state (sometimes necessary when parents are unfit or can't provide care and no guardian has been appointed)
  - If an adult, may be the parents or a spouse
- The nurse should check the patient's chart to determine guardianship
  - The guardian: has legal right to make decisions
  - Adult patients and their guardians: disagreement about care decisions require clarification via proper facility channels

Competence

- Sometimes a physician or nurse may doubt a patient's capacity to provide consent, even if he hasn't been judged incompetent (common with illnesses that cause temporary mental incompetence)
- The nurse should consult state laws to determine who can make health care decisions for the patient
  - Usually stipulated as the nearest relative

Right to privacy

Circumstances for disclosure of confidential information
- Suspected child abuse
- Criminal cases
- Government requests
- When public has a right to know
- If patient is imminent risk to himself or others

Reproductive and sexual rights
- Right to marry
- Right to have children
- Right to use contraception, abortion, or sterilization
- Right to follow lifestyle of their own choosing

Guardianship criteria
- For a minor: may be parents, legal or court-appointed guardian, or state
- For an adult: may be parents or spouse

Patient requests

- May be challenge to authority
- May be oppositional behavior: treatment team should be consulted

Criteria for involuntary admission

- Patient at risk for taking own life
- Patient poses threat to another person's life or property
- Mental illness alone not sufficient legal basis

Restraints and seclusion

- May be used only to prevent patient from seriously injuring himself or others
- May be used only when all other physical and psychological means have failed
- If required, only amount of restraint necessary to protect patient and staff is used

Criteria for using restraints

- Examination of patient by physician to determine need
- Written physician's order that's placed in patient's medical record before restraints are applied
- Application of restraints for specified duration (must follow state and facility regulations)

- When no relative can be found, requires court authorization
- Some patients have advance directives to address treatment preferences during times of temporary incompetence; the nurse should check the medical record and follow facility protocol in such cases

● **Responding to patient requests**
- Sometimes a patient will make an ordinary request that requires special consideration; the nurse's response would depend on the circumstances and her availability to supervise (a request to smoke a cigarette is an example)
  - If he's allowed to smoke only under supervision because of the danger of fire: the nurse may decide to stay with him while he smokes
  - If the nurse has a duty to be elsewhere: she should refuse his request, explaining why and telling him when he can smoke
  - If the nurse knows that refusal would agitate or anger him: she should consider asking another nurse to supervise the patient while he smokes
- In some cases, a patient's request is really a challenge to authority (such as requesting to smoke when a no-smoking policy is in effect); in such cases, the nurse may refuse the request, explaining the need to abide by facility policies
- If the patient's oppositional behavior is part of a pattern that includes such actions as refusing to shower, refusing go to bed by a certain time, or demanding to make an immediate phone call, the treatment team should be consulted; after a decision has been made, all health team members should enforce it consistently

● **Involuntary admission**
- A mentally ill or developmentally disabled person may be kept in a facility involuntarily if he's at risk for taking his own life or if he poses a threat to another person's life or property; however, mental illness alone isn't a sufficient legal basis for detaining a patient
- The nurse must know the laws regarding involuntary treatment in the state in which she practices and must never violate the patient's rights
  - Right to receive proper care
  - Right to treatment needed to make him less dangerous to himself or others, always using the least restrictive measures

● **Restraints and seclusion**
- Restraints and seclusion may be used only to prevent a patient from seriously injuring himself or others—and only when all other physical and psychological means are likely to fail to prevent such injuries
- If restraints are required, only the amount of restraint necessary to protect the patient and to safeguard staff and others is used
- Restraints are never used as punishment, for staff convenience, or as a substitute for treatment programs
- Use of restraints or seclusion must conform with facility policies guided by and in compliance with external regulatory boards and statutes
- Use of physical restraints typically requires certain elements
  - Examination of the patient by a physician to determine need
  - A written physician's order that's placed in the patient's medical record before restraints are applied
  - Application of the restraints for a specified duration (must follow state and facility regulations)

• Depending on the treatment facility, physical restraint may be applied without a physician's order in an emergency (such as a violent outburst with actual harm to persons); however, an order for the restraint should be obtained as soon as possible after the incident and documented carefully

NCLEX CHECKS

It's never too soon to begin your NCLEX® preparation. Now that you've reviewed this chapter, carefully read each of the following questions and choose the best answer. Then compare your responses to the correct answers.

1. The current system used for classifying and diagnosing mental disorders was established by the:
- ☐ **1.** ANA.
- ☐ **2.** state boards of nursing.
- ☐ **3.** APA.
- ☐ **4.** American Medical Association (AMA).

2. When completing the MSE of a patient, which of the following would the nurse assess? Select all that apply:
- ☐ **1.** LOC
- ☐ **2.** Mood and affect
- ☐ **3.** Effects of medication
- ☐ **4.** Current employment status
- ☐ **5.** Speech patterns
- ☐ **6.** Thought content

3. When developing a class presentation about changes that have occurred in the field of mental health, which of the following would the instructor include?
- ☐ **1.** Increase in the number of extended families providing support
- ☐ **2.** Greater understanding of the physiology of mental functioning
- ☐ **3.** Decrease in the rate of teenage depression
- ☐ **4.** Reduction in the rates of alcohol and substance abuse

4. Which theoretical model is being applied if the nurse views mental illness as a learned behavior?
- ☐ **1.** Existential model
- ☐ **2.** Social model
- ☐ **3.** Interpersonal model
- ☐ **4.** Behavioral model

5. The nurse asks a patient to remember three words: house, ball, and rain. About 10 minutes later, she asks the patient to repeat those words. Which aspect of memory is the nurse testing?
- ☐ **1.** Immediate recall
- ☐ **2.** Delayed recall
- ☐ **3.** Recent memory
- ☐ **4.** Remote memory

TOP 10

Items to study for your next test on psychiatric nursing

1. Stress and effects of stress on disease
2. Classification of mental disorders and the five axes of the *DSM-IV-TR*
3. Standards of care for psychiatric nursing
4. Phases of the nurse-patient relationship
5. Therapeutic and nontherapeutic communication techniques
6. Components of the mental status examination
7. Types of defense mechanisms
8. Interventions for suicidal ideation
9. Types of psychotherapy and behavioral health
10. Legal and ethical issues in mental health

6. The nurse observes a patient washing his hands every 5 minutes throughout the course of an interview, identifying this behavior as a characteristic of someone with:

☐ **1.** compulsions.
☐ **2.** obsessions.
☐ **3.** ideas of reference.
☐ **4.** delusions.

7. During the patient interview, the nurse notes that a patient is making excuses for his behaviors. She interprets this action as the patient's use of which defense mechanism?

☐ **1.** Reaction formation
☐ **2.** Projection
☐ **3.** Rationalization
☐ **4.** Regression

8. Which tool would the nurse use to assess a patient's orientation and recall?

☐ **1.** Beck Depression Inventory
☐ **2.** Thematic Apperception Test
☐ **3.** Mini–Mental Status Examination
☐ **4.** MMPI

9. Which of the following is the nurse least likely to include in the care plan of a client who's to receive behavioral therapy?

☐ **1.** Group therapy
☐ **2.** Assertiveness training
☐ **3.** Token economy
☐ **4.** Flooding

10. The nurse is legally required to disclose confidential patient information in which situation?

☐ **1.** When there's a suspicion of child abuse
☐ **2.** If a family member requests information
☐ **3.** When a legal guardian is chosen
☐ **4.** When the patient is a minor

ANSWERS AND RATIONALES

1. CORRECT ANSWER: 3
The APA established the system currently used for classifying and diagnosing mental disorders. The latest version, published in the *DSM-IV-TR*, emphasizes observable data and de-emphasizes subjective and theoretical impressions. The ANA is the professional organization for nurses of all disciplines. State boards of nursing establish the requirements for nursing licensure. The AMA is the professional organization for physicians.

2. CORRECT ANSWER: 1, 2, 5, 6
The MSE examines the patient's LOC, general appearance, behavior, speech, mood and affect, perceptions, intellectual performance, judgment, insight, and thought

content. Medication history, including the effects of specific drugs, and current employment status are general areas of the patient interview.

3. CORRECT ANSWER: 2

Advances in neurobiology have revolutionized our understanding of the physiologic basis of mental functioning. Changes in the traditional family structure have led to a loss of the extended family. Teenage depression rates have more than tripled in the past 20 years. Alcohol and substance abuse are proliferating and involving younger victims.

4. CORRECT ANSWER: 4

According to the behavioral model, which focuses on actions, all behavior — including mental illness — is learned. The existential model centers on a person's present experiences rather than past ones. It holds that alienation from the self causes deviant behavior and that people can make free choices about which behaviors to display. The social model proposes that the entire sociocultural environment influences mental health. The interpersonal model holds that human development results from interpersonal relationships and that behavior is motivated by avoidance of anxiety and attainment of satisfaction.

5. CORRECT ANSWER: 2

Telling the patient to remember three words and then asking him about them later tests the patient's delayed recall. Testing immediate recall involves having the patient state the three words immediately after asking him to remember them. Testing recent memory involves asking about an event that happened within the past few hours or days. Testing the patient's remote memory involves asking the patient to relate events in the distant past, such as where he was born or where he went to school.

6. CORRECT ANSWER: 1

Compulsions are repetitive behaviors that the patient feels compelled to perform in response to an obsession such as continual hand washing. Obsessions are preoccupations or constantly recurring thoughts that interfere with daily living. Ideas of reference refer to the patient's misinterpretation of another's acts in a highly personal way. Delusions are false fixed beliefs with no firm basis in reality.

7. CORRECT ANSWER: 3

Rationalization occurs when a person substitutes acceptable reasons for the real or actual reasons that are motivating his behavior. The patient makes excuses for shortcomings and avoids self-condemnation, disappointments, and criticism. Reaction formation involves the patient behaving in the opposite manner of the way that he feels. With projection, the patient attributes to others his own unacceptable thoughts, feelings, and impulses. Regression involves returning to the behaviors a patient used in an earlier, more comfortable time in his life.

8. CORRECT ANSWER: 3

The Mini–Mental Status Examination assesses the patient's orientation, registration, recall, calculation, language, and graphomotor function. The Beck Depression Inventory helps to diagnose depression and determine its severity. The Thematic Apperception Test is used to gain insight into a person's personality based on the story he creates in response to being shown a series of pictures. The MMPI is a paper and pencil test used to assess ego function and personality traits.

9. CORRECT ANSWER: 1

Group therapy is a type of psychotherapy that involves several individuals experiencing similar emotional problems who meet to discuss their concerns. Assertiveness training, token economy, and flooding are all examples of behavioral therapy.

10. CORRECT ANSWER: 1

The law requires disclosure of confidential information only in four situations: suspected child abuse, criminal cases, government requests, and when the public has a right to know. Disclosure under any other circumstances would be unethical and illegal.

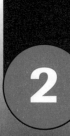

2

Disorders of children and adolescents

LEARNING OBJECTIVES

After studying this chapter, you should be able to:

- Explain the major theories of growth and development.
- Identify the characteristics of mentally healthy young people.
- List the most common psychiatric disorders that affect youth.
- Describe the signs and symptoms of psychiatric disorders in children and adolescents.
- Discuss the treatment options for children and adolescents with psychiatric disorders.

CHAPTER OVERVIEW

Because children and adolescents are in a state of rapid change and growth, a wide range of behavior is considered normal for them. Nonetheless, many children and adolescents experience emotional and mental distress that's more severe than the normal ups and downs of growing up are. Although some get better over time, others have serious and persistent problems that affect their daily activities—problems that require professional help.

Not long ago, most clinicians believed depression and certain other psychiatric disorders began only after childhood. Now we know these problems can start in early childhood and can affect the way a child develops. Unfortunately, it can be hard to tell whether a child or an adolescent has a psychiatric disorder or is demonstrating normal—if extreme—behavior for his age and developmental stage.

Key facts about mental health in children and adolescents

- Wide range of behavior is considered normal
- Many experience emotional and mental distress more severe than normal
- Problems can start in early childhood and affect development
- Sometimes difficult to differentiate psychiatric disorder and normal, but extreme, behavior

Key risk factors for mental illness in children

- Low birth weight
- Physical problems
- Family history of mental or addictive disorders
- Multigenerational poverty
- Separation from caregivers
- Abuse and neglect

Psychosocial consequences of psychiatric disorder

- May stigmatize child
- May be frightening or offensive to other children, making child social outcast
- Family members may feel guilty or embarrassed
- Family members may feel frustrated due to lack of knowledge or inability to cope
- Frustration may escalate and lead to verbal or physical abuse of child

MENTAL ILLNESS IN CHILDREN

● **Incidence**
- According to the National Institute of Mental Health, about 1 in 10 children and adolescents in the United States suffer from mental illness severe enough to cause impairment
- Fewer than one in five mentally ill children receive treatment—even though many of these disorders can be treated effectively with psychotherapy and drug therapy
- Psychiatric disorders occur in children and adolescents of all social classes and backgrounds

● **Risk factors**
- Low birth weight
- Physical problems
- Family history of mental or addictive disorders
- Multigenerational poverty
- Separation from caregivers
- Abuse and neglect

● **Psychosocial consequences**
- A child or adolescent with a psychiatric disorder has many challenges to overcome
  - May stigmatize a child—in some cases for his entire life
  - May be frightening or offensive to other children, making him a social outcast
- Family members may lack adequate knowledge of psychiatric disorders and may feel guilty or embarrassed at having a disturbed child
  - May be frustrated by lack of understanding or inability to cope with the child's behavior
  - May lead to escalation of frustration and possible verbal or physical abuse of the child
- A child whose behavior disrupts the family or who can't be integrated into the family unit may require temporary or permanent placement in a structured facility; this decision may be influenced by social, financial, religious, and cultural considerations
- Although most children and adolescents with psychiatric disorders can attend regular schools, those with severe disorders sometimes benefit from special classes or special educational facilities; such classes may be out of reach financially for some families

● **Childhood development**
- Understanding childhood disruptions and mental health problems requires familiarity with patterns of normal child development
- A child moves from infancy through childhood to adolescence in an orderly manner
- As the child grows, the personality develops; personality formation is influenced by both genetic and environmental factors
- Freud, Erikson, and Piaget proposed developmental theories to describe the progressive stages of childhood and adolescence (see *Theories of growth and development*)

Theories of growth and development

Several theorists, including Sigmund Freud, Erik Erikson, and Jean Piaget, explain how children develop intellectually, emotionally, sexually, socially, and spiritually.

FREUD: PSYCHOSEXUAL DEVELOPMENT

Freud theorized that the human mind consists of three major entities — id, ego, and superego. The id seeks instant gratification. The ego orients the person to reality, intercepting impulses from the id. The superego (conscience) develops during childhood — the product of rewards and punishments bestowed on the individual.

According to Freud, a child must master each developmental stage before he can move on to the next one.

- **Oral phase (birth to age 1):** The infant is totally dependent and narcissistic and starts to become aware of the self as an individual. Ego development begins.
- **Anal phase (ages 1 to 3):** The child learns to postpone immediate gratification and to manipulate surroundings. Episodes of negativity, rebellion, and conflict may occur. The superego begins to develop.
- **Phallic phase (ages 3 to 6):** The child becomes aware of gender and develops cooperation and socialization skills.
- **Latency period (ages 6 to 12):** As the child identifies with peers, parents become less important. Intellectual curiosity increases.
- **Adolescence (age 12 and older):** The child establishes close relationships with the opposite sex and devotes energy toward work, achievement, and interpersonal relationships. He moves away from emotional ties with family members.

ERIKSON: PSYCHOSOCIAL DEVELOPMENT

Erikson's theory of human development purports that major personality changes occur throughout life cycles. Passage from one stage to another depends on successfully gaining the skills of the preceding stage. Unlike other theorists, he suggests that new experiences may provide opportunities to cope with deficits in earlier stages.

- **Trust vs. mistrust (birth to age 1):** The infant derives a sense of security from gratification of needs.
- **Autonomy vs. shame and doubt (ages 1 to 3):** The child begins to view the self as a person apart from the parents.
- **Initiative vs. guilt (ages 3 to 6):** The child starts to behave assertively as he's guided to explore and investigate the world.
- **Industry vs. inferiority (ages 6 to 12):** Accomplishment occurs and a sense of responsibility develops as the child masters tasks and social skills.
- **Identity vs. role diffusion (ages 12 to 18):** The adolescent develops a sense of personal and role identity.

PIAGET: COGNITIVE DEVELOPMENT

Piaget's cognitive theory of development describes successive stages of mental activity that occur during childhood. By successfully encountering new experiences, the child adapts and progresses to the next stage.

- **Sensorimotor stage (birth to age 2):** The infant's world focuses on the self. He experiences and understands the world through the senses and motor movements.
- **Preoperational stage (ages 2 to 7):** The child develops language and egocentric thought, and begins symbolic play.
- **Concrete operations stage (ages 7 to 11):** The child develops the concepts of time, space, categories, numbers, and reversibility.
- **Formal operations stage (ages 12 to 15):** The adolescent begins to think abstractly and logically, and envision options and possibilities.

Freud's theory of psychosexual development

- Oral phase
- Anal phase
- Phallic phase
- Latency period
- Adolescence

Erikson's theory of psychosocial development

- Trust vs. mistrust
- Autonomy vs. shame and doubt
- Initiative vs. guilt
- Industry vs. inferiority
- Identity vs. role diffusion

Piaget's theory of cognitive development

- Sensorimotor stage
- Preoperational stage
- Concrete operations stage
- Formal operations stage

Assessment aspects of child development

- Trusting parents and appropriate caregivers
- Viewing world as safe place where needs will be met
- Having age-appropriate sense of reality
- Perceiving personal environment realistically
- Demonstrating positive sense of self
- Handling age-appropriate stress and frustration effectively
- Showing age-appropriate coping skills
- Demonstrating mastery of developmental tasks
- Communicating or expressing feelings and ideas
- Having useful and satisfying relationships

Communication guidelines

- Keep verbal communication brief, and use simple language.
- Ask direct questions when seeking specific information.
- Use body language to reinforce statements, and help child express ideas and feelings.
- Give feedback when appropriate, based on child's developmental stage.
- Talk about reality by focusing on the "here and now."
- Speak quietly but firmly when reinforcing behavioral limits.
- Avoid arguments.
- Make expectations clear.
- Role-model effective ways of communicating.

- Nurses need to understand the characteristics of normal growth and development to identify abnormal behavior in mentally ill children; this understanding involves assessing the child's development with regard to certain aspects
  - Trusting parents and appropriate caregivers
  - Viewing the world as a safe place where needs will be met
  - Having an age-appropriate sense of reality
  - Perceiving the personal environment realistically
  - Demonstrating a positive sense of self
  - Handling age-appropriate stress and frustration effectively
  - Showing age-appropriate coping skills
  - Demonstrating mastery of developmental tasks
  - Communicating or expressing feelings and ideas
  - Having useful and satisfying relationships

COMMUNICATION

General information

- When caring for a child or an adolescent with a psychiatric disorder, the first task is to establish rapport
- Demonstrating empathy and understanding is key
- The child may be frightened at first
- Initiating conversation by asking about toys, hobbies, pets, and other subjects he's interested in helps to break the ice

Guidelines to enhance communication

- Keep verbal communication brief, and use simple language
- Ask direct questions when seeking specific information
- Use body language to reinforce statements, and help the child express ideas and feelings
- Give feedback when appropriate, based on the child's developmental stage
- Talk about reality by focusing on the "here and now"
- Speak quietly but firmly when reinforcing behavioral limits
- Avoid arguments
- Make expectations clear
- Role-model effective ways of communicating

ASSESSMENT AND DIAGNOSIS

General information

- To assess a child or adolescent for a psychiatric disorder, evaluate the family as well
- Begin by collecting biographic data, including the ages of all family members, from the parents
- Gather information about the family's health, education, housing, economic situation, and religious, ethnic, and cultural background; keep in mind that various factors, including sociocultural factors, influence a child's display of emotions
- Document your description of the parents, including any marital problems

Assessing the mental status of a child or an adolescent

When evaluating the mental status of a child or adolescent, be sure to assess:

- physical appearance (including whether the patient looks his age)
- hygiene and grooming
- attention level and behavior during the interview
- understanding of his role in the interview
- speech or language development
- intellectual functioning
- judgment
- insight into self and the situation
- mannerisms, tics, and other involuntary movements
- mood and affect
- anxiety level
- obvious obsessive or compulsive behaviors
- frustration tolerance
- impulsiveness
- acting out or oppositional behavior
- verbal or physical aggression
- thought disorders, hallucinations, or delusions.

ESPECIALLY FOR ADOLESCENTS

If the patient is an adolescent, also evaluate for:

- depression
- communication problems
- difficulty expressing feelings
- low self-esteem
- unmet needs for attention and affection
- emotional closeness to peers
- relationship difficulties
- overachievement or underachievement
- noncompliance with family or school rules
- ineffective support system
- limited coping or problem-solving skills
- limited social skills
- impulsive behavior
- procrastination
- lack of leisure skills
- academic or employment problems
- discomfort with sexual feelings or inappropriate sexual behaviors
- money problems
- drug and alcohol use.

Guidelines for parental and child interviews

- Ask parents about how they view child's problem.
- Evaluate each parent's attitude.
- Obtain child's developmental history.
- Ask about services and agencies involved in family's or child's care.
- Interview child after interviewing parents.
- Include assessment of child's mental status.

● Parental interview

- Ask the parents what their concerns are
- Question how they view their child's problem and what they think might have caused it
- Evaluate each parent's attitude toward the child and his condition
- Obtain the child's developmental history from the parents
- Find out which, if any, services and agencies are involved in the family's or child's care

● Child interview

- Interview the child after interviewing the parents
- Include an assessment of his mental status (see *Assessing the mental status of a child or an adolescent*)

● Medical diagnosis

- A child with signs or symptoms of a psychiatric disorder should be evaluated by a physician
- Based on findings, the physician may recommend further evaluation by a specialist in child behavioral problems, such as a psychiatrist, psychologist, social worker, or advanced practice psychiatric nurse

Making a diagnosis

- Child should be evaluated by a physician.
- Physician may recommend further evaluation by specialist in child behavioral problems.

Characteristics of ADHD

- Neurobiological disorder
- Marked by developmentally inappropriate inattention, impulsiveness and, in some cases, hyperactivity
- May progress to conduct disorder
- Affects at least twice as many boys as girls
- Some children aren't diagnosed until they enter school
- Many symptoms continue into adulthood

Common causes of ADHD

- Genetic influence
- Typically found in at least one other close relative
- Other relatives may have symptoms that don't meet diagnostic criteria

Risk factors for ADHD

- Drug exposure in utero
- Birth complications
- Low birth weight
- Lead poisoning

- Evaluation by a specialist needs to be focused
  - Considering the child's developmental level, social and physical environment, and reports from parents and teachers
  - Ruling out other possible causes for the child's signs and symptoms
  - If appropriate, making a diagnosis according to criteria established by the American Psychiatric Association (APA)
- As for adults, psychiatric disorders in children and adolescents are classified and diagnosed according to the APA's *Diagnostic and Statistical Manual of Mental Disorders*, Fourth Edition, Text Revision

ATTENTION DEFICIT HYPERACTIVITY DISORDER

Defining characteristics

- A neurobiological disorder, attention deficit hyperactivity disorder (ADHD) is marked by developmentally inappropriate inattention, impulsiveness and, in some cases, hyperactivity
- The child's behavior may cause problems at school, in the home, and in the community and may influence his emotional development and social skills
- Unless identified and treated properly, ADHD may progress to conduct disorder, academic and job failure, depression, relationship problems, and substance abuse
- ADHD affects at least twice as many boys as girls; most children experience signs and symptoms by age 4
- Some children aren't diagnosed until they enter school; ADHD affects roughly 3% to 5% of school-age children in the United States, amounting to as many 2 million children—an average of one in every classroom
- Until recently, experts thought children outgrew ADHD by adolescence, but many symptoms continue into adulthood, causing frustrating dreams and emotional pain; approximately 2% to 4% of adults are affected

Causes

- No known biological basis
- Suggested genetic influence; at least one-third of men who had ADHD in their youth have children with the disorder
  - Typically found to exist in at least one other close relative
  - In some cases, may have a relative with symptoms that don't necessarily meet diagnostic criteria but that have a negative impact on parenting skills

Risk factors

- Drug exposure in utero
- Birth complications, such as toxemia, hypoxia, or head trauma
- Low birth weight
- Preexisting neurologic conditions, such as cerebral palsy or epilepsy
- Lead poisoning
- Multiple stressful events
- Child abuse

Signs and symptoms

- Inattention: hallmark symptom
- Short attention span

    – Focusing deliberate, conscious attention on tasks (he tends to get bored easily, tiring of tasks after just a few minutes)
    – Organizing and completing a task (he tends to lose things, be forgetful, and make careless mistakes)
    – Learning something new (because of his easy distraction, he's often reluctant to engage in tasks that call for sustained mental effort)
- Highly impulsive
    – Acting before thinking
    – Interrupting others (blurting out inappropriate remarks or answering a question before the person has finished asking it)
    – Having difficulty waiting his turn and waiting for things he wants
    – Grabbing other children's toys or striking out physically when upset
- Hyperactivity
    – Seeming to be always in motion and can't sit still
    – Trying to do several things at once
    – In school, fidgeting or squirming in seat, roaming around the room, or talking excessively
    – Having trouble engaging in quiet activities and finding it impossible to sit through a class
    – Incessantly tapping pencils, wiggling feet, or touching everything
- Behaviors intensified with boredom, unstructured situations, or required concentration for an extended period

Diagnosis
- Complete medical evaluation, with emphasis on a neurologic examination, hearing, and vision
- A psychiatric evaluation to assess intellectual ability, academic achievement, and potential learning disorder problem
- Speech and language evaluations
- Hinges on specific characteristic behaviors
    – Must appear before age 7, continue for at least 6 months, and be more frequent or severe than in that of other children the same age
    – Must create a real handicap in at least two areas of the child's life (such as school, home, or social settings)
    – Child must be overly active at school *and* unable to function well elsewhere

Treatment
- Focuses on coordinating the child's psychological and physiologic needs
- Psychotherapy to reduce ADHD symptoms and teach the child ways to modify behavior
- Such drugs as methylphenidate (Ritalin) to ease inattention, impulsiveness, and hyperactivity (see *Pharmacologic options for treating ADHD,* pages 46 and 47)
- Individualized educational plan with special services that support his strengths and minimize problems stemming from his vulnerabilities
- Family education to explain expectations, effects of medications, and need for additional structure

Nursing interventions
- Develop a trusting and accepting relationship with the child.
- Encourage him to talk about problems, difficulties, and feelings
- Assess his risk for injury related to hyperactivity and gross motor behaviors

---

Key signs and symptoms of ADHD

- Inattention (hallmark symptom)
- Short attention span
- Highly impulsive
- Hyperactivity

Diagnosing ADHD

- Hinges on specific characteristics behaviors
- Must appear before age 7 and continue for at least 6 months
- Symptoms must be more frequent or severe than seen in other children of same age
- Must create real handicap in at least two areas of child's life
- Child must be overly active at school *and* unable to function well elsewhere

Key treatment options for ADHD

- Coordination of child's psychological and physiologic needs
- Psychotherapy to reduce symptoms and teach child ways to modify behavior
- Such drugs as methylphenidate to ease inattention, impulsiveness, and hyperactivity
- Individualized educational plan, with special services that support child's strengths and minimize problems stemming from his vulnerabilities
- Family education to explain expectations, effects of medications, and need for additional structure

Pharmacologic options for treating ADHD

- Dextroamphetamine
- Methylphenidate
- Pemoline

Key nursing interventions for a patient with ADHD

- Develop trusting and accepting relationship with child.
- Encourage him to talk about problems, difficulties, and feelings.
- Assess his risk for injury.
- Maintain safe, calm environment that minimizes stimulation and distractions.
- Discuss with him disruptive behaviors, patterns of losing control, and consequences of disruptive behaviors.
- Teach him how to make choices and select appropriate ways of behaving.
- Monitor his activities and help him set limits, stay calm, and take opportunities to control undesirable behaviors.
- Schedule frequent breaks to help him control impulsiveness and minimize hyperactive behaviors.
- Help him learn how to take his turn, wait in line, and follow rules.

Pharmacologic options for treating ADHD

Three central nervous system stimulants have been used effectively to control symptoms of attention deficit hyperactivity disorder (ADHD) in both children and adults — dextroamphetamine (Dexedrine), methylphenidate (Ritalin), and pemoline (Cylert). For many patients, these drugs dramatically reduce hyperactivity and improve their ability to focus, learn, and work.

DRUG	ADVERSE REACTIONS	
Dextroamphetamine	• Anorexia • Weight loss or decrease in expected weight gain • Diarrhea • Insomnia • Hyperactivity	• Restlessness • Headache • Mild blood pressure elevation • Dizziness • Mild depression • Skin rash
Methylphenidate	• Anorexia • Nausea • Weight loss or decrease in expected weight gain • Temporary growth delay • Stomachache • Abdominal pain • Headache	• Insomnia • Transient motor tics • Mild blood pressure elevation • Social withdrawal • Rebound hyperactivity or irritability • Nervous habits
Pemoline	• Anorexia • Nausea • Weight loss or decrease in expected weight gain • Temporary growth delay • Stomachache • Seizures • Insomnia • Tourette syndrome	• Mild blood pressure elevation • Headache • Mild depression • Skin rash • Irritability • Elevated liver enzymes • Jaundice • Dry mouth

- Maintain a safe, calm environment that minimizes stimulation and distractions and helps the child remain in control
- Help the child determine acceptable and unacceptable behaviors
- Discuss with him disruptive behaviors, patterns of losing control, and consequences of disruptive behaviors
- Teach him how to make choices and select appropriate ways of behaving
- Monitor his activities and help him set limits, stay calm, and take opportunities to control undesirable behaviors
- Schedule frequent breaks to help him control impulsiveness and minimize hyperactive behaviors
- Teach the parents that hunger, thirst, fatigue, and other physical problems may trigger hyperactivity
- Help the child learn how to take his turn, wait in line, and follow rules
- Work with him to divide tasks into attainable steps so he's more likely to complete them successfully
- Give him opportunities to participate in activities with peers

CONTRAINDICATIONS	NURSING INTERVENTIONS
• Use of monoamine oxi-dase inhibitor therapy within previous 14 days (may cause a hyperten-sive crisis) • Tartrazine allergy	• Give first dose on awakening, followed by second dose in 4 to 6 hours. • Discuss concurrent use of prescription and over-the-counter (OTC) drugs with child's primary health care provider. • Monitor growth and development regularly. • Monitor sleep patterns. • Be aware that stimulant drugs have the potential for abuse.
• Tourette syndrome • Diabetes mellitus • Kidney disease • Cardiovascular disease	• Give with meals to minimize anorexia. • Administer at least 6 hours before bedtime. • Monitor growth and development regularly. Weigh the child two to three times weekly. • Monitor growth parameters. • Monitor vital signs. • Monitor for tics. • Monitor for depression. • Be aware that stimulant drugs have the potential for abuse.
• Age younger than 6 years • Impaired liver function • Epilepsy	• Give with food in the morning to minimize anorexia. • Monitor growth and development regularly. • Tell parents that therapeutic effects take 3 to 4 weeks to ap-pear. • Monitor vital signs. • Discuss concurrent use of OTC drugs with the child's primary health care provider. • Know that higher doses decrease seizure threshold. • Advise parents to withhold the child's drug over vacations and holidays. • Be aware that stimulant drugs have the potential for abuse.

• Provide positive feedback for improvement as he starts to take steps to man-age problematic behaviors

AUTISTIC DISORDER

● **Defining characteristics**
   • Autistic disorder is a pervasive developmental disorder characterized by inap-propriate responses to the environment; pronounced impairments in lan-guage, communication, and social interaction; and repetitive interests and be-haviors
   • The autistic child has disordered thinking (possibly severe learning diffi-culties and impaired intelligence) and difficulty understanding and us-ing language
      – Has difficulty understanding the feelings of others and the world around him

Characteristics of autistic disorder
• Inappropriate responses to envi-ronment
• Pronounced impairments in lan-guage, communication, and so-cial interaction
• Repetitive interests and behaviors
• Disordered thinking
• Difficulty understanding feelings of others and world around him
• Repetitive, self-injurious, or oth-er abnormal behaviors
• Occurs in 10 to 12 of every 10,000 children

Common causes of autistic disorder

- No known common cause
- May be from abnormal brain structure or function
- Possible genetic predisposition

Key signs and symptoms of autistic disorder

- During infancy: appearance of hearing failure
- Regression at age 2 after seemingly normal development
- Young children: impaired language development and difficulty expressing their needs
- Indifference toward others
- Delayed and impaired verbal and nonverbal communication
- Lack of intonation and expression in speech
- Repetitive rocking motions
- Hand flapping
- Dislike of changes in daily activities and routines
- Self-injurious behaviors, such as head banging, hitting, or biting
- Unusual fascination with inanimate objects, such as fans and air conditioners
- Dislike of touching and cuddling
- No fear of danger

Diagnosing autistic disorder

- Usually diagnosed by age 3
- Standardized rating scale for evaluation
- Tests for certain genetic and neurologic problems

– Typically appears aloof from others and lacks interest in social interactions
– Seems to prefer inanimate objects to human companionship, and may grow inappropriately attached to such objects
- In many cases, an autistic child will demonstrate repetitive, self-injurious, or other abnormal behaviors that seem strange when compared with those of other children; however, the child's physical appearance (size, shape) is otherwise normal
- Autistic disorder occurs in 10 to 12 of every 10,000 children and is up to five times more common in boys than it is in girls; it begins in childhood and lasts throughout life

Causes
- No known single cause
- May stem from abnormalities in brain structure or function
- Medical problems and a genetic predisposition; couples with one autistic child have a 7% chance of having another
- Possible links between autism and pregnancy or delivery complications and such environmental factors as viral infections, infant vaccines, metabolic imbalances, and exposure to environmental chemicals

Signs and symptoms
- During infancy: appearance of hearing failure of child
- Regression at age 2 after seemingly normal development
- Young children: impaired language development and difficulty expressing their needs
- Indifference toward others
- Delayed and impaired verbal and nonverbal communication
- Abnormal speech patterns, such as echolalia (repeating words or phrases spoken by others)
- Lack of intonation and expression in speech
- Repetitive rocking motions
- Hand flapping
- Insistence on sameness
- Dislike of changes in daily activities and routines
- Self-injurious behaviors, such as head banging, hitting, or biting
- Unusual fascination with inanimate objects, such as fans and air conditioners
- Dislike of touching and cuddling
- Frequent outbursts and tantrums
- Little or no eye contact with others
- Increased or decreased sensitivity to pain
- No fear of danger

Diagnosis
- No definitive diagnostic tool; usually diagnosed by age 3 — after first ruling out other disorders that resemble autism (neurologic disorders, hearing loss, speech problems, and mental retardation)
- Autism identifying methods by an autism specialist
  – Standardized rating scale to help evaluate the child's social behavior and language
  – Tests for certain genetic and neurologic problems (may be ordered)
  – Interviews with the parents to elicit information about the child's behavior and early development (reviewing family videotapes, photos, and baby

Screening tools for autism

Although no single behavioral or communication test can detect autism, several screening instruments can be used as aids in diagnosing the disorder.

CHILDHOOD AUTISM RATING SCALE

The Childhood Autism Rating Scale is a 15-point scale based on observed behavior. It evaluates the child's relationship to other people, including body use, adaptation to change, listening response, and verbal communication.

CHECKLIST FOR AUTISM IN TODDLERS

The Checklist for Autism in Toddlers screens for autism in children age 18 months. A short questionnaire, it has two sections – one completed by the parents and the other by the child's physician.

AUTISM SCREENING QUESTIONNAIRE

The Autism Screening Questionnaire is a 40-item screening scale used with children age 4 and older. It evaluates communication skills and social functioning.

SCREENING TEST FOR AUTISM IN 2-YEAR-OLDS

The Screening Test for Autism in 2-Year-Olds uses direct observation to study behavioral features in children younger than age 2. It identifies three skills areas important in diagnosing autism: play, motor imitation, and joint attention.

> ### Screening tools for autistic disorder
>
> - Childhood Autism Rating Scale
> - Checklist for Autism in Toddlers
> - Autism Screening Questionnaire
> - Screening Test for Autism in 2-Year-Olds

albums may help parents recall when the child reached certain developmental milestones)
- Developmental screening to reveal behaviors suggestive of autism
  - Failure to babble, coo, or gesture (point, wave, or grasp) by age 12 months
  - Failure to say single words by age 16 months and to say two-word phrases on his own by age 24 months
  - Loss of language or social skills at any age (see *Screening tools for autism*)
- After evaluation and testing, diagnoses is based on clear evidence of poor or limited social relationships; underdeveloped communication skills; and repetitive behaviors, activities, and interests

● Treatment
- A combination of early intervention, special education, family support and, in some cases, medication to help some autistic children lead more normal lives
- Early intervention and special education programs
  - Increase the child's capacity to learn, communicate, and relate to others
  - Reduce the severity and frequency of disruptive behaviors
- No drug shown to treat autistic disorder successfully; however, some drugs used to help manage symptoms
  - Stimulants (such as methylphenidate): may reduce inattentiveness, impulsivity, and overactivity in some children; however, stimulants may also increase the child's internal preoccupation, stereotypical behavior, and social withdrawal
  - Selective serotonin reuptake inhibitors (SSRIs): may be useful in managing compulsive behavior, irritability, and withdrawal
  - Lithium: helps reduce certain mood disorders associated with autism

> ### Key treatment options for autistic disorder
>
> - Early intervention
> - Special education
> - Family support
> - Drugs to manage symptoms: Stimulants, SSRIs, lithium

Teaching tips for caring for a child with autism

- Use close, face-to-face contact.
- Maintain regular, predictable daily routine.
- Use picture board showing daily activities.
- Prepare child for changes in routine.
- Avoid situations known to trigger outbursts.
- Recognize behaviors that precede temper tantrums.
- Make the home safer.
- Prevent injury.
- Be aware that punishment may worsen self-injurious behavior.
- Give tangible rewards.
- Instruct parents about any medications.
- Provide referrals.

 TIME-OUT FOR TEACHING

Caring for a child with autism

Caring for an autistic child at home is often a stressful endeavor for parents. It requires maintaining rigid schedules, detailed planning for any anticipated changes, close supervision of their child, and a great deal of patience. These tips may be helpful.

- To promote communication, advise the parents to have close, face-to-face contact with the child.
- Teach them to maintain a regular, predictable daily routine, with consistent times for waking up, dressing, eating, attending school, and going to bed.
- Suggest that they use a picture board showing the activities that will occur during the day, to help the child make transitions more easily.
- If the child's routine must be changed, instruct the parents to prepare the child for the changes.
- Advise the parents to avoid situations known to trigger outbursts.
- Teach the parents how to recognize the behaviors that precede temper tantrums such as increased hand

flapping. Instruct them to intervene before a tantrum occurs.
- Instruct the parents on ways to make the home safer—for instance, by installing locks and gates so the child can't wander unsupervised.
- If the child's behavior is self-injurious, advise the parents about ways to prevent injury.
- Inform the parents that punishment may worsen self-injurious behavior.
- Help the parents devise a plan to improve behavior by giving tangible rewards for desired behavior.
- Instruct the parents on any medications the child is taking.
- Provide referrals for early intervention, home care assistance, and support groups, as needed.

- Other drugs under investigation, including risperidone (Risperdal) and buspirone (BuSpar): may help ease explosive outbursts
- Family counseling to help the parents better understand the disorder and assist them with coping strategies and behavior modification therapies
- Home care to assist with the child's physical or behavioral management in the home; if the child's disruptive behavior persists, alternative residential placement may be necessary
- Special schools that use behavior modification; however, educational mainstreaming preferred

● Nursing interventions

- Choose your words carefully when speaking to a verbal autistic child; the child is likely to interpret words concretely and may interpret a harmless request as a threat
- Offer emotional support and information to the parents; suggest they meet with parents of other autistic children for advice on coping with tantrums, toilet training, and other problems (see the teaching tips offered in *Caring for a child with autism*)

Key nursing interventions for a patient with autistic disorder

- Choose words carefully when speaking to child.
- Offer emotional support and information to parents.

CONDUCT DISORDER

● **Defining characteristics**
- Aggressive behavior is the hallmark
  - Fights, bullies, intimidates, and assaults others physically or sexually
  - Has poor relationships with peers and adults
  - Violates others' rights and society's rules
- A child with conduct disorder rarely performs at the level predicted by IQ or age, causing academic, social, and developmental problems
  - May perform poorly at school or work
  - May be expelled from school and have problems with the law
  - If removed from the home, may have difficulty staying in an adoptive or foster family or a group home, further complicating his development
- Among children ages 9 to 17, the prevalence is approximately 1% to 4%
  - Occurs in both males and females, but more common in males
  - Typical onset before age 18
  - Early onset (occurring before age 10): predominantly affects males; associated with a worse prognosis and greater likelihood of developing antisocial personality disorder in adulthood (25% to 50% of highly antisocial children become antisocial adults)
- A child with conduct disorder is also at risk for sexually transmitted diseases, rape, teenage pregnancy, injuries, substance abuse, depression, suicidal thoughts, suicide attempts, and suicide

● **Causes**
- Unknown
- Suggested biological (including genetic) and psychosocial components in studies of twins and adopted children
- ADHD occurring in 30% to 50% of children with conduct disorder

● **Risk factors**
- Various social factors that lead to lack of attachment to the parents or family unit — and eventually, to lack of regard for societal rules
  - Early maternal rejection
  - Separation from parents, with no adequate alternative caregiver available
  - Early institutionalization
  - Family neglect, abuse, or violence
  - Frequent verbal abuse from parents, teachers, or other authority figures
  - Parental psychiatric illness, substance abuse, or marital discord
  - Large family size, crowding, and poverty
- Physical factors and other conditions
  - Neurologic damage caused by low birth weight or birth complications
  - Underarousal of the autonomic nervous system
  - Learning impairments
  - Insensitivity to physical pain and punishment

● **Signs and symptoms**
- Aggressive behavior (most common indication)
  - Fighting with family members and peers
  - Speaking to others in a nasty manner
  - Being cruel to animals

Characteristics of conduct disorder

- Aggressive behavior (hallmark symptom)
- Child rarely performs at level predicted by IQ or age

Key causes of conduct disorder

- Unknown
- May have biological and psychosocial components in twins and adopted children

Key risk factors for conduct disorder

- Early maternal rejection
- Separation from parents, with no adequate alternative caregiver available
- Early institutionalization
- Family neglect, abuse, or violence
- Frequent verbal abuse from parents, teachers, or other authority figures
- Parental psychiatric illness, substance abuse, or marital discord
- Large family size, crowding, and poverty

Key signs and symptoms of conduct disorder

- Aggressive behavior
- Destruction of property
- Deceitfulness or theft
- Disregard for rules

Diagnosing conduct disorder

- Requires team approach
- Educational assessment
- Neurologic exam if history of head trauma or seizures

Key treatment options for conduct disorder

- Psychotherapy to help with developing problem-solving skills, decreasing disruptive symptoms, and modifying behavior
- Drugs to treat neurologic difficulties
- Educational strategies to encourage and help child continue with school
- Early identification of at-risk children
- Parental instruction to teach how to deal with child's demands
- Juvenile justice system, if needed, to provide structured rules and means for monitoring and controlling child's behavior

Key nursing interventions for a child with conduct disorder

- Work to establish trusting relationship with child and family.
- Provide clear behavioral guidelines.
- Talk to him about making acceptable choices.
- Teach him effective problem-solving skills.
- Help him to identify personal needs and best strategies for meeting them.
- Teach him how to express anger.
- Monitor him for anger as well as for signs that he's internalizing anger.

– Engaging in precocious sexual activity
– Abusing others sexually
- Other indicators: destruction of property, deceitfulness or theft, and disregard for rules
    – Vandalizing or destroying property
    – Cheating in school
    – Skipping classes
    – Smoking cigarettes
    – Using drugs or alcohol
    – Stealing or shoplifting

Diagnosis
- Complete team approach—including medical and psychiatric evaluations, feedback from parents, a school consultant's recommendations, a case manager's plan, and a probation officer's report, important because antisocial behaviors tend to be underreported
- Educational assessments to determine if there are cognitive deficits, learning disabilities, or problems in intellectual functioning
- A neurologic examination if there's a history of head trauma or seizures

Treatment
- Focuses on coordinating the child's psychological, physiologic, and educational needs
    – Psychotherapy to help with developing problem-solving skills, decreasing disruptive symptoms, and modifying behavior
    – Drugs to treat neurologic difficulties
    – Educational strategies to encourage and help the child continue with school
- Early identification of at-risk children
- Parental instruction to teach how to deal with the child's demands
    – May need to learn to reinforce appropriate behaviors and to use harsh punishment for inappropriate behaviors
    – Should be encouraged to find ways to bond more strongly with child
- Juvenile justice system, if needed, to provide structured rules and a means for monitoring and controlling the child's behavior

Nursing interventions
- Work to establish a trusting relationship with the child and family; be sure to convey that you accept him
- Provide clear behavioral guidelines, including consequences for disruptive and manipulative behavior
- Talk to him about making acceptable choices
- Teach him effective problem-solving skills, and have him demonstrate them in return
- Help him to identify personal needs and the best strategies for meeting them
- Identify abusive communication, such as threats, sarcasm, and disparaging comments; encourage the child to stop using them
- Teach him how to express anger appropriately through constructive methods to release negative feelings and frustrations
- Monitor him for anger as well as for signs that he's internalizing anger, as shown by depression or suicidal ideation

- Work on helping the child accept responsibility for behavior rather than blaming others, becoming defensive, and wanting revenge
- Teach him effective coping skills and social skills
- Use role-playing so he can practice ways of handling stress and gain skill and confidence in managing difficult situations

MAJOR DEPRESSION

● Defining characteristics

- Mood changes are normal; however, when a sad mood persists and causes difficulty eating, sleeping, or concentrating, clinical depression may be present
- Depression can have widespread effects on a child's adjustment and functioning
  - Child may feel unloved, pessimistic, or even hopeless about the future (possibly thinking life isn't worth living)
  - Increases the child's risk for physical illness and psychosocial difficulties that persist long after the depressive episode resolves
- Major depression (also called *unipolar depression*) is a syndrome of persistently sad or irritable mood accompanied by disturbances in sleep and appetite, lethargy, and inability to experience pleasure
  - Characterized by one or more major depressive episodes, defined as episodes of depressed mood lasting at least 2 weeks
  - May occur as a single episode of depression followed by complete recovery (experienced by about half of all depressed patients) or depression that recurs at least once
  - Usually marked by episodes lasting an average of 7 to 9 months
- Depressed children and adolescents are typically sad and lose interest in activities that used to please them
  - Irritability that may lead to aggressive behavior
  - Difficulty making decisions and concentrating
  - Lack of energy or motivation
  - Neglect of appearance and hygiene
- Roughly 2% to 3% of children and more than 8% of adolescents in the United States suffer from depression
  - Associated with an earlier onset than it has been in past decades
  - With early onset: may persist, recur, and continue into adulthood (possibly with more severe episodes)
- Depressed adolescents are at increased risk for substance abuse and suicidal behavior
  - Suicide attempts: typically peak during the midadolescent years
  - Incidence of death from suicide: increases steadily throughout adolescent years
  - Suicide: third leading cause of death among adolescents

● Possible causes

- Controversial and not fully understood
- Possible genetic, familial, biochemical, physical, psychological, and social causes
- Patient history: specific personal loss or severe stress that probably interacts with a depression predisposition

---

Characteristics of major depression

- Also called *unipolar depression*
- Persistently sad or irritable mood accompanied by disturbances in sleep and appetite, lethargy, and inability to experience pleasure
- One or more major depressive episodes, defined as episodes of depressed mood lasting at least 2 weeks
- May occur as single episode of depression followed by complete recovery (experienced by about half of all depressed patients) or depression that recurs at least once
- Usually marked by episodes lasting an average of 7 to 9 months

Possible causes of major depression

- Genetic
- Familial
- Biochemical
- Physical
- Psychological
- Social
- Imbalances in major neurotransmitters

- Imbalances in the major neurotransmitters serotonin, norepinephrine, dopamine, acetylcholine, and gamma-aminobutyric acid
- Computed tomography (CT) and positron emission tomography (PET) scans: show abnormally slow activity in the prefrontal cortex and temporal lobes of depressed patients; suggest faulty glucose metabolism in prefrontal cortex and temporal lobes
- Link to genetic abnormalities involving chromosomes 4, 11, 18, and 21; family history of depression increases risk
- Certain medical conditions
  - Neurologic problems, such as brain tumor, brain trauma, multiple sclerosis, Parkinson's disease, and Huntington's disease
  - Cardiovascular disease
  - Acquired immunodeficiency syndrome
  - Electrolyte imbalances (especially calcium, magnesium, sodium, and potassium)
  - Endocrine disorders, such as Addison's disease, Cushing's syndrome, thyroid disorders, diabetes mellitus, and parathyroid disorders
  - Nutritional imbalances, such as deficiencies in B and C vitamins, iron, zinc, and protein

● Risk factors
- Family history of depression
- Excessive stress
- Abuse or neglect
- Physical or emotional trauma
- Loss of a parent
- Loss of a relationship
- Other psychiatric disorders
- Other chronic illness
- Other developmental, learning, or conduct disorders

● Signs and symptoms
- Commonly goes unrecognized by the child's family, physician, and teachers; mistaken for normal mood swings typical of a particular developmental stage
- Based on age
  - Children and young adolescents: may have difficulty identifying and describing their emotional states; may act out their feelings, which may be interpreted as misbehavior
  - Older adolescents: may relate feelings in more concrete terms; any indication of hopelessness or suicide requires close attention
- Differs from depression in adults
  - Psychotic features: less common in depressed children and adolescents
  - Anxiety symptoms (such as reluctance to meet people) and physical symptoms (such as aches and pains, stomachache, and headache): more common in depressed children and adolescents
- Persistent sadness
- Irritable, cranky mood
- Physical complaints, such as headache or stomachache
- Crying for no apparent reason
- Inability to concentrate or make decisions
- Withdrawal from peers and social situations
- Restlessness, fidgeting, or frequent moving

- Boredom with daily activities
- Difficulty sleeping, or sleeping more than usual
- Disorganization with periods of agitation
- Fatigue or lack of energy
- Rejection of self or others
- Not caring about self, others, or activities
- Sense of worthlessness
- Verbal or physical fights with others
- Thoughts of death, suicidal ideation, suicide attempts, and high-risk behaviors
- Struggling with normal developmental adjustments
- Absence of expected weight increase for growth and developmental stage

Diagnosis

- Patient self-reports, interviews, and observations
- Team approach—including a medical and psychiatric evaluation, a school consultant's recommendations, and feedback from parents
- Screening tools
  - Children's Depression Inventory—ages 7 to 17
  - Beck Depression Inventory—adolescents
  - Center for Epidemiologic Studies Depression Scale—adolescents
- Comprehensive diagnostic evaluation by a mental health professional for positive screenings; should include interviews with the child, parents and, when possible, other informants (such as teachers and social services personnel)

Treatment

- Psychotherapy (particularly cognitive-behavioral therapy), medication, or a combination
- Targeted interventions involving the home or school environment
- Interpersonal therapy, focusing on working through disturbed relationships that may contribute to depression
- Continuing psychotherapy for several months after symptom remission to help patients and families strengthen the skills they learned during the acute phase of depression
  - Coping with depression's aftereffects
  - Addressing environmental stressors
  - Understanding how the child's thoughts and behaviors could contribute to a relapse
- Antidepressant drugs: effective for adults; controversial for children
  - Until recently, considered too risky because of insufficient evidence about the safety and efficacy of psychotropic drugs in youth
  - Use of SSRIs—such as fluoxetine (Prozac), which was recently approved for children older than age 8—now considered safe and effective for short-term treatment (see *Pharmacologic options for treating depression,* pages 56 and 57)
  - May be a first-line treatment for children and adolescents who have severe symptoms that would make effective psychotherapy difficult, those who can't undergo psychotherapy, or those with psychosis or chronic or recurrent depressive episodes
- Requires close observation for clinical worsening or suicide attempts
- Drug therapy after symptom remission to combat recurrence
  - Should be discontinued gradually over a period of 6 weeks or longer, as appropriate

Pharmacologic options for treating major depression

- Fluoxetine
- Paroxetine
- Sertraline

Pharmacologic options for treating depression

A child or adolescent with major depressive disorder may receive a selective serotonin reuptake inhibitor (SSRI). This chart details the adverse reactions, contraindications, and nursing interventions for three SSRIs.

DRUG	ADVERSE REACTIONS	
Fluoxetine (Prozac)	• Anorexia • Nausea • Appetite changes • Dry mouth • Headache • Nervousness • Fatigue	• Tremor • Dizziness • Seizures • Chest pain • Skin rash • Blurred vision • Flulike reaction
Paroxetine (Paxil)	• Anorexia • Appetite changes • Dry mouth • Diarrhea • Headache • Insomnia • Nervousness	• Tremor • Dizziness • Orthostatic hypotension • Skin rash • Urinary hesitancy or frequency • Blurred vision • Elevated liver enzymes
Sertraline (Zoloft)	• Anorexia • Nausea • Appetite changes • Dry mouth • Headache • Insomnia • Nervousness • Fatigue • Emotional lability • Tremor • Dizziness	• Seizures • Chest pain • Cough • Blood pressure changes • Tachycardia • Skin rash • Blurred vision • Flulike reaction • Liver problems

Key nursing interventions for a child with major depression

- Maintain a safe, secure environment.
- Sustain child's typical routine.
- Monitor child for dangerous or self-destructive behavior.
- Provide appropriate times to eat, rest, sleep, and play or relax.
- Develop an agreement or contract with child.
- Help him talk about problems and stressors.
- Work on age-appropriate strategies for solving problems.

Nursing interventions

- Structure and maintain a safe, secure environment
- Find ways to sustain the child's typical routine
- Monitor him for dangerous or self-destructive behavior
- Work with him to address his needs
- Provide appropriate times to eat, rest, sleep, and play or relax
- Develop an agreement or contract with the child that he'll seek out staff if he feels desperate or suicidal
- Teach him to talk things out rather than act things out
- Discuss concerns and issues that upset or bother him
- Help him talk about problems and stressors
- Work on age-appropriate strategies for solving problems
- Encourage him to express his feelings openly
- If he has suffered a major loss, talk about the loss, what it means to him, and how to grieve for it
- Provide physical outlets for energy and aggression release (such as sports, music, or art) to help the child express feelings and develop healthy coping skills

CONTRAINDICATIONS	NURSING INTERVENTIONS
• Kidney problems • Liver problems • Diabetes mellitus • Suicidal ideation	• Give in the morning. • Supervise patients at risk for suicide. • Monitor weekly for weight changes. • Monitor for safety because drug may cause dizziness.
• Kidney problems • Liver problems • Diabetes mellitus	• Instruct patients that drug need not be taken with food. • Supervise patients at risk for suicide. • Monitor weekly for weight changes.
• Liver problems • Concurrent use of a monoamine oxidase inhibitor	• Tell patients to take drug with food. • Supervise patients at risk for suicide. • Monitor weekly for weight changes. • Monitor patients with a history of seizure disorder.

- Help him rethink negative statements about self and identify and build on current strengths
- Have him identify supportive people and learn ways to talk to these people about his feelings and needs.

MENTAL RETARDATION

● **Defining characteristics**
- Mental retardation refers to below-average general intellectual functioning, with associated deficits in communication, social skills, self-care, and adaptive behavior
- Mental retardation affects roughly 1% to 3% of the population
    - Occurs before age 18
    - If mild, may not be recognized until school age or later
    - In 30% to 40%, predisposing factors can't be determined
- A child with mental retardation has low intelligence, defined as an IQ below 70

Characteristics of mental retardation

- Below-average general intellectual functioning, with associated deficits in communication, social skills, self-care, and adaptive behavior
- Low intelligence, defined as an IQ below 70

Classifying mental retardation

- Mild (IQ 50 to 70)
- Moderate (IQ 35 to 49)
- Severe (IQ 20 to 34)
- Profound (IQ below 20)

Classifying mental retardation

The functioning level of a child or adolescent with mental retardation varies with the degree of retardation.

MILD RETARDATION (IQ 50 TO 70)

- Self-care ability: The child may be able to live somewhat independently with monitoring or assistance with life changes, challenges, or stressors (such as personal illness or the death of a loved one).
- Educational level: The child can achieve fourth- to sixth-grade reading skills and may master vocational training.
- Social skills: The child can learn and use social skills in structured settings.
- Psychomotor skills: The child can develop average to good skills but may have minor coordination problems.
- Living situation: The child must live with the family or in community housing.
- Economic situation: The child may hold a job if closely supervised, and can budget or manage money with guidance.

MODERATE RETARDATION (IQ 35 TO 49)

- Self-care ability: Typically, the child requires close supervision and must be monitored when performing certain independent activities.
- Educational level: The child can achieve up to second-grade skills and may be trained in skills to participate in a sheltered workshop setting.
- Social skills: The child has some speech limitations and difficulty following expected social norms.
- Psychomotor skills: The child may have difficulty with gross motor skills and may have limited vocational opportunities.
- Living situation: The child must live in a sheltered situation.
- Economic situation: The child may learn to handle a small amount of pocket money as well as how to make change.

SEVERE RETARDATION (IQ 20 TO 34)

- Self-care ability: The child requires complete supervision but may be able to perform simple hygiene skills, such as brushing teeth and washing hands.
- Educational level: The child rarely participates in academic training but may learn some simple skills.
- Social skills: The child has limited verbal skills and tends to communicate needs nonverbally or by acting them out.
- Psychomotor skills: The child has poor psychomotor skills, with limited ability to perform simple tasks even under direct supervision.
- Living situation: The child must live in a highly structured and closely supervised setting.
- Economic situation: The child may be taught how to use money and help with shopping.

PROFOUND RETARDATION (IQ BELOW 20)

- Self-care ability: The child requires constant assistance and supervision.
- Educational level: The child can't benefit from academic training but may master simple self-care skills.
- Social skills: The child has little speech development and little to no social skills.
- Psychomotor skills: The child lacks both fine and gross motor skills and needs constant care and supervision.
- Living situation: The child must live in a highly structured, closely supervised setting.
- Economic situation: The child must depend on others for money management.

      – Learns and develops slowly for his age, taking longer than normal to learn how to speak, walk, dress, and eat
      – Has problems due to inability to handle the expected activities of daily living appropriate for age and culture
- Mental retardation is classified as mild, moderate, severe, or profound; the degree of impairment varies with the classification (see *Classifying mental retardation*)

Causes
- Single dominant gene problems: neurofibromatosis or tuberous sclerosis
- Chromosomal disorders: trisomy 21, fragile X syndrome, or Klinefelter's syndrome
- Inborn errors of metabolism: phenylketonuria (PKU) or hyperglycinemia
- Problems during embryonic development: maternal illness (such as diabetes or toxemia) or maternal infection (such as rubella, herpes simplex, or human immunodeficiency virus)
- Pregnancy and perinatal factors: prematurity, maternal-neonate blood group incompatibility, brain trauma, or oxygen deprivation
- Infancy or early childhood problems: severe malnutrition, head trauma, meningitis, encephalitis, or poisoning from lead, medication, or toxic chemical exposure (prenatal or postnatal)
- Environmental problems: poor parenting, abuse and neglect, sensory deprivation, poor nurturance, or poor social or language development
- Preexisting mental disorders: autistic disorder

Signs and symptoms
- Suspected by family members if the motor, language, and self-help skills fail to develop or are developing much more slowly than those of the child's peers
- Failure to achieve developmental milestones
- Deficiencies in cognitive functioning such as inability to follow commands or directions
- Failure to achieve intellectual developmental markers
- Reduced ability to learn or to meet academic demands
- Expressive or receptive language problems
- Psychomotor skill deficits
- Difficulty performing self-care activities
- Neurologic impairments
- Medical problems, such as seizures
- Negativity and low self-esteem
- Irritability when frustrated or upset
- Depression or labile moods
- Acting-out behavior
- Persistence of infantile behavior
- Lack of curiosity
- Deviations in normal adaptive behaviors reflect the severity of mental retardation

Diagnosis
- Centers on a comprehensive personal and family medical history, a complete physical examination, and thorough developmental assessment and intelligence testing

Common causes of mental retardation
- Single dominant gene problems
- Chromosomal disorders
- Inborn errors of metabolism
- Problems during embryonic development
- Pregnancy and perinatal factors
- Infancy or early childhood problems
- Environmental problems
- Preexisting mental disorders

Key signs and symptoms of mental retardation
- Failure to achieve developmental milestones
- Deficiencies in cognitive functioning
- Failure to achieve intellectual developmental markers
- Psychomotor skill deficits
- Neurologic impairments
- Depression or labile moods
- Deviations in normal adaptive behaviors

Diagnosing mental retardation

- Developmental screening tests to assess age-appropriate adaptive behaviors
- Examination for underlying organic problems, including neurologic, chromosomal, and metabolic disorders
- Referral to neurologist or neuropsychologist for testing if brain injury or another neurologic cause is suspected

Key treatment options for mental retardation

- Behavior management
- Environmental supervision
- Monitoring of child's developmental needs and problems
- Programs that maximize speech, language, cognitive, psychomotor, social, self-care, and occupational skills
- Ongoing evaluation for overlapping psychiatric disorders
- Family therapy
- Early intervention programs for children younger than age 3
- Training in independent living and job skills

Key nursing interventions for a patient with mental retardation

- Determine child's strengths and abilities.
- Monitor child's developmental levels.
- Teach child about natural and normal feelings and emotions.
- Provide for child's safety needs.
- Provide consistent, supervised environment.
- Take safety precautions.
- Keep communication brief.

- Developmental screening tests to assess age-appropriate adaptive behaviors
  - Standardized IQ test, Denver Developmental Screening Test, or Bayley Scale of Infant Development: measure intellectual functioning and learning ability
  - Standardized tests, such as the Vineland Behavior Scales or the American Association on Mental Retardation's Adaptive Behavior Scale: measure social maturity and adaptive skills
- Examination for underlying organic problems, including neurologic, chromosomal, and metabolic disorders; if discovered early, conditions (such as hyperthyroidism and PKU) can be treated and the progression of retardation can be stopped — or in some cases, partially reversed
- Referral to a neurologist or neuropsychologist for testing if brain injury or another neurologic cause is suspected

● **Treatment**
- Focuses on coordinating the child's psychological and physiologic needs; drugs rarely indicated unless the child has an overlapping mental disorder
- Behavior management
- Environmental supervision
- Monitoring the child's developmental needs and problems
- Programs that maximize speech, language, cognitive, psychomotor, social, self-care, and occupational skills
- Ongoing evaluation for overlapping psychiatric disorders, such as depression, bipolar disorder, and ADHD
- Family therapy to help parents develop coping skills and deal with guilt or anger
- Early intervention programs for children younger than age 3 with mental retardation
  - Provide day schools to train the child in basic skills, such as bathing and feeding
  - Offer extracurricular activities and social programs to help the child gain self-esteem
- Training in independent living and job skills (typically starts in early adulthood, depending on the degree of mental retardation)
  - Helps those with mild retardation gain skills needed to live independently and hold a job
  - Helps those with moderate to profound retardation who require supervised community living

● **Nursing interventions**
- Determine the child's strengths and abilities, and develop a care plan to maintain and enhance capabilities
- Monitor the child's developmental levels and initiate supportive interventions, such as speech, language, or occupational skills, as needed
- Teach him about natural and normal feelings and emotions
  - Enhanced positive feelings about himself and his daily accomplishments
  - Lack of child's physical or emotional distress

- Provide for his safety needs
  - Consistent, supervised environment
  - Safety precautions (be prepared to intervene if child injures himself)
- Keep communication brief, simple, and consistent
- Teach the child adaptive skills, such as eating, dressing, grooming, and toileting; demonstrate and help him practice self-care skills
- Work to increase his compliance with conventional social norms and behaviors
  - Adequate environmental stimulation
  - Supportive limits on activities
  - Redirected energy

NCLEX CHECKS

It's never too soon to begin your NCLEX preparation. Now that you've reviewed this chapter, carefully read each of the following questions and choose the best answer. Then compare your responses to the correct answers.

1. When communicating with a child, which approach would be most effective? Select all that apply:

- ☐ **1.** Use simple language to ascertain the problem.
- ☐ **2.** Ask questions indirectly to obtain specific information.
- ☐ **3.** Talk about reality, focusing on the present.
- ☐ **4.** Avoid using body language to reinforce ideas.
- ☐ **5.** Speak quietly but firmly when reinforcing behavioral limits.

2. Which of the following would the nurse be least likely to assess in a child with ADHD?

- ☐ **1.** High degree of organization in accomplishing tasks
- ☐ **2.** Blurting out of answers before questions have been asked
- ☐ **3.** Difficulty engaging in leisure-type activities
- ☐ **4.** Failure to follow through with instructions

3. Which information would the nurse include when teaching the parents of a child who's receiving methylphenidate?

- ☐ **1.** Monitor the child's blood glucose level because the drug increases the risk of diabetes.
- ☐ **2.** Monitor the child's growth closely because the drug may interfere with growth and development.
- ☐ **3.** Have the child undergo IQ testing because the drug may decrease intelligence.
- ☐ **4.** Have the child's hearing tested because the drug can cause hearing loss.

4. In which degree of mental retardation would a child be classified if his IQ was determined to be 30?

- ☐ **1.** Mild
- ☐ **2.** Moderate
- ☐ **3.** Severe
- ☐ **4.** Profound

TOP 10

Items to study for your next test on disorders of children and adolescents

1. Growth and development theories
2. Child and adolescent metal status evaluation
3. Signs and symptoms of ADHD
4. Treatment of and nursing interventions for ADHD
5. Defining characteristics and signs and symptoms of autistic disorder
6. Risk factors and key indicators for conduct disorder
7. Differences between childhood and adolescent depression and adult depression
8. Possible causes of mental retardation
9. Classification of mental retardation
10. Nursing interventions for child with mental retardation

5. When talking to a group of parents of school-age children and adolescents, the nurse identifies some of the characteristics associated with childhood depression. Which statement by the group indicates their understanding of the issues discussed?

☐ **1.** "Children can readily describe their feelings of depression."

☐ **2.** "Acting out by children rarely indicates that they are depressed."

☐ **3.** "The link between depression and substance abuse in adolescents is unclear."

☐ **4.** "Aches and pains are more common in depressed children than they are in depressed adults."

6. The diagnosis of ADHD hinges on which specific features?

☐ **1.** Academic difficulties that begin at age 12

☐ **2.** Behaviors that appear before age 7, continue for at least 6 months, and are more frequent or severe than those are in other children the same age

☐ **3.** Poor social skills throughout adolescent years

☐ **4.** Behaviors that appear after age 12 and continue for at least 12 months

7. Which area is a priority concern for the parents of an autistic child who engages in head banging?

☐ **1.** Stimulant administration

☐ **2.** Home safety measures

☐ **3.** Face-to-face communication

☐ **4.** Regular routines

8. The nurse is caring for a 10-year-old child with major depression. Which drug would she expect to administer?

☐ **1.** Methylphenidate

☐ **2.** Haloperidol (Haldol)

☐ **3.** Fluoxetine

☐ **4.** Risperidone

9. When developing a care plan for a child with an IQ of 47, the nurse would expect the child to be capable of:

☐ **1.** some degree of independence in self-care activities.

☐ **2.** money budgeting with guidance.

☐ **3.** communicating needs nonverbally.

☐ **4.** participating in a sheltered workshop setting.

10. The nurse recognizes that, according to Piaget's stages of cognitive development, children usually begin to think abstractly and logically during:

☐ **1.** formal operations stage.

☐ **2.** concrete operations stage.

☐ **3.** preoperational stage.

☐ **4.** sensorimotor stage.

ANSWERS AND RATIONALES

1. CORRECT ANSWER: 1, 3, 5

When communicating with a child, the nurse should keep verbal communication brief, use simple language, talk about reality (focusing on the here and now), and speak quietly but firmly when reinforcing behavioral limits. She should use direct questions to obtain specific information. Body language helps to reinforce ideas about what has been said and encourages the child's expression of ideas and feelings.

2. CORRECT ANSWER: 1

The child with ADHD typically has difficulty organizing tasks and following through with instructions—both due to problems involving inattention. Blurting out answers before questions have been asked suggests impulsivity, which is a criterion for diagnosing ADHD. Difficulty engaging in leisure-type activities indicates that the child is hyperactive, another diagnostic criterion for ADHD.

3. CORRECT ANSWER: 2

The child's physical growth should be monitored because methylphenidate may cause weight loss and temporary interference with growth and development. The drug doesn't affect glucose levels, intelligence, or hearing.

4. CORRECT ANSWER: 3

A child who has an IQ of 30 is considered severely retarded. Children with mild retardation have an IQ of 50 to 70, moderate between 35 to 49, severe between 20 to 34, and profound below 20.

5. CORRECT ANSWER: 4

Depression in children is more commonly expressed as physical symptoms such as aches and pains, and as anxiety symptoms such as a reluctance to meet others. Children and adolescents usually have difficulty expressing how they feel. As a result, they act out their feelings, which may be interpreted as misbehavior. Depression in adolescents increases the risk for substance abuse and suicidal behavior.

6. CORRECT ANSWER: 2

Characteristic behaviors of ADHD must appear before age 7, continue for at least 6 months, and be more frequent or severe than they are in other children the same age. The behaviors must create a real handicap in at least two areas of the child's life (such as school, home, or social settings). Poor social skills characterizes autism.

7. CORRECT ANSWER: 2

Safety is the priority for the autistic child who engages in head banging. Parents should be instructed on ways to prevent injury and making the home safe for the child. Stimulants (which may be useful in reducing the child's inattentiveness, impulsivity, and hyperactivity), face-to-face communication, and regular routines are all important for the child with an autistic disorder. However, safety is the priority concern.

8. CORRECT ANSWER: 3

Fluoxetine is an antidepressant approved for use in children age 8 and older who are diagnosed with major depression; it requires close monitoring when used in children. Methylphenidate is a stimulant typically used to treat ADHD. Haloperidol and risperidone are antipsychotic agents that may be used to treat Tourette syndrome.

9. CORRECT ANSWER: 4

The child with an IQ of 47 is moderately retarded and can achieve up to second-grade skills; therefore, he's probably capable of being trained in skills that would allow him to participate in a sheltered workshop setting. A child with mild retardation may be able to live somewhat independently with some degree of monitoring or assistance with life changes, and may be able to budget or manage money with guidance. A child who's severely retarded has limited verbal skills and tends to communicate his needs nonverbally or by acting them out.

10. CORRECT ANSWER: 1

Abstract and logical thinking is characteristic of Piaget's formal operations stage (ages 12 to 15). In the concrete operations stage (ages 7 to 11), the child develops the concepts of time, space, categories, numbers, and reversibility. In the preoperational stage (ages 2 to 7), the child develops language and egocentric thought and begins symbolic play. In the sensorimotor stage (birth to age 2), the infant focuses on the self and experiences the world through senses and motor movements.

3

Disorders of elderly people

LEARNING OBJECTIVES

After studying this chapter, you should be able to:

- Describe the role and responsibilities of the geropsychiatric nurse.
- Identify the mental status changes of older adulthood.
- Discuss the care settings for older adults with psychiatric disorders.
- Explain the diagnosis, treatment, and nursing interventions for older adults with age-related cognitive decline, Alzheimer's dementia, and vascular dementia.

CHAPTER OVERVIEW

Americans are living longer, with the vast majority surviving to at least age 65. Likewise, the elderly population is increasing. In fact, the U.S. population older than age 65 is expected to double from approximately 35 million in 2000 (13% of the total population) to 70 million in 2030 (20% of the population).

A significant number of older adults are disabled — sometimes severely — by psychiatric disorders, such as depression, anxiety, and dementia. As the life expectancy of Americans continues to rise, the number of older adults experiencing mental disorders will keep growing. Unfortunately, many health care professionals lack the training to identify these disorders, whose symptoms may mimic those of other medical conditions.

Incidence of mental disorders in elderly people

- Memory complaints: about 55% to 80%
- Moderate to severe memory impairment: about 4% in those ages 65 to 69; about 36% in those age 85 and older

Barriers to treatment of elderly people

- Belief that senility, depression, and hopelessness are natural conditions of aging that can't or don't need to be treated
- Reluctance to discuss psychological symptoms, dwelling on physical problems instead
- Preference for primary care with many primary care providers lacking the training to diagnose and treat psychiatric disorders in older adult
- Complexity of treatment, even if provider is properly trained
- Reluctance by providers to inform elderly patients that they have a mental disorder
- Time pressures on — or reimbursement failure for — costs of treatment

ELDERLY PEOPLE AND MENTAL HEALTH

● **Incidence of mental disorders and elderly people**
- Nearly 20% of older Americans experience mental disorders that aren't a part of normal aging
  - Memory complaints: about 55% to 80% of elderly persons report subjective complaints; may be more related to depression than declining memory
  - Moderate to severe memory impairment: occurs in about 4% of those ages 65 to 69; about 36% of those age 85 or older
  - Severe symptoms of depression: occurs in nearly one out of every four persons age 85 or older
  - Suicide: accounts for 20% of all suicides in the Unites States (highest rate)
- Despite the substantial need for mental health services, older adults make little use of them
  - Some deny existence of their mental disorders; of those who acknowledge existence, only about half seek treatment, and only a fraction of those receive specialty mental health services
  - Often overlooked by health care providers, who fail to identify the characteristic signs and symptoms
- Barriers to treatment are prevalent
  - Belief that senility, depression, and hopelessness are natural conditions of aging that can't or don't need to be treated
  - Reluctance to discuss psychological symptoms, dwelling on physical problems instead
  - Preference for primary care with many primary care providers lacking the training to diagnose and treat psychiatric disorders in the older adult
  - Complexity of treatment, even if the provider is properly trained
  - Reluctance by providers to inform elderly patients that they have a mental disorder
  - Time pressures on — or reimbursement failure for — the costs of treatment

● **Neurobiological changes of normal aging**
- Normal aging brings certain changes in mental functioning
- Most older adults experience slight declines in intelligence, learning ability, short-term memory, and reaction time, which grow more significant by about age 75
- Physical changes in the brain occur with age
  - A 20% decrease in the brain's weight by age 90
  - Selective loss of 5% to 20% of neurons (brain cells)
  - Neuron shrinkage
  - About 15% to 20% decline in synapses (communication areas between two neurons) in the frontal lobes
- Cognition, which involves intelligence, language, learning, and memory, declines with age; cognitive deficits are a prominent feature of many mental and physical disorders seen in adults
  - May manifest as mental deficits in a patient who previously didn't show such deficits
  - May result from any condition that alters or destroys brain tissue and, in turn, impairs cerebral functioning

- Vocabulary changes with age, with changes increasing slightly until about age 75 and then declining
- Fluid intelligence (ability to solve novel problems) declines over time; research shows it can be enhanced through training in cognitive skills and problem-solving strategies
- Mental processing capacity (ability to understand text, make inferences, and pay attention) decreases with age
- Certain cognitive processes show little or no decline with age
  - Implicit memory (information that can't be brought to mind but that can affect behavior)
  - Prospective memory (remembering things you need to do)
  - Highly practiced expert skills, such as typing or playing bridge or chess
  - Picture recognition
- Studies show that working memory and long-term memory decline with aging
  - Working memory: used for tasks (such as keeping a phone number in mind just long enough to write it down) as well as in planning, organizing, and rehearsing
  - Long-term memory: responsible for storing information on a relatively permanent basis
- Aging affects *recall* (process of bringing an experience back into consciousness) more than it affects *recognition* (ability to recognize someone or something through remembering)
- Age-related cognitive changes lead to slower learning so teaching may be required
  - Repeating new information frequently
  - Practicing new skills and habits until they become automatic (reduces the memory load of new information)
  - Allowing additional time for learning and practice sessions
- Four variables influence high cognitive performance in older adults
  - Educational level (strongest predictor; suggests education affects brain function early in life and foreshadows sustained production later in life)
  - Activity level
  - Peak pulmonary flow rate
  - Self-efficacy (person's judgment of his ability to reach a specific goal)

DEPRESSION IN OLDER ADULTS

● General information
- Late-life depression can have serious consequences, including increased illness and death from suicide
- Depression typically results from losses
  - Deaths of friends and loved ones
  - Loss of physical capacities
  - Loss of social status and self-esteem
- About 800,000 older Americans are widowed each year

● Bereavement
- *Bereavement* — the natural response to a loved one's death — causes sorrow, anxiety, crying, agitation, insomnia, and appetite loss

Neurobiological changes of normal aging
- Slight declines in intelligence, learning ability, short-term memory, and reaction time, which grow more significant by about age 75
- A 20% decrease in brain's weight by age 90
- Selective loss of 5% to 20% of neurons
- Neuron shrinkage
- About 15% to 20% decline in synapses
- Decline in cognition
- Changes in vocabulary, increasing slightly until about age 75, then declining
- Decline in fluid intelligence
- Decrease in mental processing capacity
- Little or no decline of certain cognitive processes, such as implicit memory, prospective memory, highly practiced expert skills, and picture recognition

Influences on high cognitive performance in older adults
- Educational level
- Activity level
- Peak pulmonary flow rate
- Self-efficacy

Causes of depression in older adults
- Deaths of friends and loved ones
- Loss of physical capacities
- Loss of social status and self-esteem

Key facts about bereavement

- Important risk factor for depression
- Bereavement-related depression commonly coexists with traumatic grief

Key signs and symptoms of bereavement-related depression

- Frequent thoughts of death
- Sense of worthlessness
- Guilt about things other than the actions he took
- Pronounced slowing of psychomotor functions
- Prolonged, marked functional impairment

Symptoms of pathologic grief

- Extreme decline in functioning
- Harming oneself or others
- Changes in interpersonal relationships

Symptoms of posttraumatic stress disorder

- Insomnia
- Exaggerated startle response
- Angry outbursts
- Hypervigilance

Bereavement red flags

Bereavement is common among older adults who survive family members and friends. Sometimes, however, bereavement can turn into a major depressive disorder. Suspect a depressive disorder if your patient experiences:
- frequent thoughts of death
- sense of worthlessness
- guilt about things other than the actions he took — or failed to take — at the time of the loved one's death
- pronounced slowing of psychomotor functions
- prolonged, marked functional impairment.

NOT-SO-HARMLESS HALLUCINATIONS
Some bereaved people hallucinate, thinking they've heard the dead person's voice or seen that person's face. Some report that they've seen their deceased spouses in a crowd or heard them call their name while drifting off to sleep. Such hallucinations are common among bereaved people.
   A patient who has other types of hallucinations, however, may be suffering a serious mental disorder and needs help.

- Symptoms possibly coincide with major depression, but by themselves, they aren't necessarily mental illness
- Bereavement is an important risk factor for depression
  - Clinically significant depression: occurs in roughly 10% to 20% of widows and widowers during the first year of bereavement
  - Persistent and chronic depression: occurs without treatment, leading to further disability and health impairment (possibly including altered endocrine and immune function)
  - Bereavement symptoms lasting 2 months or more: places older adult at higher risk for adjustment disorder or major depressive disorder
  - Bereavement symptoms lasting less than 2 months: possibly warrants clinical attention because it's a highly stressful condition that increases the likelihood of mental and somatic (physical) disorders (see *Bereavement red flags*)
- Bereavement-related depression commonly coexists with traumatic grief
- Symptoms of traumatic grief are extremely disabling, causing health and functional impairments as well as persistent thoughts of suicide
  - Symptoms exhibited in pathologic grief (extreme decline in functioning, harming oneself or others, changes in interpersonal relationships)
  - Symptoms of posttraumatic stress disorder (insomnia, an exaggerated startle response, angry outbursts, hypervigilance)
- Nurses caring for grieving elderly patients, especially those in long-term care facilities, should be aware of the grieving process and the benefits of grief counseling (see *Guiding patients through grief*)
  - Helps avert severe depression and suicidal behavior (about half of all newly admitted patients are at increased risk for depression)
  - May involve suicide prevention strategies

Guiding patients through grief

To help elderly patients work through their grief, you need to recognize the signs and symptoms of grief and its phases. Grief refers to a sequence of mood changes that occur in response to an actual or perceived loss, such as a loved one's death or a change in family role, residence, or body image caused by illness or injury.

Acute grief typically lasts 1 to 2 years. Prolonged grieving may persist for up to 12 years.

GRIEVING STAGES

Usually, successful adaptation requires progressing through grieving stages. Discrete stages of grieving are listed below. But patients don't necessarily move through the stages in an orderly way. They may experience several stages at once or may even regress.

- *Disequilibrium.* The patient has feelings of shock and disbelief, followed by a numbed sensation. He may cry and feel anger and guilt.
- *Disorganization.* Restlessness and the inability to organize and complete tasks are common. The patient typically experiences loss of self-esteem; profound feelings of loneliness, fear, and helplessness; preoccupation with the image of the lost person or object; feelings of unreality; and emotional distance from others.
- *Reorganization.* The patient establishes new goals and interpersonal relationships. He begins to test new behaviors and expand his sense of identity.

PATHOLOGIC GRIEF

The patient who can't cope with change risks developing a maladaptive or pathologic grief reaction. Stay alert for such warning signs as:
- prolonged, excessive activity with no sense of loss
- physical symptoms similar to those that the deceased person experienced

- psychosomatic illness
- progressive social isolation
- extreme hostility
- wooden or formal conduct
- activity detrimental to social or economic well-being
- manic episodes
- depression
- substance abuse or other self-destructive behavior.

COPING WITH GRIEF

To help your patient cope with grief in a positive way, take these steps:
- Explain the normal stages of grieving, emphasizing that a wide range of feelings and behaviors may occur.
- Establish rapport and build trust.
- Convey a caring attitude to encourage the patient to express his feelings.
- Discuss the patient's loss and the concrete changes that have resulted.
- Encourage him to express sadness, guilt, or anger. If he becomes angry with you, don't get defensive.
- Help him to determine what realistic changes he needs to make.
- Suggest that he use more adaptive ways of coping and make concrete plans for the future.
- Urge him to review and share both good and bad memories. Gradually help him shift his focus from sharing memories to coping with the present and planning for the future.

Stages of grief
- Disequilibrium
- Disorganization
- Reorganization

Key warning signs of pathologic grief
- Prolonged, excessive activity with no sense of loss
- Physical symptoms similar to those of deceased person
- Psychosomatic illness
- Progressive social isolation
- Extreme hostility
- Manic episodes
- Depression

Coping with grief
- Explain normal stages of grieving.
- Establish rapport and build trust.
- Convey caring attitude.
- Discuss patient's loss.
- Encourage patient to express sadness, guilt, or anger.
- Help patient determine what realistic changes he needs to make.
- Suggest that patient use more adaptive ways of coping.
- Urge patient to review and share both good and bad memories.

Key facts about geropsychiatric nurse

- Works as part of mental health care team
- Has firm background in behavioral and social sciences
- Possesses thorough knowledge of pathophysiology, psychopharmacology, and normal aging process
- Must be familiar with community resources in area that help older adults maintain highest possible wellness level

Key facts about advanced geropsychiatric practice

- Usually requires master's degree in nursing and advanced certification in a specialty area
- May involve some type of prescriptive authority

GEROPSYCHIATRIC NURSING

● General information

- Geropsychiatric nursing is one of the newest and fastest growing nursing specialties
  - Addresses the unique mental health care needs of elderly patients
  - Blends expertise from four specialties: gerontologic nursing; psychiatric nursing; medical-surgical nursing; and community health nursing
- The geropsychiatric nurse works as part of the mental health care team — typically as a case manager — and provides the bulk of hands-on patient care
  - Has a firm background in the behavioral and social sciences
  - Possesses a thorough knowledge of pathophysiology, psychopharmacology, and the normal aging process
- The geropsychiatric nurse must be familiar with the community resources in the area that help older adults maintain the highest possible wellness level

● Advanced practice

- Geriatric and geropsychiatric advanced practice nurses (APNs) provide various specialty services to older adults with physical and mental health needs
  - Usually requires a master's degree in nursing and advanced certification in a specialty area, such as clinical nurse specialist (CNS) or nurse practitioner
  - In many states, may involve some type of prescriptive authority (nurses typically work in physicians' group practices, hospitals, or independent practices)
- Geriatric APNs serve as resources for the care of elderly adults, including those with mental health problems
  - See patients on site
  - Intervene as needed with research-based, advanced clinical nursing skills
- Geropsychiatric APNs combine a strong background in medical-surgical nursing and psychiatric nursing with patient education
  - May be certified to provide psychotherapy
  - May have the authority to prescribe medications
- Because of their accessibility, APNs may be more capable than other health care professionals in meeting the special mental health care needs of older adults
  - May be necessary because of unavailability of board-certified geropsychiatrists (such as in long-term care facilities and certain geographic areas)
  - May be preferred by patients themselves (many older adults shy away from psychiatrists because of their negative preconceptions about them)

ASSESSMENT AND TREATMENT

● Assessment considerations

- Assessing and diagnosing psychiatric disorders in elderly patients can be challenging, especially because disorders may present differently in older adults than in younger ones
  - More likely to report physical symptoms of depression than psychological ones

– In some cases, full criteria for depressive disorders not met based on somatic complaints reported
- Coexisting medical disorders are common in older adults and may mask or mimic psychopathology
- Some mental disorders may be confused with nonpathologic types of age-related cognitive decline
- Obtaining an accurate patient history is crucial; it may be necessary to obtain the history from family or caregivers when the patient's cognitive status is poor

Treatment considerations

- Treatment may include medication, psychotherapy, support groups, and sociocultural supports
- Ideally, a multidisciplinary team approach is used, with the patient (when able) and his family helping to set goals and make decisions about treatment options
  – Typically includes nurse, physician, psychologist or psychiatrist, pharmacist, dietitian, social worker, and other professionals (such as a physical therapist or activity therapist or chemical dependency counselor) as needed
  – Requires early referrals for optimal results
- All patients, including older adults, have a right to confidentiality in matters related to health care
  – Includes obtaining a signed informed consent from the patient (or a family member or guardian, if the patient is incapacitated) before information can be shared with other health care professionals or facilities
  – Involves never disclosing patient's identity to the public

Outpatient therapy

- Outpatient therapy is usually provided by experienced mental health professionals, such as psychiatrists, psychologists, psychotherapists, social workers, or psychiatric or geropsychiatric APNs; a multidisciplinary approach helps ensure comprehensive care
- Therapy can be provided to individuals, couples, families, or groups
- Insurance may cover a portion of short-term outpatient psychotherapy costs

Support groups

- Support groups give older adults a chance to discuss how their illnesses affect their lives and to help each other by sharing workable solutions
- The support group usually consists of patients (and family members) with a common problem
- A mental health professional facilitates the group, monitoring and focusing the discussion
- Support groups typically meet in churches, senior centers, hospitals, schools, and other public meeting places
- These groups may be free or may charge a nominal fee

Types of care settings

- General hospitals
- Patients' homes
- Outpatient clinics
- Partial hospitalization programs
- Short-term rehabilitation
- Adult day care
- Long-term care facilities

Role of geropsychiatric nurse in home care

- Must be prepared to draw on her medical-surgical, community health, and psychiatric nursing experience
- Must be flexible
- Must be familiar with physical assessment techniques, commonly prescribed medications, crisis de-escalation, and community services for the elderly
- May serve as care coordinator

CARE SETTINGS

General information
- Nurses must be prepared to meet older adults' psychiatric needs in a variety of settings
- Settings may include general hospitals, patients' homes, outpatient clinics, partial hospitalization programs, short-term rehabilitation, adult day care, and long-term care facilities

Home care
- The home is one of the newest delivery settings for geropsychiatric nursing care
  - May be needed upon being discharged from the hospital, a partial hospitalization program, a rehabilitation budget center, or a group home
  - May be needed to enable the patient to remain in his home
- Services provided in the home are expanding rapidly and currently include medication management, psychotherapy, detoxification, and dementia care
- The geropsychiatric nurse must be prepared to draw on her medical-surgical, community health, and psychiatric nursing expertise to meet home care patients' needs
  - Flexibility, frequent communication with other treatment team members, and respecting the patient's right to choose his own lifestyle
  - Familiarity with physical assessment techniques; commonly prescribed medications (especially cardiac, hypertensive, and psychiatric drugs) and their interactions; crisis de-escalation; and community services for elderly people
  - In some cases, serving as the care coordinator if the patient is receiving simultaneous services from a community mental health clinic, case management agency, and community support program
- The elderly home care patient may be vulnerable to crime and abuse; the home care nurse is responsible for assessing any suspected abuse and reporting it to the authorities
  - Includes crimes against the patient, threats of crime, or other unusual situations
  - Requires listening carefully to the patient's complaints or suspicions (even though the patient has a mental disorder, his descriptions of threatening situations may be reality-based)

Long-term care
- Admission to a nursing home or other long-term care facility can cause situational depression; the patient will need help adjusting to the change of environment and close monitoring for signs of depression
  - For those admitted to short-term rehabilitation programs: may need reminders that stay is only temporary and that the goal is to return home
  - For those with chronic mental health problems such as Alzheimer's disease: may require placement in a specialized unit that provides a low-stimulus environment with trained staff who assist in activities of daily living (ADLs), nutrition, and safety
- Psychiatric services provided to older adults in long-term care facilities are regulated by the Omnibus Budget Reconciliation Act (OBRA) of 1987, which has certain mandates

- Monitoring use of physical restraints and chemical restraints (psychotropic drugs) in skilled nursing facilities
- Treating older nursing home residents who have been diagnosed with a primary psychiatric disorder for that disorder by a mental health professional
- Screening new residents in skilled nursing facilities for mental illness before admission
- Having professional mental health consultants available in skilled nursing facilities to monitor patient behavior, work with staff, and manage psychotropic medications
- Many nursing homes designate one nursing staff member as the first-line, in-house mental health nursing specialist
    - Must be available on short notice to help with a specific patient or answer a complicated question
    - Doesn't require the depth of knowledge, background, or experience of an APN; however, if a particular clinical problem continues, worsens, or requires in-depth assessment, the patient should be referred to an APN for telephone consultation or monthly rounds
- An increasing number of geropsychiatric CNS's are working as consultants for long-term care facilities
    - Share their expertise with attending physicians, nursing staff, and families
    - In many cases, can successfully manage behavior problems in the facility without the need for a psychiatrist
    - May be preferred by the patient (or family) over seeing a psychiatrist in an unfamiliar office

Hospital emergency department (ED)

- An older adult may be taken to an ED for a medical emergency, a suicide attempt, or an episode of violent or threatening behavior
- A geriatric patient with a history of acting-out behavior should undergo a thorough physical assessment with baseline diagnostic tests, including electrocardiography, complete blood count with differential, chemistry panel, thyroid function, syphilis serology, and urinalysis
- Intervention aims to keep the patient from harming himself or others; provide rapid tranquilization or sedation; and avoid overmedication and toxicity
- Some hospitals have hired community liaison nurses to address the problems of caring for the mentally ill in the ED
    - Work collaboratively with other staff; act as link among crisis intervention, outreach, and continuity-of-care staff
    - Can provide valuable information to the intervention team and expedite rapid referrals

Inpatient geropsychiatric units

- Inpatient geropsychiatric units are used to evaluate patients for suspected dementia or depression and to stabilize aggressive or suicidal patients
- Efforts focus on rapid evaluation to rule out physical illness, rapid mood stabilization, and discharge planning
- Stays on these units are typically brief, reflecting the trend toward community-based health care

● **Partial hospitalization**
  • Psychiatric partial hospitalization provides intense, structured, multidisciplinary therapy for patients who have more acute needs than outpatients do
    – Serves as adjuncts for patients who have used up their allotted insurance coverage for inpatient days but still need intensive treatment
    – Located close to patient's home (usually, patients are driven to site in the morning, then returned home later that day)
    – Includes specialty psychiatric programs (such as chemical dependency programs)
    – Provides training and education in such skills as medication management, stress management, and ADLs
  • Nursing care focuses
    – Stabilizing lifestyle changes to help the patient stay well
    – Preparing the patient and his family to adapt to living with mental illness and to cope with the real world

● **Adult day care**
  • Adult day care centers are available for elderly patients with chronic mental disorders
    – Provide structured activities, personal care, recreation, socialization, nutritional support, and health care
    – Typically include social services and caregiver support
  • Adult day care offers respite for family members and other caregivers
    – Allows them to maintain their jobs or to have time away from caregiving responsibilities
    – Helps postpone or avoid institutionalizing the older adult

● **Community education programs**
  • Senior centers, hospitals, and churches sponsor public education programs on mental illness
  • Depression and anxiety screening programs encourage older adults and their families to learn more about mental health and help connect them with skilled practitioners for treatment
  • Many community and psychiatric specialty hospitals offer free educational programs on psychiatric issues, such as family dynamics, depression, and anxiety

DRUG THERAPY

● **General information**
  • Because of their slower metabolic rates, older adults are at increased risk for adverse reactions, interactions, toxicity, and other drug-related problems
    – More vulnerable to adverse effects of psychotropic drugs, including tardive dyskinesia (motor disorder causing involuntary jerky movements of the face, tongue, jaws, trunk, and limbs)
    – May experience worsening of a coexisting medical disorder
  • Older patients receiving medications commonly need frequent dosage and scheduling adjustments and close monitoring

- Some older adults have multiple drug prescribers who may not be aware that the patient is seeing other practitioners; consequently, the patient may be taking concurrent multiple medications for coexisting illnesses—a practice called *polypharmacy*
- Caring for an older adult who's receiving multiple medications involves certain actions
  - Maintaining a thorough, up-to-date list of all the medications the patient uses (including prescription and nonprescription drugs)
  - Evaluating the patient's use of nutritional and herbal supplements, such as St. John's wort, especially when the patient is receiving prescribed antidepressants
  - Monitoring the patient closely for adverse effects; an assessment scale to check for tardive dyskinesia and other adverse drug effects may be useful (see *Dyskinesia Identification System: Condensed User Scale,* pages 76 to 79)

Dosage concerns
- Generally, dosages for older adults should start at 25% of the amount used for younger adults, then be increased gradually as tolerated
- The physician may order monitoring of blood or urine drug levels to ensure that the patient isn't getting a toxic dose
- Older adults may not achieve adequate blood drug levels due to lower dosages and slower administration schedules

Compliance issues
- Compliance with drug treatment can be a challenge in elderly patients, especially those with moderate to severe cognitive deficits
  - With poor vision, may misread instructions or mistake one drug for another
  - With cognitive impairment, may not remember whether they have taken all of their doses
- Other challenges to compliance may include a poor physician-patient relationship, inadequate patient teaching about the necessity of or procedure for taking drugs, a large number of daily dosages, and multiple drugs taken at the same time

Administration concerns
- Psychotropic drugs (such as antidepressants, sedatives, tranquilizers, or lithium) may cause oversedation in an older adult
- Because of diminished kidney and liver functions, drugs take longer to be metabolized and excreted in older people
  - May not respond to a psychotropic drug immediately
  - May inadvertently receive more of the medication, which can cause drug accumulation and possible adverse effects ranging from a hangover feeling to near-coma
- Older patients who receive psychotropic medications are also at high risk for falls—especially if they have other illnesses or mobility problems
- Problems may arise if psychotropic medications are discontinued before surgery and then resumed a few days later, leading to possible withdrawal symptoms

(Text continues on page 80.)

Strategies for avoiding dangers of polypharmacy
- Maintain thorough, up-to-date list of all medications patient uses (including prescription and nonprescription drugs).
- Evaluate patient's use of nutritional and herbal supplements, especially when patient is receiving prescribed antidepressants.
- Monitor patient closely for adverse effects.

Key facts about dosages for older adults
- Dosages should start at 25% of amount used for younger adults, then be increased gradually as tolerated.
- Physician may order monitoring of blood or urine drug levels to ensure that patient isn't getting toxic dose.
- Older adult may not achieve adequate blood drug levels due to lower dosages and slower administration schedules.

Key facts about drug administration in older adults
- Psychotropic drugs may cause oversedation in older adults.
- Because of diminished kidney and liver functions in older adults, drugs take longer to be metabolized and excreted.
- Older patients who receive psychotropic medications are also at high risk for falls.
- Problems may arise if psychotropic medications are discontinued before surgery and then resumed a few days later.

Dyskinesia Identification System:
Condensed User Scale

Name _Marjorie Jenkins_
Stewart Memorial hospital
(facility)

Exam type (check one)
☑ 1. Baseline
☐ 2. Annual
☐ 3. Semi-annual
☐ 4. D/C – 1 month
☐ 5. D/C – 2 month
☐ 6. D/C – 3 month
☐ 7. Admission
☐ 8. Other

**Dyskinesia Identification System:
Condensed User Scale (DISCUS)**

*Current psychotropics/anticholinergic
and total mg/day*
Haldol, 0.5 mg P.O. __/__ mg
_____ _____ mg
_____ _____ mg

Cooperation (check one)
☐ 1. None
☑ 2. Partial
☐ 3. Full

Assessment
DISCUS item and score *(circle one score for each item)*

Face	1. Tics	0	①	2	3	4	NA
	2. Grimaces	⓪	1	2	3	4	NA
Eyes	3. Blinking	⓪	1	2	3	4	NA
Oral	4. Chewing/lip smacking	⓪	1	2	3	4	NA
	5. Puckering/sucking/ thrusting lower lip	⓪	1	2	3	4	NA
Lingual	6. Tongue thrusting/ tongue in cheek	⓪	1	2	3	4	NA
	7. Tonic tongue	⓪	1	2	3	4	NA
	8. Tongue tremor	⓪	1	2	3	4	NA
	9. Athetoid myokymic/ lateral tongue	⓪	1	2	3	4	NA
Head/	10. Retrocollis/torticollis	⓪	1	2	3	4	NA
Neck/ Trunk	11. Shoulder/hip torsion	⓪	1	2	3	4	NA
Upper limb	12. Athetoid/myokymic finger-wrist-arm	⓪	1	2	3	4	NA
	13. Pill rolling	⓪	1	2	3	4	NA
Lower limb	14. Ankle flexion/ foot tapping	⓪	1	2	3	4	NA
	15. Toe movement	⓪	1	2	3	4	NA

Comments _____   15-item score __/____

Rater's signature and title   Exam date _5/14/05_
Angela Bavaro, RN _____   Next exam date _12/14/05_

Scoring

0 Not present (movements not observed, or some movements observed but not considered abnormal)

1 Minimal (abnormal movements difficult to detect, or movements easy to detect but occurring only once or twice in a short, nonrepetitive manner)

2 Mild (abnormal movements easy to detect and occurring infrequently)

3 Moderate (abnormal movements easy to detect and occurring frequently)

4 Severe (abnormal movements easy to detect and occurring almost continuously)

NA Not assessed (or not able to assess)

Evaluation

1. Greater than 90 days' neuroleptic exposure

                             Yes   No

2. Scoring/intensity level met   Yes   No

3. Other diagnostic conditions   Yes   No

    (If yes specify) _____

4. Last exam date _____

    Last total score _____

    Last conclusion _____

    Preparer's signature and title for items 1 to 4
    (if different from physician) _____

5. Conclusion *(circle one)*

    A. No tardive dyskinesia (TD); if scoring prerequisite met, list other diagnostic condition or explain in comments.

    B. Probably TD

    C. Masked TD

    D. Withdrawal TD

    E. Persistent TD

    F. Remitted TD

    G. Other (specify in comments)

6. Comments _____

                  _____

                  _____

Physician's signature _____

Date _____

(continued)

Diagnoses for TD

Prerequisites for diagnosis
- History of at least 3 months' total cumulative neuroleptic exposure
- Total score of 5 or more
- No other conditions responsible for the involuntary movements

Diagnosis
- Based on current exam and relationship to previous exam
- Can shift depending on presence of movements

Dyskinesia Identification System:
Condensed User Scale *(continued)*

SIMPLIFIED DIAGNOSES FOR TARDIVE DYSKINESIA
Prerequisites

The three prerequisites for diagnosing TD are as follows, although exceptions may occur.

1. A history of at least 3 months' total cumulative neuroleptic exposure. (Include amoxapine and metoclopramide in all categories below as well.)

2. Scoring/intensity level. Total score of 5 or more. Also be alert for any change from baseline or scores below 5 that have at least a moderate (3) or severe (4) movement on any item or at least two mild (2) movements on two items located in different body areas.

3. Other conditions are not responsible for the abnormal involuntary movements.

Diagnoses

The diagnosis is based on the current exam and its relation to the last exam. It can shift depending on whether movements are present or not, whether movements are present for 3 months or more (6 months for a semi-annual assessment), and whether neuroleptic dosage changes occur and affect movements.

- No TD (Movements not present on this exam, or movements present but caused by some other condition. The last diagnosis must be "No TD," "Probable TD," or "Withdrawal TD.")
- Probable TD (Movements present on this exam for the first time, or for the first time in 3 months or more. The last diagnosis must be "No TD" or "Probable TD.")
- Persistent TD (Movements present on this exam and have been present for 3 months or more with this exam or present at some point in the past. The last diagnosis can be any except "No TD.")
- Masked TD (Movements not present on this exam, but this is due to a neuroleptic dosage increase or restart after an earlier exam when movements were present. Or, movements not present due to the addition of a non-neuroleptic medication to treat TD. The last diagnosis must be "Probable TD," "Persistent TD," "Withdrawal TD," or "Masked TD.")
- Remitted TD (Movements are not present on this exam, but persistent TD has been diagnosed and no neuroleptic dosage increase or restart has occurred. The last diagnosis must be "Persistent TD" or "Remitted TD." If movements re-emerge, the diagnosis shifts back to "Persistent TD.")
- Withdrawal TD (Movements are not present while patient receives neuroleptics or at the last dosage level, but are seen within 8 weeks after neuroleptic reduction or discontinuation. The last diagnosis must be "No TD" or "Withdrawal TD." If movements continue for 3 months or more after neuroleptic reduction or discontinuation, the diagnosis shifts to "Persistent TD." If movements don't continue for 3 months or more after the reduction or discontinuation, the diagnosis shifts to "No TD.")

INSTRUCTIONS

1. The rater completes the Assessment according to the standardized exam procedure. If the rater also completes the Evaluation items 1 to 4, he must also sign the preparer box. The form is given to the physician. Or, the physician may perform the assessment.

2. The physician completes the Evaluation section. The physician is responsible for the entire Evaluation section and its accuracy.

3. A physician should examine any person who meets the three prerequisites or has movements not explained by other factors. He should obtain any neurologic assessments or differential diagnostic tests that may be needed.

4. File form according to facility policy or procedure.

OTHER CONDITIONS (PARTIAL LIST)

1. Age
2. Blind
3. Cerebral palsy
4. Contact lenses
5. Dentures, no teeth
6. Down syndrome
7. Drug intoxication (specify)
8. Encephalitis
9. Extrapyramidal adverse effects (specify)
10. Fahr's syndrome
11. Heavy metal intoxication (specify)
12. Huntington's disease
13. Hyperthyroidism
14. Hypoglycemia
15. Hypoparathyroidism
16. Idiopathic torsion dystonia
17. Meige syndrome
18. Parkinson's disease
19. Stereotypies
20. Sydenham's chorea
21. Tourette syndrome
22. Wilson's disease
23. Other (specify)

Instructions for Dyskinesia Identification System: Condensed User Scale

- Rater completes form according to exam procedure.
- Rater or physician may complete the evaluation section.
- Form should be filed according to facility policy.

Characteristics of ARCD

Gradual deterioration
- Memory
- Learning
- Attention
- Concentration
- Thinking
- Language use
- Other mental functions

Common causes of ARCD

- Faulty inhibitory mechanism in patient's working memory

Key signs and symptoms of ARCD

- Subjective complaints, including inability to remember appointments or solve complex problems
- Noted poor hygiene, inappropriate dress, or weight loss
- Signs of depression (stooped posture, shuffling gait, poor eye contact, and abnormal movements), hostility, resistance, and defensiveness

Diagnosing ARCD

- By neuropsychological and cognitive testing
- By assessment
- Physical appearance
- Remote, recent, and immediate memory
- Speech characteristics
- Higher language skills
- Alertness level

AGE-RELATED COGNITIVE DECLINE

● **Defining characteristics**
- Age-related cognitive decline (ARCD) refers to an objectively identified decrease in cognitive functioning related to aging that's within normal limits and not attributable to a specific mental disorder or neurologic condition
- ARCD is characterized by a gradual deterioration
  – Memory
  – Learning
  – Attention
  – Concentration
  – Thinking
  – Language use
  – Other mental functions
- Deterioration of cognition may be noted
  – Slowed ability to perform cognitive tasks, even when given unlimited time to complete them
  – Problems with timing in complex situations such as when approaching a traffic interchange on a freeway at high speed
- Some older adults have greater memory and cognitive problems than others do, but their symptoms aren't severe enough to qualify as Alzheimer's disease; they're considered to have mild cognitive impairment or a mild neurocognitive disorder

● **Causes**
- Faulty inhibitory mechanism in working memory (the type of memory that enables individuals to ignore irrelevancies)
  – May cause the older adult to heed irrelevant details and to interpret context incorrectly
  – May find irrelevancies too distracting to ignore

● **Risk factors**
- Advancing age
- Female gender
- Heart failure
- History of myocardial infarction

● **Signs and symptoms**
- Subjective complaints, including an inability to remember appointments or solve complex problems
- Noted poor hygiene, inappropriate dress, or weight loss from others (family, caregivers, health care providers)
- Signs of depression (stooped posture, shuffling gait, poor eye contact, and abnormal movements), hostility, resistance, and defensiveness

● **Diagnosis**
- Requires a specialized professional evaluation
- Neuropsychological and cognitive testing to determine and measure the severity and rate of cognitive decline
- Various evaluations that encompass elements of the mental status examination
  – Physical appearance (may give clues to overall health and self-esteem)

- Remote, recent, and immediate memory
- Speech characteristics
- Higher language skills
- Calculation skills
- Decision-making ability
- Affective function, such as mood and anxiety level
- Motor function (may indicate depression, affective illness, or behavioral disturbances)
- Social skills (may suggest cognitive deficits or psychosocial impairment)
- Responses to questions (may suggest cognitive or psychological impairment)
- Orientation (may reflect cognitive deficits)
- Degree of contact with reality (may indicate delusions, paranoia, hallucinations, or illusions)
- Alertness level (may indicate undetected medical disturbances)
- Based on the criteria in the *Diagnostic and Statistical Manual of Mental Disorders,* Fourth Edition, Text Revision (*DSM-IV-TR*)

Treatment
- Various drugs, vitamins, herbs, and dietary therapies (currently being investigated) to treat cognitive decline
- Close monitoring by a physician because any new medical problems could further impair cognitive function
- Interdisciplinary management, including psychiatrists, social workers, and other health care professionals to provide sociocultural support and counseling as needed

Nursing interventions
- Reduce and eliminate factors that may worsen confusion, such as dehydration, malnutrition, and difficulty sleeping
- Carefully monitor the patient's fluid and electrolyte and nutritional status
  - Adequate fluid intake
  - A well-balanced diet
- Promote normal sleep-rest activities; avoid giving sedative-hypnotic drugs when possible
- Promote optimal vision and hearing
  - Keeping rooms well lit
  - Cleaning cerumen out of ears
  - Promoting frequent eye and ear examinations
  - Ensuring that hearing aids are in good working order and positioned properly in the ear
- Reduce unnecessary stimulation, and make the environment as stable as possible; avoid changing the patient's room and moving furniture or possessions around
- Provide frequent, meaningful sensory input and reorientation
  - Placing a large clock and calendar in every room
  - Providing outdoor activities or a bed by the window
  - Orienting the patient with all activities and conversations (frequently telling him your name and what you're going to be doing)
- Encourage the patient to participate in therapeutic groups, such as those centered on reality orientation, remotivation, reminiscence, recreational therapy, pet therapy, music therapy, and sensory training

Characteristics of dementia of the Alzheimer's type

- Irreversible disease marked by global, progressive impairment of cognitive functioning, memory, and personality
- Most common cause of dementia among people age 65 and older
- Affects an estimated 4 million Americans
- Sixth leading cause of death among white women age 85 and older

Common causes of dementia of the Alzheimer's type

- Significant loss of neurons and volume in brain regions devoted to memory and higher mental functioning
- Neurofibrillary tangles
- Buildup of amyloid
- Accumulation of beta amyloid, an insoluble protein, which forms sticky patches (neuritic plaques) surrounded by debris of dying neurons
- Environmental factors: infection, metals, and toxins
- Excessive amounts of metal ions, such as zinc and copper, in brain

- Frequently assess his need for medications, paying close attention to dosages (may need adjustments), adverse effects, and possible drug interactions
- Check on the patient frequently because he may be prone to falls, wandering, and self-poisoning
- Take extra safety measures regarding bath water and food temperature to avoid accidental burns

DEMENTIA OF THE ALZHEIMER'S TYPE (LATE ONSET)

● **Defining characteristics**
- Alzheimer's-type dementia is an irreversible disease marked by global, progressive impairment of cognitive functioning, memory, and personality
- The most common cause of dementia among people age 65 and older, Alzheimer's disease affects an estimated 4 million Americans
  - Sixth leading cause of death among white women age 85 and older
  - Carries an average duration (from onset of symptoms to death) of 8 to 10 years
  - As aging population increases, incidence likely to continue growing unless a cure or effective prevention is discovered
- Typically, memory loss is the earliest symptom of Alzheimer's disease
- As the disease progresses, symptoms progressively interfere with the patient's social and occupational functioning

● **Causes**
- Unknown; may be a link to specific biological factors triggered by various environmental and genetic factors
- Brain-imaging techniques: significant loss of neurons and volume in the brain regions devoted to memory and higher mental functioning
- Abnormalities found on biopsy
  - Neurofibrillary tangles (twisted nerve cell fibers that are the damaged remains of microtubules—support structures that permit nutrients to flow through neurons); key component is an abnormal form of the tau protein, which aids in assembling microtubules; the defective tau appears to block the actions of the normal version
  - A buildup of amyloid (a sticky protein)
- Accumulation of beta amyloid, an insoluble protein, which forms sticky patches (neuritic plaques) surrounded by the debris of dying neurons
  - May be linked to decreased levels of acetylcholine, a neurotransmitter crucial to memory and learning
  - May damage the brain's sodium, potassium, and calcium channels, disrupting the electrical charges that allow messages to pass between neurons
  - Research focusing on oxidation and inflammatory processes to determine toxicity of beta amyloid to nerve cells
    - Release of oxygen-free radicals when beta amyloid breaks down
    - Binding of the unstable chemicals to other molecules through the process of oxidation

Alzheimer's disease and apolipoprotein E

Apolipoprotein E (Apo E), a plasma protein involved in cholesterol transport, is a current focus of research on Alzheimer's disease. The Apo E gene comes in three major types — Apo E4, Apo E3, and Apo E2.

APO E AND BETA AMYLOID
Studies show the greatest number of deposits of beta amyloid (a protein) in people with the Apo E4 gene. People with Apo E3 have fewer beta amyloid deposits, and those with Apo E2 have fewer still.

Because significant beta amyloid accumulations are characteristic of Alzheimer's disease, Apo E4 may be a major risk factor for late-onset Alzheimer's disease.

ONE COPY OR TWO?
Everyone inherits a copy of one type of the Apo E gene from each parent. According to some researchers, the number of Apo E4 copies inherited affects the risk of Alzheimer's disease:

- People with no copies of Apo E4 have a 9% to 20% chance of developing Alzheimer's disease by age 85.
- People with one copy of the gene have a 25% to 60% chance.
- People with two copies have a 50% to 90% chance.

NO FOREGONE CONCLUSIONS
Nonetheless, Alzheimer's disease isn't inevitable, even in people with two Apo E4 copies. In addition, most people with late-onset Alzheimer's disease don't even carry the Apo E4 gene.

Increasingly, researchers are speculating that many cases of Alzheimer's disease stem from a combination of genetic factors involved in beta amyloid production or degradation.

Key facts about beta amyloid accumulation
- May be linked to decreased levels of acetylcholine
- May damage brain's sodium, potassium, and calcium channels
- Research focuses on oxidation and inflammatory processes to determine toxicity of beta amyloid to nerve cells
- Oxygen-free radicals are released when beta amyloid breaks down
- Unstable chemicals bind to other molecules through process of oxidation
- Oxidant overproduction creates too many immune factors that trigger inflammatory response, causing severe damage to cells and tissue

---

- Overproduction of oxidants (produces too many immune factors that trigger an inflammatory response, causing severe damage to cells and tissue)
- Genetic factors (play a role in buildup of beta amyloid found in the brain); a major research focus on apolipoprotein E, which aids cholesterol transport and nerve cell repair (see *Alzheimer's disease and apolipoprotein E*)
- Environmental factors: infection, metals, and toxins (may trigger oxidation, inflammation, and the Alzheimer's disease process — especially in people with genetic susceptibility)
  - May be a link between a genetic susceptibility to Alzheimer's disease and the actions of certain viruses — particularly when the immune system is weakened
  - No specific virus definitively linked to Alzheimer's disease, although research is focusing on herpesvirus 1 and *Chlamydia pneumoniae*
- Excessive amounts of metal ions, such as zinc and copper, in the brain
  - May change the chemical architecture of beta amyloid, making it more harmful
  - May involve mildly acidic environment, which seems to help metals bind to beta amyloid (an acidic environment and higher zinc and copper levels commonly result from the inflammatory response to local injury)
- Other possible factors being researched
  - Deficiencies of vitamins B_6, B_{12}, and folate: possible risk factor due to increased levels of homocysteine (amino acid that may interfere with nerve cell repair)

Key signs and symptoms of dementia of the Alzheimer's type

- Decreased intellectual function
- Personality changes
- Impaired judgment
- Changes in affect

Stage 1
- Agitated or apathetic mood
- Attempts to cover up symptoms
- Deterioration in personal appearance
- Decline in recent memory
- Poor concentration
- Depression
- Wandering

Stage 2
- Confabulation
- Continuous, repetitive behaviors
- Increased apraxia, agnosia, and aphasia
- Decreasing ability to understand or use language
- Disorientation to person, place, and time
- Failure to recognize family members

Stage 3
- Severe decline in cognitive functioning
- Compulsive touching and examination of objects
- Decreased response to stimuli
- Deterioration in motor ability

– Early depression: common genetic factors seen in those with early depression and Alzheimer's disease
– Serious head injury: possible link between injury in early adulthood and later development of Alzheimer's disease
– Education level: increased risk in those with less education than in those who remain mentally active (possibly because learning may stimulate increased neuron growth, resulting in greater brain reserve)

● **Signs and symptoms**
- Decreased intellectual function, personality changes, impaired judgment, and changes in affect
- Stage 1
    – Agitated or apathetic mood
    – Attempts to cover up symptoms
    – Deterioration in personal appearance
    – Decline in recent memory
    – Poor concentration
    – Depression
    – Disorientation to time
    – Sleep disturbances
    – Inability to retain new memories
    – Mild asphasia
    – Susceptibility to falls
    – Transitory delusions of persecution
    – Wandering
- Stage 2
    – Bowel and bladder incontinence
    – Confabulation (filling of memory gaps with fabrications that the patient believes to be facts)
    – Continuous, repetitive behaviors
    – Increased apraxia, agnosia, and aphasia
    – Decreasing ability to understand or use language
    – Disorientation to person, place, and time
    – Failure to recognize family members
    – Inability to retain new information
    – Inability to perform ADLs without assistance
    – Increased appetite without weight gain
    – Socially unacceptable behavior
    – Tantrums
    – Sundowning (increased disorientation and agitation with nightfall)
- Stage 3
    – Severe decline in cognitive functioning
    – Compulsive touching and examination of objects
    – Decreased response to stimuli
    – Deterioration in motor ability
    – Emaciation
    – Nonresponsiveness

● **Diagnosis**
- Difficult to obtain direct pathologic evidence
- Diagnosis in a living patient: ruling out other possible causes of dementia as based on the criteria in the *DSM-IV-TR*

- Tests to aid diagnosis
  - Cognitive assessment evaluation (typically shows cognitive impairment in Alzheimer's disease)
  - Functional dementia scale (may indicate the degree of dementia)
  - Magnetic resonance imaging (MRI) of the brain (typically shows structural and neurologic changes)
  - Mini–Mental Status Examination (MMSE) (reveals disorientation and cognitive impairment)
  - Spinal fluid analysis (may show increased beta amyloid deposits)

Treatment

- No cure for Alzheimer's disease; certain drugs prescribed to improve or stabilize symptoms
- Several care strategies and activities to minimize or prevent behavioral problems
- Institutional placement (should be delayed until absolutely necessary)
- Drugs
  - Anticholinesterase agents, such as donepezil (Aricept), rivastigmine (Exelon), galantamine (Reminyl), and memantine (Namenda), to improve cognitive functioning
  - Antipsychotic agents, such as haloperidol (Haldol) and risperidone (Risperdal), to calm agitated behavior
  - Benzodiazepines, such as alprazolam (Xanax), to ease anxiety
- Agents under investigation for treating Alzheimer's disease: estrogen, nonsteroidal anti-inflammatory agents, vitamin E, selegiline (Carbex, Eldepryl), and ginkgo biloba; a vaccine is being studied in mice
- Hyperbaric oxygen treatment and tissue transplantation
- Brief psychotherapy techniques, such as reality orientation and memory retraining, to aid patients during certain stages
- Alzheimer's disease prevention, targeting individuals at increased genetic risk; may involve prophylactic nutritional agents (such as vitamin E) or cholinergic- or amyloid-targeting interventions

Nursing interventions

- Protect the patient from injury; remove hazardous items or potential obstacles to help maintain a safe environment
- Monitor the patient's food and fluid intake because he's at risk for poor nutrition
- To the extent possible, have the patient follow a regular exercise routine, maintain normal social contacts with family and friends, and continue intellectual activities
- Encourage the patient to see his physician every 3 to 6 months
- Speak to the patient calmly, using a soft, low-pitched voice
- State your expectations simply and completely
- Minimize confusion by maintaining consistent, structured verbal and nonverbal communication
- If the patient discusses an event that isn't happening or people who are no longer alive, affirm his emotions without adding to or refuting the fantasy (for example, if he talks about his dead mother coming to his birthday party, you might say, "Birthdays are fun")
- Add orienting details to every conversation (for example, frequently tell the patient your name and what you're going to be doing)

Diagnosing dementia of the Alzheimer's type

- Cognitive assessment evaluation
- Functional dementia scale
- MRI of brain
- MMSE
- Spinal fluid analysis

Key treatment options for dementia of the Alzheimer's type

- No cure
- Drugs, such as anticholinesterase agents, antipsychotic agents, and benzodiazepines

Key nursing interventions for a patient with dementia of the Alzheimer's type

- Protect patient from injury.
- Monitor patient's food and fluid intake.
- Have patient follow regular exercise routine.
- Encourage patient to see his physician every 3 to 6 months.
- Speak to patient calmly.
- State your expectations simply.
- Minimize confusion.
- Provide outdoor activities.
- Provide frequent meaningful sensory input.
- Increase patient's social interaction.

- Place a large clock and calendar in every room
- Provide outdoor activities or a bed by the window
- Redirect him to appropriate activities when behavior problems occur
- Decrease environmental stimuli, such as noise, excessive artificial light, and television use
- Provide frequent meaningful sensory input
- Increase the patient's social interaction to provide stimuli; however, avoid placing him in large rooms with many people, such as dining rooms or group activity rooms
- Check the patient for adverse drug effects and drug interactions
- Advise the patient and his family that scientific evidence generally doesn't support claims that certain nonprescription products can improve mental functioning
- Instruct the family to always check with the physician before the patient begins nonprescription agents, especially if he has heart or liver problems or is taking a drug for heart problems, hypertension, diabetes, or mental illness
- Give the patient and his family information about community resources, support groups, and placement in a long-term care facility (if necessary)
- Refer the patient to health care professionals skilled in caring for patients with Alzheimer's disease
- Teach the patient and his caregivers stress-management techniques
- Provide support and education to home caregivers, referring them to respite services and social services as needed

VASCULAR DEMENTIA

Defining characteristics
- Also called *multi-infarct dementia*, vascular dementia is a condition characterized by an irreversible alteration in brain function that results from damage or destruction of brain tissue such as blood clots that block small vessels in the brain
  - Impairs cognitive functioning, memory, and personality
  - Doesn't affect level of consciousness
  - Affects localized parts of the brain, sparing some brain function
  - May cause slight brain damage, with barely noticeable symptoms; however, as more small vessels are blocked over time, mental decline becomes obvious
- Vascular dementia typically starts between ages 60 and 75
  - Accounts for about 10% to 20% of all dementias; approximately 20% of patients have both vascular dementia and Alzheimer's disease
  - Affects more men than women
  - Has a more abrupt onset than dementia of the Alzheimer's type

Causes
- Small focal deficits (typically caused by a series of small strokes)
  - Tends to progress in stages, causing patchy distribution of cognitive problems
  - Lesions usually found in the frontal and subcortical parts of the brain
- Contributing factors
  - Advanced age

Characteristics of vascular dementia
- Also called *multi-infarct dementia*
- Irreversible alteration in brain function that results from damage or destruction of brain tissue such as blood clots that block small vessels in brain
- Impairs cognitive functioning, memory, and personality
- Doesn't affect level of consciousness
- Affects localized parts of brain, sparing some brain function
- May cause slight brain damage, with barely noticeable symptoms; however, as more small vessels are blocked over time, mental decline becomes obvious

Common causes of vascular dementia
- Small focal deficits
- Contributing factors such as advanced age, cerebral emboli or thrombi, diabetes, heart disease, hypertension, TIAs

- Cerebral emboli or thrombosis
- Diabetes
- Heart disease
- High blood cholesterol level
- Hypertension (leading to stroke)
- Transient ischemic attacks

Signs and symptoms

- Occur more abruptly than those associated with Alzheimer's disease; also are more episodic, with multiple remissions
- Confusion
- Problems with recent memory
- Wandering or getting lost in familiar places
- Loss of bladder or bowel control
- Inappropriate emotional reactions such as laughing or crying inappropriately
- Difficulty following instructions
- Problems handling money
- Depression
- Dizziness
- Neurologic symptoms lasting only a few days
- Slurred speech
- Leg or arm weakness

Diagnosis

- Cognitive assessment scale (shows deterioration in cognitive ability)
- Global deterioration scale (indicates degenerative dementia)
- MMSE (reveals disorientation and difficulty with recall)
- MRI or computed tomography scan (shows structural, vascular, and neurologic changes in the brain)
- An abbreviated mental examination to detect memory problems and aid differential diagnosis, treatment, and rehabilitation
    - Requires periodic re-examination
    - Inaccuracy of test possible if the patient is affected by depression
- Based on criteria established in *DSM-IV-TR*

Treatment

- Specific therapies to treat the underlying condition (such as hypertension, high cholesterol, or diabetes), including dietary interventions, medications, and smoking cessation
- Carotid endarterectomy to remove blockages in the carotid artery
- Drug therapy, such as aspirin, to decrease platelet aggregation and prevent clots

Nursing interventions

- Monitor the patient's environment to prevent overstimulation
    - Reducing unnecessary stimulation
    - Making the environment as stable as possible
    - Avoiding changing the patient's room and moving furniture or possessions around
- Minimize factors that may contribute to confusion, such as dehydration, malnutrition, and difficulty sleeping
- Orient the patient to his surroundings to ease his anxiety

Key signs and symptoms of vascular dementia

- Occur more abruptly than those associated with Alzheimer's disease
- More episodic
- Multiple remissions

Diagnosing vascular dementia

- Cognitive assessment scale
- Global deterioration scale
- MMSE
- MRI or computed tomography scan
- An abbreviated mental examination to detect memory problems and aid differential diagnosis, treatment, and rehabilitation

Key treatment options for vascular dementia

- Carotid endarterectomy
- Drug therapy such as aspirin

Key nursing interventions for a patient with vascular dementia

- Reduce unnecessary stimulation.
- Make environment as stable as possible.
- Avoid changing patient's room and moving furniture or possessions.
- Minimize factors that may contribute to confusion.
- Orient patient to his surroundings to ease his anxiety.

– Providing frequent, meaningful sensory input
– Placing a large clock and calendar in every room
– Mentioning orienting details in every conversation (frequently telling the patient your name and what you're going to be doing)
- Check the patient often because he may be prone to falls, wandering, and self-poisoning
- Take extra safety measures regarding food and bath water temperature to avoid accidental burns
- Teach the patient and family members about proper diet, weight control, and exercise to reduce cardiovascular risk factors
- Frequently assess the patient's need for medications, paying close attention to dosages (may need adjustments), adverse effects, and possible drug interactions

NCLEX CHECKS

It's never too soon to begin your NCLEX preparation. Now that you've reviewed this chapter, carefully read each of the following questions and choose the best answer. Then compare your responses to the correct answers.

1. When reviewing population statistics for a class on the older adult, which statement would the nurse identify as true? Select all that apply:
- **1.** The vast majority of persons are living to at least age 60.
- **2.** The incidence of mental disorders typically peaks between ages 65 and 69.
- **3.** The population of those older than age 65 is expected to double by 2030.
- **4.** Older adults have the highest suicide rate of all groups in the United States.
- **5.** Approximately 25% of those age 85 and older experience severe depression.

2. Which finding related to aging would the nurse expect to assess in an older adult?
- **1.** Increased ability to make inferences
- **2.** Inability to recognize pictures
- **3.** Decreased fluid intelligence
- **4.** Increased working memory

3. An older adult who's experiencing grief due to the recent loss of her spouse appears restless and unable to organize specific tasks. She states, "I feel so helpless and alone." Further questioning reveals that she avoids talking to her friends on the phone and has stopped going to her local church meetings. The nurse interprets these findings as an indication of:
- **1.** prolonged grieving.
- **2.** the disorganization stage of grief.
- **3.** pathologic grief.
- **4.** the disequilibrium stage of grief.

TOP 10

Items to study for your next test on disorders of elderly people

1. Barriers to treatment for elderly persons with mental disorders
2. Neurobiological changes of normal aging
3. Common causes of depression in older adults
4. Bereavement and grief in older adults
5. Advanced practice roles and geropsychiatric nurses
6. Care settings
7. Drug therapy issues and concerns related to older adults
8. Defining characteristics and signs and symptoms of ARCD
9. Signs and symptoms of the three stages of dementia of the Alzheimer's type
10. Causes of and contributing factors for vascular dementia

4. When working in a community center for older adults, the nurse would integrate knowledge that age-related declines in intelligence, learning ability, short-term memory, and reaction time may grow more significant by about age:

- ☐ **1.** 60.
- ☐ **2.** 65.
- ☐ **3.** 70.
- ☐ **4.** 75.

5. The history of a patient reveals gradually occurring global impairments of cognitive functioning, memory, and personality. Which disorder would the nurse most likely suspect as the patient's problem?

- ☐ **1.** ARCD
- ☐ **2.** Alzheimer's-type dementia
- ☐ **3.** Vascular dementia
- ☐ **4.** Tardive dyskinesia

6. Which method is most appropriate when teaching an older adult?

- ☐ **1.** Audiotapes
- ☐ **2.** Pictures
- ☐ **3.** Television programs
- ☐ **4.** Musical recordings

7. A patient with a primary psychiatric disorder is a resident of a long-term facility. Based on the knowledge of OBRA requirements, the nurse would expect the patient to receive treatment from which provider?

- ☐ **1.** Neurologist
- ☐ **2.** Geropsychiatric CNS
- ☐ **3.** Mental health professional
- ☐ **4.** Psychiatrist

8. Which drug would the nurse expect the physician to prescribe to improve cognitive functioning in an older patient with Alzheimer's-type dementia?

- ☐ **1.** Donepezil
- ☐ **2.** Haloperidol
- ☐ **3.** Risperidone
- ☐ **4.** Alprazolam

9. When teaching a group of family members about Alzheimer's disease, which statement demonstrates the nurse's knowledge about the disease's cause?

- ☐ **1.** "It's caused by damage to the brain from a series of small strokes."
- ☐ **2.** "Advancing age and high blood cholesterol levels are contributing factors."
- ☐ **3.** "The problem results from typical age-related changes in memory."
- ☐ **4.** "Researchers are attempting to identify the exact cause of this problem."

10. Which intervention would the nurse include when developing a care plan for a patient with Alzheimer's disease or vascular dementia?

- ☐ **1.** Speak to the patient in a loud voice.
- ☐ **2.** Keep the television on throughout the day's activities.
- ☐ **3.** Frequently tell the patient what's going to happen.
- ☐ **4.** Place the patient in a group activity room with about 10 people.

ANSWERS AND RATIONALES

1. CORRECT ANSWER: 3, 4, 5

The population of those older than age 65 is expected to double by 2030, and approximately one in four (25%) of those age 85 and older experience severe depression. Additionally, older adults have the highest suicide rate of all groups in America. Life expectancy is increasing, with most persons living to at least age 65. The incidence of mental disorders increases with increasing age, such that a little more than 33% (roughly one-third) of those age 85 and older experience problems.

2. CORRECT ANSWER: 3

With aging, fluid intelligence—the ability to solve novel problems—declines with age. The ability to make inferences (part of mental processing capacity) and working memory also decrease with age. Picture recognition shows little or no decline with age.

3. CORRECT ANSWER: 2

The patient is exhibiting signs and symptoms associated with the disorganization stage of grief, which includes restlessness; inability to organize and complete tasks; loss of self-esteem; profound feelings of loneliness, fear, and helplessness; feelings of unreality and emotional distance from others. Prolonged grieving is a grief reaction that lasts beyond 2 years (in this situation, the patient's loss is recent). Pathologic grief is demonstrated by an extreme decline in functioning, harming of one's self or others, and changes in interpersonal relationships. The disequilibrium stage of grief involves feelings of shock and disbelief, followed by a numbed sensation. Crying and feelings of anger and guilt may also occur.

4. CORRECT ANSWER: 4

Most older adults experience slight declines in intelligence, learning ability, short-term memory, and reaction. By about age 75, these changes grow more significant.

5. CORRECT ANSWER: 2

A patient with Alzheimer's-type dementia suffers global impairment of cognitive functioning, memory, and personality. The dementia occurs gradually, but with a continuous decline. ARCD is characterized by deterioration in memory, learning, attention, concentration, thinking, language use, and other mental functions. Although the changes usually emerge gradually, they aren't severe enough to qualify as Alzheimer's disease. Vascular dementia impairs cognitive functioning, memory, and personality, but it doesn't affect the level of consciousness. It's caused by damage to or destruction of brain tissue. Tardive dyskinesia is an adverse effect of antipsychotic medications as manifested by repetitive, involuntary, purposeless movements.

6. CORRECT ANSWER: 2

Because picture recognition doesn't seem to be affected by aging, using pictures can help older adults with memory and learning. Audiotapes, television programs, and musical recordings may be less effective teaching aids because of the sensory deficits experienced by many older adults.

7. CORRECT ANSWER: 3

OBRA guidelines stipulate that residents of a long-term care facility who have a primary psychiatric disorder must receive treatment from a mental health professional. This professional may in fact be a neurologist, a geropsychiatric CNS, or a psychiatrist. However, OBRA doesn't identify a specific provider; qualification to provide care is the only prerequisite.

8. CORRECT ANSWER: 1

Donepezil is an anticholinesterase agent used to improve cognitive functioning in patients with Alzheimer's disease. Haloperidol and risperidone are antipsychotic agents that may be used to calm the patient's agitation. Alprazolam is a benzodiazepine that may be used to treat the patient's anxiety.

9. CORRECT ANSWER: 4

Currently, the exact cause of Alzheimer's disease isn't known, but researchers suspect it's linked to specific biological factors that are triggered by various environmental and genetic factors. Vascular dementia involves brain damage due to small strokes; aging and high cholesterol levels are considered contributing factors. Typical age-related changes in memory are associated with ARCD.

10. CORRECT ANSWER: 3

For the patient with Alzheimer's disease or vascular dementia, the nurse should frequently orient the patient and tell him what she's going to be doing. The nurse should speak slowly in a soft, low-pitched voice and minimize environmental stimuli, such as noise, excessive artificial light, and television use. The nurse should increase the patient's social interaction to provide stimuli but avoid placing him in large rooms with many people to avoid overstimulating him.

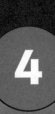

Schizophrenic disorders

CHAPTER OVERVIEW

Schizophrenia refers to a group of severe, disabling psychiatric disorders marked by withdrawal from reality, illogical thinking, possible delusions and hallucinations, and other emotional, behavioral, or intellectual disturbances. These disturbances may affect everything from speech, affect, and perception to psychomotor behavior, interpersonal relationships, and sense of self.

Patients with schizophrenia may have difficulty distinguishing reality from fantasy. Their speech and behavior may frighten or mystify those around them.

UNDERSTANDING SCHIZOPHRENIA

● **General information**
- Schizophrenia is a disabling disease characterized by disturbed thinking, disorganized speech and, in many cases, odd—sometimes frightening—behavior
- Comprising a group of disorders, schizophrenia can be classified according to its five subtypes: catatonic, paranoid, disorganized, residual, and undifferentiated
- A patient's subtype may change over time
- Schizophrenia strikes over 2 million Americans each year; about 1% of the population (1 in every 100 persons) develops schizophrenia during their lifetime
- More prevalent than Alzheimer's disease, diabetes insipidus, and multiple sclerosis, the disease affects men and women equally
- In the United States, schizophrenics occupy one in every four hospital beds and account for about 20% of all Social Security disability days

● **Effects of the disorder**
- The patient's overall disability depends mainly on the severity of cognitive impairment
  - May impair the patient's ability to hold a job, stay in school, maintain relationships, and even perform self-care
  - In some cases, leaves the patient unemployable, socially isolated, and estranged from family and friends
- Many schizophrenics neglect their personal hygiene and ignore their health needs; subsequently, their life expectancy is about 10 years shorter than that of the general population
- Approximately 10% of schizophrenics commit suicide, typically within the first 10 years of illness

● **Disease onset and course**
- Symptoms of schizophrenia usually arise gradually, but in some patients they emerge over just a few days or 1 week
- The most common age of onset is late adolescence—although earlier and later onsets aren't unusual
  - In males: typically starts in the late teens or early 20s
  - In females: may start in the mid-20s or early 30s
- Between periods of exacerbation, some patients have no disability, while others need continuous institutional care
- With each acute episode, the prognosis worsens
- Few schizophrenics experience just a single psychotic episode
  - Only about one in five recovers completely
  - Most continue to suffer at least some lifelong symptoms
- The outcome for patients with this disorder has improved with safer and better treatments
  - About one-third: achieve significant and lasting improvement
  - Another third: improve somewhat but have intermittent relapses and residual disabilities
  - Remaining third: are severely and permanently incapacitated
  - About 30%: unresponsive to medication, despite adherence or compliance

---

Classifying schizophrenia
- Catatonic
- Disorganized
- Paranoid
- Residual
- Undifferentiated

Effects of schizophrenia
- May impair patient's ability to hold a job
- In some cases, leaves patient unemployable
- Many schizophrenics neglect their personal hygiene
- Approximately 10% of schizophrenics commit suicide

Onset and course of schizophrenia
- Symptoms of schizophrenia usually arise gradually
- Most common age of onset is late adolescence
- Between periods of exacerbation, some patients have no disability, while others need continuous institutional care
- With each acute episode, prognosis worsens

- Other factors promote a good prognosis
  - Late or sudden disease onset
  - Female gender
  - Good pre-illness functioning
  - Minimal cognitive impairment
  - Paranoid subtype with many positive symptoms (such as delusions and hallucinations)
  - Family history of mood disorder (rather than schizophrenia)
- Some factors are linked to a poor outcome
  - Early age at onset
  - Poor pre-illness functioning
  - Family history of schizophrenia
  - Disorganized subtype with many negative symptoms (such as apathy, blunted affect, and anhedonia)
- New discoveries into possible causes and cutting-edge brain-imaging techniques hold the promise of further insights and therapeutic advances

PSYCHOSOCIAL AND ECONOMIC ISSUES

General information
- Schizophrenia is a devastating illness—and the afflicted person isn't the only one who suffers; family, friends, and the entire community feel the effects
- Few schizophrenics seek initial treatment on their own
- Because of impaired thought processes and perceptual problems, many deny that they need help and resist seeking health care

Socioeconomic factors
- Schizophrenia statistically occurs across the board, affecting all strata of the population; however, cultural biases toward minorities may show more Blacks diagnosed with schizophrenia (White middle-class Americans are more likely to be diagnosed with a mood disorder)
- It's also more common among single persons, possibly reflecting the effects of the illness or its precursors on the person's social functioning

Impact on the family
- Schizophrenia profoundly affects the patient's family; in many cases, the patient's behavior frightens those closest to him
- Few families are adequately prepared to deal with the stressors caused by chronic schizophrenia, such as personality changes, hospitalizations, and medication noncompliance
- Some problems may stem from lack of information about the disease

Substance abuse
- An estimated 50% of schizophrenics are substance abusers
- Substance abuse may lead to noncompliance with prescribed medication, repeated illness relapses, frequent hospitalizations, declining function, and loss of social support

---

Impact of schizophrenia on family

- Schizophrenia profoundly affects patient's family
- In many cases, patient's behavior frightens those closest to him
- Few families are adequately prepared to deal with stressors caused by chronic schizophrenia
- Some problems may stem from lack of information about the disease

Results of substance abuse in schizophrenics

- Noncompliance with prescribed medication
- Repeated illness relapses
- Frequent hospitalizations
- Declining function
- Loss of social support

CAUSES OF SCHIZOPHRENIA

● **General information**
  - Schizophrenia is a complex illness whose precise cause is unknown
  - Like many diseases, it probably results from the interplay of genetic, biochemical, anatomic, and other factors

● **Genetic factors**
  - Most likely, multiple genes are involved in creating a predisposition to schizophrenia with other factors (such as prenatal infections, perinatal complications, and certain environmental stressors) seeming to influence disease development
  - How genetic predisposition is transmitted isn't clearly understood; consequently, there's no sure way to predict who will develop the disease (see *Vulnerability-stress theory*)
  - Scientists are investigating several regions of the human genome to identify the genes involved in schizophrenia; the strongest evidence points to chromosomes 13 and 6, although these findings haven't been confirmed

● **Biochemical theories**
  - Scientists strongly suspect that schizophrenics have abnormalities affecting neurotransmitters—particularly dopamine, serotonin, norepinephrine, and glutamate
  - Most studies have focused on dopamine
    - May cause disease (at least in part) due to an overactive dopamine system in the brain
    - Might explain such symptoms as hallucinations, agitation, delusional thinking, and grandiosity—forms of hyperactivity that have been linked to excessive dopamine activity
  - Recent studies have found that schizophrenics have dopamine abnormalities
    - Excess dopamine-1 (D1) receptors in the frontal part of the cerebral cortex (based on evidence using positron emission tomography, the more D1 receptors a schizophrenic has, the worse his symptoms are)

Common causes of schizophrenia

- Precise cause unknown
- Probably results from interplay of genetic, biochemical, anatomic, developmental, and other factors

Biochemical theories of schizophrenia

- Presence of abnormalities that affect neurotransmitters—particularly dopamine, serotonin, norepinephrine, and glutamate
- Dopamine may cause disease due to overactive dopamine system in the brain
- Overactive dopamine system might explain such symptoms as hallucinations, agitation, delusional thinking, and grandiosity
- Excess D1 receptors in frontal part of cerebral cortex may affect severity of disease

---

Vulnerability-stress theory

Some experts believe schizophrenia occurs when a biologically susceptible person experiences an environmental stressor. According to the vulnerability-stress theory, a stressful event (such as the death of a loved one, job loss, or divorce) can trigger symptom onset in a vulnerable person.

FETAL FOREBODINGS
What causes this vulnerability in the first place? Some researchers blame such factors as:
- genetic predisposition
- viral infections of the central nervous system

- illness or complications during pregnancy, delivery, or the neonatal period. For instance, the offspring of women who get influenza during the second trimester of pregnancy or experience maternal-fetal Rh incompatibility during a second or subsequent pregnancy are at increased risk for developing schizophrenia.

Structural brain abnormalities in schizophrenics

- Enlarged ventricles
- Higher ventricle-to-brain volume ratio
- Reduced size of certain brain regions
- Abnormal brain functions, including decreased metabolic activity in some brain regions

Developmental theories of schizophrenia

- Results from faulty connections formed by neurons during fetal development
- Errors may lie dormant until puberty

Other possible causes of schizophrenia

- Maternal influenza
- Birth trauma
- Head injury
- Huntington's chorea
- Cerebral tumor
- Stroke
- Systemic lupus erythematosus

– Higher percentage of active dopamine receptors than that of healthy people
– Increased number of dopamine receptors in the basal ganglia (masses of gray matter in the cerebral hemispheres and upper brainstem)
- Other neurotransmitters (norepinephrine, serotonin, acetylcholine, and gamma-aminobutyric acid) and endorphins may also play a role in the development of schizophrenia
  – High norepinephrine levels linked to positive symptoms of schizophrenia
  – Some cognitive symptoms possibly associated with abnormalities of glutamate (neurotransmitter involved in dopamine breakdown as well as learning and memory; aids neuron migration during brain development and may play a role in the structural brain abnormalities found in some schizophrenics)

Structural brain abnormalities

- Abnormal brain structures may account for some cases of schizophrenia; however, it's important to note that not all schizophrenics have structural brain abnormalities; moreover, such abnormalities do occur in those without the disease
- Postmortem examinations of schizophrenics' brains have found small changes in the distribution or number of brain cells
- In living schizophrenic patients, neuroimaging techniques have uncovered certain changes
  – Enlarged ventricles
  – Higher ventricle-to-brain volume ratio
  – Reduced size of certain brain regions
  – Abnormal brain functions, including decreased metabolic activity in some brain regions

Developmental factors

- Developmental neurobiologists suspect that schizophrenia results from faulty connections formed by neurons during fetal development
- Errors may lie dormant until puberty, at which point normally occurring brain changes may interact adversely with the faulty connections
- Researchers are trying to identify which prenatal factors influence the apparent abnormality
- Proposed vulnerability markers for schizophrenia include psychophysiologic deficits in eye tracking, information processing, attention, and sensory inhibition (see *Psychophysiologic markers of schizophrenia*)

Other possible causes

- Many physical conditions have been linked to schizophrenia
  – Maternal influenza during the second trimester of pregnancy
  – Birth trauma
  – Head injury
  – Epilepsy (especially of the temporal lobe)
  – Huntington's chorea
  – Cerebral tumor
  – Stroke
  – Systemic lupus erythematosus

Psychophysiologic markers of schizophrenia

Adding to an already convincing body of evidence showing a genetic influence on schizophrenia, researchers have found abnormal eye-tracking movements in about 40% to 80% of schizophrenic patients and in 25% to 40% of their first-degree relatives.

NOT SO SMOOTH PURSUIT

When tracking a moving object, such as a baseball in flight, the human eye uses a movement called *smooth pursuit*. The neuromuscular system produces pursuit movement by adjusting the moving eyeball's velocity to that of the object being viewed. This adjustment allows a stable image to be reflected onto the retina.

In schizophrenics, smooth-pursuit eye movements are interrupted inappropriately by rapid eye movements, such as those used to read or look around. Although this genetically driven abnormality doesn't directly relate to the cause or effects of schizophre-

nia, it may serve as a genetic marker and a predictor of possible disease development.

OTHER ABNORMALITIES

Studies also show that schizophrenics are more likely to have abnormal results on cognition and attention tests as well as deficient sensory gating (blocking of an incoming sensory message when other stimuli are occupying the person's attention). These markers, also found in first-degree relatives of schizophrenics, may signal vulnerability before the overt onset of illness.

Psychophysiologic markers of schizophrenia

- Interruption of smooth-pursuit eye movements by rapid eye movements may serve as a genetic marker or predictor
- May also see abnormal cognitive and attention test results as well as deficient sensory gating, which may signal vulnerability

- Myxedema
- Parkinsonism
- Wilson's disease (rare inherited disorder of poor copper metabolism)
- Alcohol abuse
- Some postmortem studies of patients with schizophrenia have found degenerative changes involving neurons and neuroglia (supportive cells of the nervous system), suggesting involvement of a healed viral or inflammatory infection associated with or related to disease development

SYMPTOM CATEGORIES

- **General information**
  - Behaviors and functional deficiencies seen in schizophrenia vary widely among patients
  - Assessment findings depend partly on the disease subtype, prevailing symptom cluster, and illness phase (See *Recognizing schizophrenia,* page 98)
  - The signs and symptoms of schizophrenia are typically categorized into three groups: positive, negative, and disorganized
  - Symptom clusters may vary throughout the course of illness; however, a single symptom cluster usually predominates at any one time
  - Positive and negative symptoms have been linked to brain abnormalities
    - Positive symptoms: associated with temporal lobe abnormalities
    - Negative symptoms: linked to abnormalities in the frontal cortex and ventricles

Categorizing signs and symptoms of schizophrenia

- Positive: associated with temporal lobe abnormalities
- Negative: linked to abnormalities in frontal cortex and ventricles
- Disorganized

Characteristic signs and symptoms of schizophrenia

- Speech abnormalities
- Thought distortions
- Poor social interactions
- Regression
- Ambivalence
- Echopraxia

Positive symptoms of schizophrenia

- Hallucinations
- Delusions

Recognizing schizophrenia

During the assessment interview, you may note characteristic signs and symptoms in a patient with schizophrenia. Remember that specific findings vary with the schizophrenia subtype — catatonic, paranoid, disorganized, undifferentiated, residual — and other factors.

SPEECH ABNORMALITIES
The patient's speech may include:
- clang associations — words that rhyme or sound alike, used in an illogical, nonsensical manner (for example, "It's the rain, train, pain")
- echolalia — meaningless repetition of words or phrases
- loose association and flight of ideas — rapid succession of incomplete ideas that aren't connected by logic or rationality
- word salad — illogical word groupings (for example, "She had a star, barn, plant")
- neologisms — bizarre words that have meaning only for the patient.

THOUGHT DISTORTIONS
Stay alert for evidence of:
- overly concrete thinking — inability to form or understand abstract thoughts
- delusions — false ideas or beliefs accepted as real by the patient

- hallucinations — false sensory perceptions with no basis in reality
- thought blocking — sudden interruption in the train of thought
- magical thinking — a belief that thoughts or wishes can control other people or events.

SOCIAL INTERACTIONS
Note whether the patient exhibits:
- poor interpersonal relationships
- withdrawal and apathy — lack of interest in objects, people, or surroundings.

OTHER FINDINGS
In some schizophrenics, you also may assess:
- regression — return to an earlier developmental stage
- ambivalence — coexisting strong positive and negative feelings, leading to emotional conflict
- echopraxia — involuntary repetition of movements observed in others.

- Patients with negative symptoms and cognitive dysfunction also have demonstrated diminished activation in the prefrontal cortex and mesolimbic regions

● **Positive symptoms**
- Positive symptoms are deviant symptoms — symptoms that are present but should be absent
  - Indicate the patient has lost touch with reality
  - Primarily include delusions and hallucinations
- Hallucinations are the most common feature of schizophrenia
  - Involve hearing, seeing, smelling, tasting, or feeling touched by things that aren't actually there
  - May manifest as voices the patient hears (such as voices that comment on his behavior, converse with one another, make critical and abusive comments, or command or direct the patient to do certain things)
- Delusions are erroneous beliefs that may grow out of misinterpreted experiences and cannot be changed by logic or persuasion
  - May cause the patient to think that someone is reading his thoughts, plotting against him, or monitoring his behavior

– May cause him to think that he can control the minds of other people
- Delusions fall into several categories
  – *Persecutory delusion:* patient thinks he's being tormented, followed, tricked, or spied on
  – *Reference delusion:* patient may think that passages in books, newspapers, television shows, song lyrics, or other environmental cues are directed at him
  – *Delusions of thought withdrawal or thought insertion:* patient believes others can read his mind, his thoughts are being transmitted to others, or outside forces are imposing their thoughts or impulses on him

● Negative symptoms
- Negative (deficit) symptoms reflect the absence of normal characteristics
  – Apathy: lack of interest in people, things, and activities
  – Lack of motivation: renders the patient uninterested or unable to start and follow through with activities
  – Blunted affect: flattening of the emotions in which patient's face may appear immobile and inexpressive; as schizophrenia progresses, blunted affect may grow more pronounced
  – Poverty of speech: speech that is brief and lacks content; patient gives curt replies to questions, creating the impression of inner emptiness
  – Anhedonia: diminished capacity to experience pleasure
  – Asociality: avoidance of people and relationships; the patient may withdraw socially, feeling safe when alone or being entirely self-absorbed

● Disorganized symptoms
- Disorganized symptoms reflect the patient's abnormal thinking and ability to communicate and his strange behavior
  – Thought disorder: confused thinking and speech, ranging from mildly disorganized speech to incoherent ramblings; includes making loose associations, jumping from one idea to another, and wandering farther and farther from the original topic (patient may have trouble carrying on conversations with others)
  – Bizarre behavior: may include childlike silliness, laughing or giggling, agitation, and inappropriate appearance, hygiene, or conduct; may move slowly, repeat rhythmic gestures, or walk in circles; may be unable to make sense of everyday sights, sounds, and feelings

DISEASE PHASES

● General information
- Schizophrenia usually progresses through three distinct phases
  – Prodromal
  – Active
  – Residual

● Prodromal phase
- The prodromal phase may arise a year or so before the first hospitalization

---

Categorizing delusions
- Persecutory
- Reference
- Thought withdrawal or thought insertion

Negative symptoms of schizophrenia
- Reflect absence of normal characteristics
- Apathy
- Lack of motivation
- Blunted affect
- Poverty of speech
- Anhedonia
- Asociality

Disorganized symptoms of schizophrenia
- Reflect patient's abnormal thinking and ability to communicate
- Thought disorder
- Bizarre behavior

Phases of schizophrenia
- Prodromal
- Active
- Residual

Prodromal phase of schizophrenia

- May arise a year or so before first hospitalization
- Patient shows clear decline from his previous level of functioning

Active phase of schizophrenia

- Commonly triggered by stressful event
- Patient has acute psychotic symptoms
- Functional deficits worsen
- Prognosis worsens with each acute episode

Residual phase of schizophrenia

- Illness pattern may become established, disability levels may stabilize, or late improvements may appear
- Usually characterized by stabilization of disease
- Rarely marked by full remission
- Blunted affect and impaired role functioning possibly more pronounced
- Persistence of some psychotic symptoms (such as hallucinations)

Key facts about course of schizophrenia

- Varies among patients
- Can be mild, moderate, or severe and unstable; patient with mild course is usually stable
- During first 5 years of illness, patient's level of functioning may deteriorate
- Acute episodes are followed by residual impairment
- After first 5 years, disability level tends to plateau

- The person shows a clear decline from his previous level of functioning
  - May withdraw from friends, hobbies, and other interests
  - May exhibit peculiar behavior, neglect personal hygiene and grooming, and lack energy and initiative
  - May see a deterioration in the patient's work or school performance

● Active phase

- The active phase is commonly triggered by a stressful event
- The patient has acute psychotic symptoms, such as hallucinations, delusions, incoherence, or catatonic behavior
- Functional deficits worsen
- Symptomatic periods may occur episodically (with identifiable exacerbations and remissions) or continuously (with no identifiable remissions)
- Up to one-third of schizophrenics have just one acute episode and no more; others have repeated, acute exacerbations of the active phase
- Prognosis worsens with each acute episode

● Residual phase

- During the residual phase, which follows the active phase, the illness pattern may become established, disability levels may stabilize, or late improvements may appear
  - Usually characterized by stabilization of disease, with residual impairment
  - Rarely marked by full remission and return to pre-illness level of functioning
- Symptoms resemble those of the prodromal phase
  - Blunted affect and impaired role functioning possibly more pronounced
  - Persistence of some psychotic symptoms (such as hallucinations) but without strong affect

DISEASE COURSE

● General information

- The course of schizophrenia varies among patients
- Often noncompliance with the prescribed antipsychotic drug regimen is associated with relapses, but treatment-compliant patients can also relapse
- During the first 5 years of the illness, the patient's level of functioning may deteriorate
  - Social and work skills may decline
  - Cognitive deficits are more pronounced
  - Self-care neglect may worsen progressively
  - Negative symptoms may grow more severe
- In the most common disease course, acute episodes are followed by residual impairment
- During the first few years of schizophrenia, impairment between episodes commonly increases
- After the first 5 years, the disability level tends to plateau; some evidence suggests that illness severity may lessen later in life, particularly among women

● Mild course

- The patient with a mild disease course is usually stable

- The patient always complies with drug treatment, has just one or two major relapses by age 45, and experiences only a few mild symptoms
- **Moderate course**
  - Typically, the patient with a moderate disease course takes medications as prescribed most of the time but isn't fully compliant
  - The patient has several major relapses by age 45 and increased symptoms during stressful periods
  - Between relapses, the patient's symptoms persist
- **Severe, unstable course**
  - The patient with a severe disease course doesn't comply with the prescribed medication regimen — or discontinues it entirely
  - The patient has frequent relapses and is stable only for brief periods between relapses
  - The patient experiences bothersome symptoms and needs help with activities of daily living (ADLs)
  - The patient is also likely to have other problems (such as substance abuse) that make recovery more difficult

DIAGNOSIS

- **General information**
  - A mental status examination, psychiatric history, and careful clinical observation form the basis for diagnosing schizophrenia
  - For a thorough evaluation, the patient should undergo physical and psychiatric examinations to rule out other possible causes of symptoms — including physical disorders, substance-induced psychosis, and primary mood disorders with psychotic features
  - Official diagnosis is based on the criteria established in the *Diagnostic and Statistical Manual of Mental Disorders,* Fourth Edition, Text Revision (*DSM-IV-TR*)
- **Diagnostic test results**
  - No diagnostic test definitively confirms schizophrenia
  - Tests may be ordered to rule out disorders that can cause psychosis, including vitamin deficiencies, uremia, thyrotoxicosis, and electrolyte imbalances
  - Computed tomography (CT) scans and magnetic resonance imaging (MRI) may show enlarged ventricles and other findings characteristic of schizophrenia
    - Structural brain abnormalities found on CT scans in up to 40% of schizophrenics; abnormalities include lateral ventricular enlargement (common in males but not in females), enlargement of the sulci or fissures on the cerebral surface, and atrophy of the cerebellum
    - Abnormalities in the brain's amygdala, limbic system, frontal cortex, temporal lobes, hippocampus, basal ganglia, and thalamus seen on MRIs
    - Decreased blood flow to the thalamus; may cause a flood of sensory information
  - Ventricular-brain ratio (VBR) analysis may find an elevated VBR in schizophrenic patients
  - Brain scans reveal functional cerebral asymmetries in a reverse pattern when compared to that found in normal healthy persons

Treatment goals in schizophrenia

- Reducing severity of psychotic symptoms
- Preventing recurrences of acute episodes and associated functional decline
- Meeting patient's physical and psychosocial needs
- Helping patient to function at highest level possible

Drug therapy in schizophrenia

- Drugs are mainstay of treatment

Types of antipsychotics
- Conventional
- Clozapine
- Atypical

Benefits of antipsychotics

- Reduce positive symptoms, such as hallucinations and delusions
- Ease thought disorders
- Relieve anxiety and agitation
- Maximize patient's level of functioning

TREATMENT

● General information

- Regardless of which schizophrenia subtype the patient has, antipsychotic (neuroleptic) drugs are the mainstay of treatment, helping to prevent a relapse of acute symptoms
  - With continuous prophylactic antipsychotic drug therapy, about 30% of patients relapse within 1 year
  - Without prophylactic drugs, relapse rate climbs to 70% to 80%
- Psychotic symptoms are usually present an average of 12 to 24 months before patients receive their first medical treatment
  - Interval between symptom onset and first treatment closely tied to severity of negative symptoms
  - Generally, treatment beginning soon after diagnosis yields better, quicker response
- Treatments are needed, in addition to drug therapy
  - Psychosocial treatment and rehabilitation
  - Compliance promotion programs
  - Vocational counseling
  - Supportive psychotherapy
  - Appropriate use of community resources
- In rare cases, some patients with schizophrenia also may be candidates for electroconvulsive therapy (ECT)
- There are treatment goals for the schizophrenic patient
  - Reducing the severity of psychotic symptoms
  - Preventing recurrences of acute episodes and the associated functional decline
  - Meeting the patient's physical and psychosocial needs
  - Helping the patient to function at the highest level possible

● Drug therapy

- The wide choice of drug treatment options available today has improved patients' chances for remission and recovery
- Antipsychotic drugs are a critical component in symptom reduction; however, not all patients are responsive to antipsychotic medications
- Antipsychotic drugs appear to work at least in part by blocking postsynaptic dopamine or other neurotransmitter receptors
- Antipsychotics have multiple benefits
  - Reducing positive symptoms, such as hallucinations and delusions
  - Easing thought disorders
  - Relieving anxiety and agitation
  - Maximizing the patient's level of functioning
- Three categories of antipsychotics are available: conventional antipsychotics, clozapine (Clozaril), and newer atypical antipsychotics
- Regardless of the drug therapy prescribed, patients and their families need thorough teaching about drug therapy (see *Antipsychotic drug therapy*)

● Drug therapy: Conventional antipsychotics

- Conventional antipsychotics have been in use the longest; chlorpromazine (Thorazine) was the first antipsychotic used

TIME-OUT FOR TEACHING

Antipsychotic drug therapy

If your patient is receiving antipsychotic medication, be sure to include these topics in your teaching plan:
- Name of the drug
- Reason for use
- Prescribed dosage
- Frequency of administration
- Special instructions for administration such as taking drug on an empty stomach or with food
- Possible adverse effects, including sedative, anticholinergic, and extrapyramidal effects

- Dangerous signs and symptoms to report immediately, especially neuroleptic malignant syndrome
- Necessary follow-up measures such as routine blood counts for clozapine
- Safety measures to minimize orthostatic hypotension
- Need for compliance
- Signs and symptoms of relapse

- Although partially effective in managing positive symptoms of schizophrenia, conventional antipsychotics don't relieve negative symptoms
- Other conventional antipsychotics exist
    - Fluphenazine (Prolixin)
    - Haloperidol (Haldol)
    - Molindone (Moban)
    - Perphenazine (Trilafon)
    - Thioridazine (Mellaril)
    - Thiothixene (Navane)
    - Trifluoperazine (Stelazine)
- These drugs are now used less frequently, largely because of their only partial efficacy and adverse effects (see *Adverse effects of antipsychotic drugs,* page 104)
- Patients who do well on them and avoid troublesome adverse effects are usually advised to continue them, unless they are demonstrating early signs of tardive dyskinesia
- Some noncompliant patients may receive fluphenazine or haloperidol depot formulations (long-acting I.M. doses that release the drug gradually over several weeks)

● **Drug therapy: Clozapine**
- Introduced in 1990, clozapine was the first atypical antipsychotic
- It's effective in about 25% to 50% of patients who don't respond to conventional antipsychotics
- The drug controls a wider range of signs and symptoms (including negative symptoms) than conventional agents do and causes few or no adverse motor effects
- Clozapine may cause agranulocytosis—a potentially fatal blood disorder marked by a low white blood cell count and pronounced neutrophil depletion

Conventional antipsychotics

- Chlorpromazine: first antipsychotic used
- Fluphenazine
- Haloperidol
- Molindone
- Perphenazine
- Thioridazine
- Thiothixene
- Trifluoperazine

Key facts about clozapine

- First atypical antipsychotic
- Controls a wider range of signs and symptoms and causes few or no adverse motor effects
- May cause agranulocytosis

Adverse effects of antipsychotics

- Sedative, anticholinergic, and extrapyramidal effects
- Orthostatic hypotension
- Tardive dyskinesia
- Neuroleptic malignant syndrome

Adverse effects of antipsychotic drugs

Patients with schizophrenia must take antipsychotic drugs for a long time—usually for life. Unfortunately, some of these drugs may cause unpleasant adverse effects.

SEDATIVE, ANTICHOLINERGIC, AND EXTRAPYRAMIDAL EFFECTS

High-potency conventional antipsychotics (such as haloperidol) cause minimal sedation and anticholinergic effects, such as rapid pulse, dry mouth, inability to urinate, and constipation.

However, these drugs carry a high incidence of extrapyramidal (motor) effects. The most common motor effects are dystonia, parkinsonism, and akathisia.

- *Dystonia* refers to prolonged, repetitive muscle contractions that may cause twisting or jerking movements, especially of the neck, mouth, and tongue. It's most common in young males, usually appearing within the first few days of drug treatment.
- Drug-induced *parkinsonism* results in bradykinesia (abnormally slow movements), muscle rigidity, shuffling gait, stooped posture, flat facial affect, tremors, and drooling. It may emerge 1 week to several months after drug treatment begins.
- *Akathisia* causes restlessness, pacing, and an inability to rest or sit still.

Intermediate-potency conventional antipsychotics (such as molindone) have a moderate incidence of extrapyramidal effects. Low-potency agents (such as chlorpromazine) are highly sedative and anticholinergic but cause few extrapyramidal effects.

ORTHOSTATIC HYPOTENSION

Low-potency antipsychotics may cause orthostatic hypotension (low blood pressure when standing).

TARDIVE DYSKINESIA

With prolonged use, antipsychotics may cause tardive dyskinesia—a disorder characterized by repetitive, involuntary, purposeless movements. Signs and symptoms include grimacing, rapid eye blinking, tongue protrusion and smacking, lip puckering or pursing, and rapid movements of the hands, arms, legs, and trunk.

Symptoms may persist long after the patient stops taking the antipsychotic drug. With careful management, though, some symptoms eventually lessen or even disappear.

NEUROLEPTIC MALIGNANT SYNDROME

In up to 1% of patients, antipsychotic drugs cause neuroleptic malignant syndrome. This life-threatening condition leads to fever, extremely rigid muscles, and altered consciousness. It may occur hours to months after drug therapy starts or the dosage is increased.

- Patients receiving clozapine require routine blood monitoring to detect the disorder because it's reversible if caught early
- Other adverse effects of clozapine include drowsiness, sedation, hypotension, weight gain, excessive salivation, hyperglycemia, tachycardia, dizziness, and seizures

● Drug therapy: Newer atypical antipsychotics

- The introduction of newer atypical antipsychotics has given new hope to many schizophrenics

- They're called *atypical* because they work differently than the older, conventional antipsychotics do and are much less likely to cause tardive dyskinesia
- There's a wide range of atypical antipsychotics available
  - Aripiprazole (Abilify)
  - Olanzapine (Zyprexa)
  - Quetiapine (Seroquel)
  - Risperidone (Risperdal)
  - Ziprasidone (Geodon)
- Patients should take these drugs for a trial of 4 to 8 weeks to assess their efficacy
  - For acute treatment, rapid symptom resolution is the goal
  - For maintenance, patients should receive lowest dose that prevents symptoms
- Newer atypical antipsychotics offer many benefits
  - Selective affinity for brain regions involved in schizophrenia symptoms
  - Relief of positive symptoms
  - Improvement in negative symptoms that's more effective than that with conventional antipsychotics
  - Enhancement of brain's serotonin levels while stabilizing dopamine levels
  - Improvement in neurocognitive deficits
  - Greater effectiveness in treating refractory schizophrenia
  - Less likely to cause motor adverse effects
  - Little or no prolactin elevation (possible adverse effect of conventional antipsychotics)

● Drug therapy: Other drugs
- Antidepressants and anxiolytics may be used to control associated signs and symptoms in some patients
- Mood-stabilizing agents, such as lithium, carbamazepine (Tegretol), and valproic acid (Depakote), may be given to manage mood swings
- Benzodiazepines may be prescribed for patients who are substance abusers

● Psychosocial treatment and rehabilitation
- Most patients need support to overcome the illness and deal with the isolation, stigma, and fear it usually brings
- Experts recommend psychosocial treatment, rehabilitation services, and special living arrangements to aid in the various stages of recovery (see *Home is where the help is,* page 106)
- Psychosocial treatment for schizophrenic patients include key components
  - Patient and family teaching about the disease and its treatment
  - Collaborative decision making
  - Monitoring of medication therapy and symptoms
  - Assistance with obtaining prescribed medications, services, and resources (such as disability income and food stamps)
  - Supervision of financial resources, as needed
  - Training and assistance with ADLs
  - Peer support and self-help groups
  - Supportive psychotherapy

Newer atypical antipsychotics
- Aripiprazole
- Olanzapine
- Quetiapine
- Risperidone
- Ziprasidone

Other drugs for treating schizophrenia
- Antidepressants and anxiolytics: may be used to control associated signs and symptoms in some patients
- Mood-stabilizing agents, such as lithium, carbamazepine, and valproic acid: may be given to manage mood swings
- Benzodiazepines: may be prescribed for patients who are substance abusers

Components of psychosocial treatment of schizophrenia
- Patient and family teaching about disease and its treatment
- Collaborative decision making
- Monitoring of medication therapy and symptoms
- Assistance with obtaining prescribed medications, services, and resources (such as disability income and food stamps)
- Supervision of financial resources, as needed
- Training and assistance with ADLs
- Peer support and self-help groups
- Supportive psychotherapy

Residential options for a patient with schizophrenia

- Brief respite or crisis homes
- Transitional group homes
- Foster or boarding homes
- Supported or supervised apartments
- Family living
- Independent living

Home is where the help is

A stable place to live plays an important role in treating schizophrenia. Depending on the patient's geographic location, a wide range of residential options may be available.

BRIEF RESPITE OR CRISIS HOMES

Brief respite or crisis homes are intensive residential programs with on-site clinical staff who can provide 24-hour supervision and treatment. These homes may be a good choice for patients experiencing acute episodes or during the stabilization phase that follows an acute episode. For relapsing patients, these homes may help them avoid the need for hospitalization.

TRANSITIONAL GROUP HOMES

Transitional group homes are structured programs that typically offer in-house daily training in living skills and 24-hour coverage by paraprofessionals. They help stabilize patients after acute episodes or after a stay in a hospital or brief respite home.

FOSTER OR BOARDING HOMES

Foster or boarding homes are supportive group living situations run by laypersons. Usually, the staff provides supervision during the day, with one staff member sleeping over at night. These homes may be recommended for patients in long-term recovery and maintenance.

SUPPORTED OR SUPERVISED APARTMENTS

Supported or supervised apartments usually have a specially trained on-site residential manager who provides support, assistance, and supervision. Alternatively, a mental health professional or family member may provide these services.

These apartments are useful for patients in long-term recovery and maintenance. They help the patient remain autonomous while providing sufficient care to minimize his chance of relapse and reduce the need for inpatient hospitalization.

FAMILY LIVING

For some patients, living with family members may be the best long-term arrangement. For others, it may be needed only during acute episodes. Support and advocacy groups can provide families with information and support.

INDEPENDENT LIVING

During long-term recovery and maintenance, independent living is recommended for most patients. Of course, such independence may be impossible during acute episodes and for patients with a more severe disease course.

Key facts about psychotherapy

- Typically used during maintenance phase or during stabilization phase that follows an acute episode.
- Focus of individual therapy is reality-based and supportive.
- Group therapy aimed at encouraging socialization and social and coping skills and resolving interpersonal conflicts; also promotes reality testing.

Psychotherapy

- Psychodynamic individual or group psychotherapy has little value in treating schizophrenia; however, adjunctive psychotherapy may be used
  - Providing emotional support
  - Reinforcing health-promoting behaviors
  - Helping in adjustment to the illness
  - Fostering use of most of the patient's abilities
- Psychotherapy typically is used during the maintenance phase or during the stabilization phase that follows an acute episode
- The focus of individual therapy is reality-based and supportive

- Group therapy is aimed at encouraging socialization and social and coping skills and resolving interpersonal conflicts; it also promotes reality testing

Family psychotherapy and teaching
- Schizophrenia is disruptive to the family, who may benefit from discussing their experiences with their ill family member with an experienced psychotherapist or counselor
  - Reduces feelings of guilt and disappointment
  - Improves acceptance of the patient
  - Teaches the family stress-management skills and ways to assist the patient in his recovery efforts
- For patients who live with their families, psychoeducational family interventions can assist family life and possibly reduce the relapse rate

Rehabilitation
- Rehabilitation may be particularly important for patients who need to sharpen their job skills, want to work, and have only a few residual symptoms
- During the long-term recovery and maintenance phases of the illness, three types of rehabilitation programs may be used
  - Psychosocial rehabilitation programs (such as the Fountain House program): help patients improve their work skills so they can get and keep jobs
  - Psychiatric rehabilitation: teaches patients the skills they need to define and achieve their personal goals regarding education, work, socialization, and living arrangements
  - Vocational rehabilitation: involves work assessment and training to help patients prepare for full-time employment

Electroconvulsive therapy
- ECT is sometimes used in rare cases to treat patients with acute schizophrenia and those who can't tolerate or don't respond to medication
- It's effective in reducing depressive and catatonic symptoms of schizophrenia

CATATONIC SCHIZOPHRENIA

Defining characteristics
- Catatonic schizophrenia is a rare disease form in which the patient tends to remain in a fixed stupor or position for long periods, periodically yielding to brief spurts of extreme excitement
- Many catatonic schizophrenics have an increased potential for destructive, violent behavior when agitated

Signs and symptoms
- Remaining mute; refusal to move about or tend to personal needs
- Exhibiting bizarre mannerisms, such as facial grimacing and sucking mouth movements
- Rapid swings between stupor and excitement (extreme psychomotor agitation with excessive, senseless, or incoherent shouting or talking)
- Bizarre postures such as holding the body (especially the arms and legs) rigidly in one position for a long time
- Diminished sensitivity to painful stimuli
- Negative symptoms (such as those discussed earlier in the chapter)

3 types of rehabilitation for a patient with schizophrenia
- Psychosocial rehabilitation programs: help patients improve their work skills so they can get and keep jobs
- Psychiatric rehabilitation: teaches patients skills they need to define and achieve their personal goals regarding education, work, socialization, and living arrangements
- Vocational rehabilitation: involves work assessment and training to help patients prepare for full-time employment

Characteristics of catatonic schizophrenia
- Rare disease form
- Patient tends to remain in a fixed stupor or position for long periods

Key signs and symptoms of catatonic schizophrenia
- Remaining mute; refusal to move about or tend to personal needs
- Exhibiting bizarre mannerisms, such as facial grimacing and sucking mouth movements
- Rapid swings between stupor and excitement
- Bizarre postures, such as holding body rigidly in one position for a long time
- Diminished sensitivity to painful stimuli
- Negative symptoms
- Echolalia
- Echopraxia

Key nursing interventions for a patient with schizophrenia

- Establish trust and rapport.
- Maximize level of functioning.
- Promote social skills.
- Ensure safety.
- Provide reality-based activities and explanations.
- Deal with patient's hallucinations.
- Promote compliance with and monitor drug therapy.
- Encourage family involvement.

General nursing interventions for schizophrenic patients

You can use these nursing interventions when caring for a schizophrenic patient – regardless of which schizophrenia subtype he has.

ESTABLISHING TRUST AND RAPPORT

- Expect the patient to put you through a rigorous testing period before he shows evidence of trust. Don't tease or joke with him.
- Don't touch him without first telling him exactly what you're going to do. For example, clearly explain, "I'm going to put this cuff on your arm so I can take your blood pressure."
- If necessary, postpone procedures that require physical contact with hospital personnel until the patient is less suspicious or agitated.
- Use an accepting, consistent approach. Don't avoid or overwhelm the patient. Keep in mind that short, repeated contacts are best until trust has been established.
- Use clear, unambiguous language. Otherwise, the patient may interpret your words the wrong way. (For example, if you tell him, "This procedure will be done on the floor," he may become frightened, thinking he's being told to lie down on the floor.)
- Maintain a sense of hope for possible improvement, and convey this to the patient.

MAXIMIZING THE LEVEL OF FUNCTIONING

- Assess the patient's ability to carry out activities of daily living.
- Avoid promoting dependence. Meet the patient's needs, but do for him only what he can't do for himself.
- Reward positive behavior and work with him to increase his sense of personal responsibility in improving his level of functioning.

PROMOTING SOCIAL SKILLS

- Encourage the patient to engage in meaningful interpersonal relationships.
- Provide support in assisting him to learn social skills.

ENSURING SAFETY

- Maintain a safe environment with minimal stimulation.
- As needed, use physical restraints according to facility policy to ensure the patient's and others' safety.
- Monitor the patient's nutritional status. Weigh him regularly if he isn't eating. If he thinks his food is poisoned, let him fix his own food when possible, or offer him foods in closed containers that he can open. If you

Key treatment options for catatonic schizophrenia

- ECT
- Benzodiazepines

- Echolalia (repeating words or phrases spoken by others)
- Echopraxia (imitating others' movements)

● **Diagnosis**
- Ruling out other possible causes of the patient's symptoms
- Meeting the *DSM-IV-TR* criteria

● **Treatment**
- ECT and benzodiazepines (such as diazepam or lorazepam) for catatonic schizophrenics

give liquid medication in a unitdose container, allow him to open the container.

- If the patient expresses suicidal thoughts, institute suicide precautions. Document his behavior and your precautions.
- If he expresses homicidal thoughts (for example, "I have to kill my mother"), initiate homicidal precautions. Notify the doctor and the potential victim. Document the patient's comments and who was notified.

KEEPING IT REAL

- Engage the patient in reality-oriented activities that involve human contact, such as inpatient social skills training groups, outpatient day care, and sheltered workshops.
- Provide reality-based explanations for distorted body images or hypochondriacal complaints.
- Clarify private language, autistic inventions, or neologisms. Tell the patient that other people don't understand what he says.

DEALING WITH HALLUCINATIONS

- If the patient is hallucinating, explore the content of the hallucinations. If he has auditory hallucinations, determine if they're command hallucinations that place him or others at risk. Tell him you don't hear the voices but you know they're real to him.

- Avoid arguing about the hallucinations. If possible, change the subject.

PROMOTING COMPLIANCE AND MONITORING DRUG THERAPY

- Administer prescribed drugs to manage schizophrenia symptoms or ease anxiety.
- Encourage the patient to comply with the medication regimen to prevent relapse.
- If he's taking a drug that requires monitoring of blood levels, stress the importance of returning to the hospital or outpatient setting for weekly monitoring (or as ordered).
- Regularly assess the patient for adverse drug effects. Document and report these promptly.
- Instruct a patient taking a slow-release drug formulation when to return for the next dose. Urge him to keep the appointment.

ENCOURAGING FAMILY INVOLVEMENT

- Involve the patient's family in his treatment, particularly as his altered thought processes may make teaching difficult.
- Teach family members how to recognize an impending relapse (nervousness, insomnia, decreased ability to concentrate, and loss of interest). Suggest ways they can manage the patient's symptoms.

- Avoiding conventional antipsychotic drugs (they may worsen catatonic symptoms)
- Investigating atypical antipsychotic drugs to treat catatonic schizophrenia (requires further evaluation)

● Nursing interventions

- Catatonic schizophrenics benefit from the same nursing interventions used for patients with other types of schizophrenia (see *General nursing interventions for schizophrenic patients*)

Key nursing interventions for a patient with catatonic schizophrenia

- Spend time with patient.
- Tell patient directly, specifically, and precisely what needs to be done.
- Assess for signs and symptoms of physical illness.
- If patient is in bizarre posture, provide range-of-motion exercises and ambulate patient every 2 hours to prevent pressure ulcers or decreased circulation.
- Stay alert for violent outbursts.

Characteristics of disorganized schizophrenia

- Incoherent, disorganized speech and behavior
- Blunted or inappropriate affect
- May start early and insidiously

Key signs and symptoms of disorganized schizophrenia

- Incoherent, disorganized speech, with markedly loose associations
- Grossly disorganized behavior
- Blunted, silly, superficial, or inappropriate affect
- Grimacing
- Hypochondriacal complaints
- Extreme social withdrawal

Diagnosing disorganized schizophrenia

- Must meet *DSM-IV-TR* criteria
- Other causes of symptoms should be ruled out

Key treatment options for disorganized schizophrenia

- Antipsychotics
- Psychotherapy

- Spend time with the patient even if he's mute and unresponsive, to provide reassurance and support
- Remember that, despite appearances, the patient is acutely aware of his environment; assume the patient can hear — speak to him directly and don't talk about him in his presence
- Emphasize reality during all patient contacts, to reduce distorted perceptions (for example, say, "The leaves on the trees are turning colors and the air is cooler. It's fall!")
- Verbalize for the patient the message that his behavior seems to convey; encourage him to do the same
- Tell the patient directly, specifically, and concisely what needs to be done; don't give him a choice (for example, say, "It's time to go for a walk. Let's go.")
- Assess for signs and symptoms of physical illness; keep in mind that if he's mute, he won't complain of pain or physical symptoms
- Remember that if he's in a bizarre posture, he may be at risk for pressure ulcers or decreased circulation
    - Provide range-of-motion exercises
    - Ambulate every 2 hours
- During periods of hyperactivity, try to prevent him from experiencing physical exhaustion and injury
- As appropriate, meet his needs for adequate food, fluid, exercise, and elimination; follow orders with respect to nutrition, urinary catheterization, and enema use
- Stay alert for violent outbursts; if these occur, get help promptly to intervene safely for yourself, the patient, and others

DISORGANIZED SCHIZOPHRENIA

● **Defining characteristics**
- Disorganized schizophrenia is marked by incoherent, disorganized speech and behaviors and by blunted or inappropriate affect
    - May have fragmented hallucinations and delusions with no coherent theme
    - Usually includes extreme social impairment
- This type of schizophrenia may start early and insidiously, with no significant remissions

● **Signs and symptoms**
- Incoherent, disorganized speech, with markedly loose associations
- Grossly disorganized behavior
- Blunted, silly, superficial, or inappropriate affect
- Grimacing
- Hypochondriacal complaints
- Extreme social withdrawal

● **Diagnosis**
- Ruling out other causes of the patient's symptoms
- Meeting the *DSM-IV-TR* criteria

● **Treatment**
- Treatments described for other types of schizophrenia

- Antipsychotic drugs and psychotherapy (see earlier discussions of treatments for further details)

● **Nursing interventions**
- Follow the measures described in *General nursing interventions for schizophrenic patients*, pages 108 and 109

PARANOID SCHIZOPHRENIA

● **Defining characteristics**
- Paranoid schizophrenia is characterized by persecutory or grandiose delusional thought content and, possibly, delusional jealousy
- Some patients also have gender identity problems, such as fears of being thought of as homosexual or of being approached by homosexuals
- Stress may worsen the patient's symptoms
- Paranoid schizophrenia may cause only minimal impairment in the patient's level of functioning—as long as he doesn't act on delusional thoughts
- Although patients with paranoid schizophrenia may experience frequent auditory hallucinations (usually related to a single theme), they typically lack some of the symptoms of other schizophrenia subtypes—notably, incoherence, loose associations, flat or grossly inappropriate affect, and catatonic or grossly disorganized behavior
  - Tend to be less severely disabled than other schizophrenics
  - Are more responsive to treatments
- Those with late onset of disease and good pre-illness functioning (ironically, the very patients who have the best prognosis) are at the greatest risk for suicide
  - Capable of feeling grief and anguish
  - May be more prone to act in despair (based on their realistic recognition of the disease's effects and implications)

● **Signs and symptoms**
- Persecutory or grandiose delusional thoughts
- Auditory hallucinations
- Unfocused anxiety
- Anger
- Tendency to argue
- Stilted formality or intensity when interacting with others
- Violent behavior

● **Diagnosis**
- Ruling out other causes of the patient's symptoms
- Meeting the *DSM-IV-TR* criteria

● **Treatment**
- Antipsychotic drug therapy
- Psychosocial therapies and rehabilitation, including group and individual psychotherapy

● **Nursing interventions**
- Use the interventions described in *General nursing interventions for schizophrenic patients*, pages 108 and 109

Nursing interventions for a patient with disorganized schizophrenia

- Ask patient's permission to touch him, as appropriate.
- Set limits formally.
- Explore content of hallucinations, as appropriate.
- Don't combat patient's delusions with logic.

Characteristics of paranoid schizophrenia

- Persecutory or grandiose delusional thought content and, possibly, delusional jealousy
- Gender identity problems
- Stress may worsen symptoms
- Only minimal impairment in patient's level of functioning—as long as he doesn't act on delusional thoughts

Key signs and symptoms of paranoid schizophrenia

- Persecutory or grandiose delusional thoughts
- Auditory hallucinations
- Unfocused anxiety
- Anger
- Tendency to argue
- Stilted formality or intensity when interacting with others
- Violent behavior

Diagnosing paranoid schizophrenia

- Must meet *DSM-IV-TR* criteria
- Must rule out other causes for symptoms

Key treatment options for paranoid schizophrenia

- Antipsychotics
- Psychosocial therapies and rehabilitation

Key nursing interventions for a patient with paranoid schizophrenia

- Don't touch patient without telling him first exactly what you're going to be doing and before obtaining his permission to touch him.
- Set limits firmly but without anger; avoid a punitive attitude.
- If patient has auditory hallucinations, explore content of hallucinations; tell him you don't hear the voices, but you know they're real to him.
- Don't try to combat patient's delusions with logic; instead, address feelings, themes, or underlying needs associated with the delusion.
- If patient expresses suicidal thoughts or says he hears voices telling him to harm himself, institute suicide precautions; document his behavior and precautions.
- If patient expresses homicidal thoughts, institute homicide precautions.

- Build trust, and be honest and dependable; don't threaten or make promises you can't fulfill
- Be aware that brief patient contacts may be most useful initially
- When the patient is newly admitted, minimize his contact with the staff
- Don't touch the patient without telling him first exactly what you're going to be doing and before obtaining his permission to touch him
- Approach him in a calm, unhurried manner
- Avoid crowding him physically or psychologically; he may strike out to protect himself
- Respond neutrally to his condescending remarks; don't let him put you on the defensive, and don't take his remarks personally
- If he tells you to leave him alone, do leave—but make sure you return soon
- Set limits firmly but without anger; avoid a punitive attitude
- Be flexible, giving the patient as much control as possible
- Anticipate the need for reduced social contact to increase the patient's comfort level
- Consider postponing procedures that require physical contact with hospital personnel if the patient becomes suspicious or agitated
- If the patient has auditory hallucinations, explore the content of the hallucinations (what voices are saying to him, whether he thinks he must do what they command); tell him you don't hear the voices, but you know they're real to him
- Don't try to combat the patient's delusions with logic; instead, address the feelings, themes, or underlying needs associated with the delusion ("It seems you feel you've been treated unfairly"—response to persecution delusion)
- Offer simple, matter-of-fact explanations about environmental safeguards, medications, and facility policies
- If the patient expresses suicidal thoughts or says he hears voices telling him to harm himself, institute suicide precautions; document his behavior and precautions
- If he expresses homicidal thoughts, institute homicide precautions
    - Notifying the physician and potential victim
    - Documenting the patient's comments and names of those notified
- Make sure the patient's nutritional needs are met and that he's comfortable with his meal plan
    - Fixes his own food when possible (may suspect a preparer other than himself of attempting to poison him)
    - Receives foods in closed containers that he can open himself
- Monitor the patient for adverse drug reactions; document and report these promptly
- Don't tease, joke, argue with, or confront the patient; remember, his distorted perceptions will cause him to misinterpret such actions in a way that's derogatory to himself
- Let him talk about anything he wishes initially, but keep the conversation light and social; avoid engaging in power struggles

RESIDUAL SCHIZOPHRENIA

- **Defining characteristics**
  - Residual schizophrenia is a muted form of the disease that stops short of recovery
  - The patient has a history of acute schizophrenic episodes and persistence of negative symptoms such as restricted affect or poverty of speech
  - Grossly disorganized or catatonic behavior is absent, and delusions, hallucinations, and other positive symptoms no longer dominate

- **Signs and symptoms**
  - No prominent psychotic symptoms
  - Other disease characteristics: inappropriate affect, social withdrawal, eccentric behavior, illogical thinking, or loose associations

- **Diagnosis**
  - Ruling out other causes of the patient's symptoms
  - Meeting the *DSM-IV-TR* criteria

- **Treatment**
  - Treatments described for other types of schizophrenia
  - Antipsychotic drugs and psychotherapy (see earlier discussions of treatments for further details)

- **Nursing interventions**
  - Follow the measures described in *General nursing interventions for schizophrenic patients,* pages 108 and 109

UNDIFFERENTIATED SCHIZOPHRENIA

- **Defining characteristics**
  - Undifferentiated schizophrenia refers to the presence of schizophrenic symptoms, such as delusions and hallucinations, in a patient who doesn't fall into the category of paranoid, disorganized, or catatonic schizophrenia
  - Although the patient meets the general diagnostic criteria for schizophrenia, his symptoms don't conform to any of the other subtypes or he has features of more than one subtype, with no clear predominance of a particular set of diagnostic characteristics

- **Signs and symptoms**
  - Usual signs and symptoms of schizophrenia, with no evidence of the distinguishing characteristics of any specific disease subtype
  - Display positive symptoms (see pages 98 and 99)

- **Diagnosis**
  - Ruling out other causes of the patient's symptoms
  - Meeting the *DSM-IV-TR* criteria

- **Treatment**
  - Treatments described for other types of schizophrenia
  - Antipsychotic drugs and psychotherapy

Key nursing interventions for a patient with undifferentiated schizophrenia

- Ask patient's permission to touch him, as appropriate.
- Set limits formally.
- Don't combat patient's delusions with logic.
- Explore content of hallucinations, as appropriate.
- Institute suicide or homicide precautions, as needed.

TOP 10

Items to study for your next test on schizophrenic disorders

1. Schizophrenic disorder subtypes
2. Factors related to the development of schizophrenia
3. Positive symptoms of schizophrenia
4. Negative symptoms of schizophrenia
5. Disorganized symptoms of schizophrenia
6. The three phases of schizophrenia
7. The major modes of treatment for schizophrenia
8. The three categories of drugs used for schizophrenia
9. Psychosocial rehabilitation
10. Nursing interventions for patients with schizophrenia

● **Nursing interventions**
- Follow the measures described in *General nursing interventions for schizophrenic patients,* pages 108 and 109

NCLEX CHECKS

It's never too soon to begin your NCLEX preparation. Now that you've reviewed this chapter, carefully read each of the following questions and choose the best answer. Then compare your responses to the correct answers.

1. Which of the following would the nurse associate with paranoid symptoms of schizophrenia?
- ☐ **1.** Norepinephrine
- ☐ **2.** Prostaglandins
- ☐ **3.** Dopamine
- ☐ **4.** Glutamate

2. A patient with schizophrenia says, "We can, pan, scan, ran, plan." The nurse identifies this as which speech abnormality?
- ☐ **1.** Clang association
- ☐ **2.** Echolalia
- ☐ **3.** Word salad
- ☐ **4.** Neologism

3. When assessing a patient with schizophrenia, the nurse notes negative symptoms. Which findings would the nurse most likely document? Select all that apply:
- ☐ **1.** Apathy
- ☐ **2.** Delusions
- ☐ **3.** Hallucinations
- ☐ **4.** Lack of motivation
- ☐ **5.** Blunted affect
- ☐ **6.** Bizarre behavior

4. When developing a teaching plan for a group a students who are learning about possible structural brain abnormalities associated with schizophrenia, which information would the nurse include?
- ☐ **1.** Decreased size of lateral ventricles in males
- ☐ **2.** Enlargement of cerebral surface fissures
- ☐ **3.** Diminished VBR
- ☐ **4.** Cerebellar hypertrophy

5. A patient is to receive conventional antipsychotic drug therapy. Which drug would the nurse expect to administer?
- ☐ **1.** Prolixin
- ☐ **2.** Olanzapine
- ☐ **3.** Seroquel
- ☐ **4.** Risperidone

6. A patient with schizophrenia exhibits flattening of emotions. The nurse documents this finding as:
- ☐ **1.** anhedonia.
- ☐ **2.** asociality.
- ☐ **3.** blunted affect.
- ☐ **4.** regression.

7. During his assessment interview, a schizophrenic patient tells the nurse, "People are reading my mind. They're out to get me." The nurse documents that the patient is experiencing:

- ☐ **1.** delusions.
- ☐ **2.** hallucinations.
- ☐ **3.** illusions.
- ☐ **4.** magical thinking.

8. A newly admitted patient can't take care of his personal needs, shows insensitivity to painful stimuli, and exhibits negativism, rigidity, and posturing. The nurse would suspect which diagnosis?

- ☐ **1.** Paranoid schizophrenia
- ☐ **2.** Residual schizophrenia
- ☐ **3.** Undifferentiated schizophrenia
- ☐ **4.** Catatonic schizophrenia

9. A schizophrenic patient who began taking Haldol 1 week ago is exhibiting jerking movements of the neck and mouth. The nurse interprets these findings as suggesting:

- ☐ **1.** dystonia.
- ☐ **2.** tardive dyskinesia.
- ☐ **3.** akathisia.
- ☐ **4.** parkinsonism.

10. When caring for a patient with schizophrenia, which nursing intervention would be least effective?

- ☐ **1.** Exploring the content of his hallucinations
- ☐ **2.** Asking the patient to clarify his neologisms
- ☐ **3.** Rewarding the patient for positive behavior
- ☐ **4.** Performing all activities for the client so his needs are met

ANSWERS AND RATIONALES

1. CORRECT ANSWER: 3
Increased dopamine activity is associated with the paranoid (delusional) symptoms that develop in schizophrenia. High norepinephrine levels are linked to the positive symptoms of schizophrenia. Prostaglandin abnormalities have also been linked to schizophrenia, but not specifically paranoid symptoms. Glutamate is correlated with some cognitive symptoms of schizophrenia.

2. CORRECT ANSWER: 1
Words that rhyme or sound alike, used in an illogical, nonsensical manner, such as the patient's statement, reflect clang association. Echolalia involves the meaningless repetition of words or phrases — for example, the nurse might say, "How are you feeling?" and the patient repeats, "How are you feeling?" Word salad involves illogical word groupings such as, "I saw the star, the barn, plant." Neologisms are bizarre words that have meaning only for the patient — for example, "We're going kerfluktering."

3. CORRECT ANSWER: 1, 4, 5
Negative symptoms include apathy, lack of motivation, and blunted affect as well as poverty of speech, anhedonia, and asociality. Delusions and hallucinations are considered positive symptoms. Bizarre behavior is a disorganized symptom.

4. CORRECT ANSWER: 2

Structural brain abnormalities detected with diagnostic testing include enlargement of the cerebral surface fissures, enlargement of the lateral ventricles in males, elevated VBR, and cerebellar atrophy.

5. CORRECT ANSWER: 1

Prolixin is a conventional antipsychotic. Olanzapine, Seroquel, and risperidone are atypical antipsychotic agents.

6. CORRECT ANSWER: 3

Blunted affect is the flattening of emotions. The patient's face may be immobile and inexpressive, with poor eye contact. Anhedonia refers to the diminished ability to experience pleasure. Asociality refers to avoidance of relationships. Regression refers to going back to a previous stage of development.

7. CORRECT ANSWER: 1

Delusions are false ideas or beliefs accepted as real by the patient. Among schizophrenics, delusions of grandeur, persecution, and reference are common. Hallucinations are false sensory perceptions with no basis in reality. Illusions are false sensory perceptions that have some basis in reality. Magical thinking is a belief that thoughts or wishes can control other people or events.

8. CORRECT ANSWER: 4

Catatonic schizophrenia is characterized by the inability to take care of personal needs, diminished sensitivity to painful stimuli, negativism, rigidity, and posturing. Paranoid schizophrenia is characterized by preoccupation with one or more delusions or frequent auditory hallucinations. Flat affect and disorganized speech or behavior aren't prominent. Residual schizophrenia is characterized by a history of at least one schizophrenic episode and the waning or absence of delusions, hallucinations, disorganized speech, and grossly disorganized or catatonic behavior. Undifferentiated schizophrenia is characterized by delusions, prominent hallucinations, disorganized speech, grossly disorganized behavior, and negative symptoms.

9. CORRECT ANSWER: 1

Haloperidol and other high-potency conventional antipsychotics cause a high incidence of dystonia and other extrapyramidal adverse effects. Dystonia is marked by prolonged, repetitive muscle contractions that cause twisting or jerking movements, especially of the neck, mouth, and tongue. It occurs early in drug therapy. Tardive dyskinesia is a disorder characterized by repetitive involuntary purposeless movements due to prolonged use of conventional antipsychotics. Akathisia involves restlessness, pacing, and the inability to rest or sit still. Parkinsonism results in abnormally slow movements, muscle rigidity, shuffling gait, stooped posture, flat facial affect, tremors, and drooling.

10. CORRECT ANSWER: 4

The nurse should avoid promoting dependence. Instead, she should assist the patient to carry out activities of daily living, doing for him only what he can't do for himself to promote his maximum level of functioning. Exploring the content of his hallucinations and asking the patient to clarify his neologisms help to promote reality. Rewarding the patient for positive behavior aids in maximizing his level of functioning.

5

Mood
disorders

LEARNING OBJECTIVES

After studying this chapter, you should be able to:

- Differentiate between the types of mood disorders.
- Describe symptoms of bipolar and depressive disorders.
- Identify the effects of mood disorders on functioning.
- Explain the proposed causes of mood disorders.
- List drugs commonly used to treat mood disorders.
- Describe appropriate interventions for patients with various mood disorders.
- Discuss how to assess a patient's suicide risk.

CHAPTER OVERVIEW

Mood disorders are disturbances in the regulation of mood, behavior, and affect that go beyond the normal fluctuations that most people experience. In the United States, more than 20 million people suffer from mood disorders. Throughout the world, mood disorders are a leading cause of disability.

Two major mood disorders, bipolar disorders and depressive disorders, can be potentially disabling, affecting every aspect of a person's life—thought processes, emotions, behavior, spiritual health, and even physical health.

Many people with mood disorders have coexisting mental and physical disorders. For instance, about one-half of those with a major depressive disorder also suffer from an anxiety disorder.

Defining affect

- Outward expression of emotion attached to ideas, including but not limited to facial expression and vocal modulation

Abnormalities in affect

- Blunted affect: severe reduction in intensity of outward emotional expression
- Flat affect: complete or almost complete absence of outward emotional expression
- Restricted affect: reduction in intensity of outward emotional expression
- Inappropriate affect: affect that doesn't match situation or content of verbalized message
- Labile affect: rapid and easily changing affective expression that's unrelated to external events or stimuli

Classifying mood disorders

- Bipolar disorder
- Cyclothymic disorder
- Dysthymic disorder
- Major depressive disorder

Challenges in caring for patients with mood disorders

- May be mistaken for physical illnesses
- Patient may neglect self-care
- May alter family and social relationships
- Financial hardship may result
- Patient may be at risk for suicide

UNDERSTANDING MOOD DISORDERS

- **General information**
  - Mood disorders are characterized by persistent feelings that cause a wide range of emotional and behavioral problems that interfere with the patient's social and psychological functioning
  - Patients with mood disorders may exhibit various abnormalities in affect (outward expression of emotion attached to ideas, including but not limited to facial expression and vocal modulation)
    - Blunted affect—severe reduction in the intensity of outward emotional expression
    - Flat affect—complete or almost complete absence of outward emotional expression
    - Restricted affect—reduction in the intensity of outward emotional expression
    - Inappropriate affect—affect that doesn't match the situation or the content of the verbalized message (for instance, laughter when describing a loved one's death)
    - Labile affect—rapid and easily changing affective expression that's unrelated to external events or stimuli
  - Depending on the type of disorder, the patient may be prone to extremely high (manic) or extremely low (depressed) mood states and, in some cases, a combination of the two
  - Mood disorders are generally classified as four types
    - Bipolar disorder
    - Cyclothymic disorder
    - Dysthymic disorder
    - Major depressive disorder

- **Challenges in caring for patients with mood disorders**
  - Mood disorders may cause primarily somatic (physical) symptoms, so they may be mistaken for physical illnesses
  - They're viewed as social or moral problems rather than medical health problems that are appropriate to discuss with health care providers
  - Mainstream and immigrant cultures feel that depression implies moral weakness
  - The patient may neglect self-care because of lowered motivation and energy levels
  - Mood disorders may alter family and social relationships, leading to frustration, anger, and guilt; consequently, the patient may be the victim or perpetrator of abuse
  - If the patient can't work because of the mood disorder, financial hardship may result
  - A seriously depressed patient may be at risk for suicide

CAUSES

- **Genetic factors**
  - Genetics appear to play a major role in mood disorders
  - Major depressive disorder and bipolar disorders occur much more often in first-degree relatives than they do in the general population

- Studies of identical twins show that when one twin is diagnosed with major depression, the other twin has a greater than 70% chance of developing it

Biological factors

- Biological research focuses on deficiencies or abnormalities in the brain's chemical messengers — neurotransmitters, such as norepinephrine, serotonin, dopamine, and acetylcholine
- The effectiveness of drug therapy that affects neurotransmitter levels supports the theory that mood disorders have biological roots

Psychological theories

- Cognitive theory suggests that people who suffer from depression process information in a characteristically negative way
  - View themselves and the world in a negative light
  - Believe their negative perceptions will continue in the future
  - Experience cognitive distortions and thinking errors
- Behavioral theorists explain mood disorders in terms of the learned helplessness theory, in which a person's helplessness and depression develop from his experiences with negatively perceived events (such as a loved one's death or a job loss)
  - Leads to dampened motivation, self-esteem, and initiative due to perceived lack of control over life events
  - Increases risk of depression after stressful events due to a lack of social support and ineffective stress-management and problem-solving skills
- According to psychoanalytic theory, depression results from a harsh superego (the "conscience" of the unconscious mind) and feelings of loss and aggression
  - Susceptibility to depression later in life if a child experiences early losses
  - Loss interpreted by child as a form of rejection and a sign that he's unworthy of love
  - Possible feelings of aggression toward those who have rejected him, with realization that these aggressive feelings could lead to further rejection
  - Feelings pushed out of awareness and turned inward (against himself), resulting in depression

BIPOLAR DISORDERS

Defining characteristics

- Bipolar disorders (also called *manic-depressive disorders*) are mood disorders marked by severe, frequent, pathologic mood swings
- Typically, the patient experiences extreme highs (mania or hypomania) alternating with extreme lows (depression); interspersed between the highs and lows are periods of normal mood
- Mood swings usually occur across the patient's life span, with symptom-free periods between episodes
  - Residual symptoms in about one-third of patients
  - Despite treatment, chronic unremitting symptoms in a small percentage
- Variations in the pattern of highs and lows can occur (for instance, some people experience only acute episodes of mania or hypomania with severe depression)
- An estimated 3 million people in the United States have bipolar disorders; roughly half of those affected have difficulties in work performance and psychological functioning

---

Biological factors in mood disorders

- Deficiencies or abnormalities in brain's neurotransmitters, such as norepinephrine, serotonin, dopamine, and acetylcholine

Psychological theories of mood disorders

- Cognitive theory: suggests that people who suffer from depression process information in a characteristically negative way
- Behavioral theory: involves learned helplessness theory, in which a person's helplessness and depression develop from his experiences with negatively perceived events
- Psychoanalytic theory: depression results from a harsh superego (the "conscience" of the unconscious mind) and feelings of loss and aggression

Characteristics of bipolar disorders

- Also called *manic-depressive disorders*
- Marked by severe, frequent, pathologic mood swings
- Patient experiences extreme highs (mania or hypomania) alternating with extreme lows (depression)
- Periods of normal mood are interspersed between the highs and lows
- Severe episodes of mania or depression can sometimes involve psychotic symptoms

Characteristics of mania

- Elation
- Euphoria
- Agitation or irritability
- Hyperexcitability
- Hyperactivity
- Rapid thought and speech
- Exaggerated sexuality
- Delusions
- Hallucinations
- Decreased sleep

Defining hypomania

- An expansive, elevated, or agitated mood that resembles mania
- Less intense than mania and lacks psychotic symptoms

Classifying bipolar disorders

- Bipolar I disorder: classic and most severe disease form; characterized by manic episodes or mixed episodes that alternate with major depressive episodes
- Bipolar II disorder: characterized by milder episodes of hypomania that alternate with depressive episodes
- Cyclothymic disorder: history of numerous hypomanic episodes intermingled with numerous depressive episodes that don't meet criteria for major depressive episodes
- Rapid-cycling bipolar disorder: variant form that affects up to 20% of all patients diagnosed with bipolar disorder (mostly women)

– Men and women affected equally
– Women likely to have more depressive episodes; men, more manic episodes
- Onset usually occurs between ages 20 and 30
  – Symptoms sometimes appearing in late childhood or early adolescence
  – May be misdiagnosed or overlooked until documented pattern or cycle begins to emerge
- Mania is characterized by episodes of elation, euphoria, agitation or irritability, hyperexcitability, hyperactivity, rapid thought and speech, exaggerated sexuality, delusions, hallucinations, and decreased sleep
  – Impulsive behavior during manic episode can have far-reaching emotional, physical, and social consequences
    • Divorce, child abuse, joblessness, accidents, physical decompensation, bankruptcy
    • Promiscuity (increased incidence of sexually transmitted diseases and unwanted pregnancies)
    • Hyperactivity and sleep disturbances, possibly leading to exhaustion, poor nutrition, and dehydration
    • Increased risk of suicide (suicide attempt may occur impulsively during either a manic or depressive episode)
- *Hypomania* refers to an expansive, elevated, or agitated mood that resembles mania but is less intense and lacks psychotic symptoms
  – May not cause problems in social activities or work
  – May make patient feel good, with high energy, confidence, and enhanced social functioning and productivity
  – Without proper treatment, may progress to severe mania or may change to depression
- Severe episodes of mania or depression can sometimes involve psychotic symptoms
  – May include hallucinations (hearing, seeing, touching, smelling, or tasting things that aren't actually there) or delusions (false beliefs not influenced by logical reasoning or explained by a person's usual cultural concepts)
  – May result in misdiagnosis of schizophrenia (see chapter 4 for a discussion of schizophrenia)

Classification

- Bipolar I disorder is the classic and most severe disease form
  – Characterized by manic episodes or mixed episodes (with symptoms of both mania and depression) that alternate with major depressive episodes
  – Occurrence of depressive phase immediately before or after manic phase; may also be separated from manic phase by months or years
- In bipolar II disorder, the patient doesn't experience severe mania but instead has milder episodes of hypomania that alternate with depressive episodes
- In cyclothymic disorder, the patient has a history of numerous hypomanic episodes intermingled with numerous depressive episodes that don't meet the criteria for major depressive episodes
- Rapid-cycling bipolar disorder, a variant form of the disease, affects up to 20% of all patients diagnosed with bipolar disorder (mostly women)
  – Characterized by four or more distinct episodes of depression, mania, hypomania, or mixed states occurring within a 12-month period; periods of normal mood are typically brief (sometimes absent)

– Tends to develop
– Generally, the m
swings (in some
some ultra-rapic
• Experts believe that
tern, but most retur

Causes
• Precise cause unkn ob-
ably play a role
• Genetic componen ies
– Higher incider der)
among first-de gen-
eral populatio
– Autosomal-dc
• Probably stems in es,
possibly involving
• In predisposed i ssful
life events (serio
• Other possible t
– Use of antid switch
to mania)
– Sleep depri
– Hypothyroi

Signs and symptoms
• Can be difficult to diagnose and assess; findings vary with illness phase
• Manic phase
– Expansive, grandiose, or hyperirritable mood
– Increased psychomotor activity, such as agitation, pacing, or hand-wringing
– Excessive social extroversion
– Short attention span
– Rapid speech with frequent topic changes (flight of ideas)
– Decreased need for sleep and food
– Impulsivity
– Impaired judgment
– Easy distractibility
– Excessive spending
– Rapid response to external stimuli, such as background noise or a ringing telephone
– Hypersensitivity
– Promiscuity
– Possible delusions, hallucinations, paranoid thinking, and inflated sense of self-esteem, ranging from uncritical self-confidence to marked grandiosity (severe mania)
• Depressive phase
– Low self-esteem
– Overwhelming inertia
– Social withdrawal
– Feelings of hopelessness, apathy, or self-reproach

- Difficulty concentrating or thinking clearly (without obvious disorientation or intellectual impairment)
- Psychomotor retardation (sluggish physical movements and activity)
- Slowing of speech and responses
- Sexual dysfunction
- Sleep disturbances (such as difficulty falling or staying asleep, or early-morning awakening)
- Decreased muscle tone; weight loss or gain
- Slow gait
- Constipation
- Anhedonia (diminished ability to experience pleasure)
- Suicidal ideation

● Diagnosis

- Suggested by evidence of signs and symptoms
- Confirmed if *Diagnostic and Statistical Manual of Mental Disorders,* Fourth Edition, Text Revision (*DSM-IV-TR*) criteria met

● Treatment

- Lithium (Eskalith)
  - Highly effective in both preventing and relieving manic episodes; curbs accelerated thought processes and hyperactive behavior without the sedating effect of antipsychotic drugs
  - Also may prevent recurrence of depressive episodes, but ineffective for treatment of acute depression
  - Effectively decreases the risk of suicide
  - Has narrow margin of safety and small therapeutic window for efficacy; requires beginning treatment cautiously with a low dose (adjusted slowly as needed) because of possible toxicity
  - Requires frequent blood specimens to determine therapeutic levels; must maintain therapeutic blood levels for 7 to 10 days before desired mood stability occurs—at start of therapy, possible use of antipsychotic drugs for mood stabilization and symptom relief until desired effects achieved (see *Guidelines for patients receiving lithium therapy*)
- Valproic acid (Depakote)
  - May be prescribed for rapid cyclers or for patients who can't tolerate lithium; frequent blood levels needed to determine therapeutic levels
- Carbamazepine (Tegretol)
  - May be useful in treating mania, although not approved by Food and Drug Administration for bipolar disorder
  - Frequent blood levels needed to determine therapeutic levels
- Antidepressants
  - Usually prescribed to augment a mood stabilizer
  - Occasionally prescribed to treat depressive symptoms
  - Must be used cautiously; may trigger a manic episode
- Other medications: lamotrigine (Lamictal), olanzapine (Zyprexa)

● Nursing interventions (manic phase)

- Provide for the patient's dietary needs
  - Encouraging small amounts eaten frequently throughout the day (patient may jump up and walk around the room after every mouthful but will sit down again if reminded)

TIME-OUT FOR TEACHING

Guidelines for patients receiving lithium therapy

For a patient who's receiving lithium (Eskalith), blood level monitoring is crucial because of the drug's narrow therapeutic margin. In fact, lithium shouldn't be used if the patient can't have regular blood tests. In addition, because lithium is excreted by the kidneys, it shouldn't be given to patients with renal impairment.

If the doctor has prescribed lithium for your patient, be sure to include the following information in your teaching plan:

- Tell the patient that blood levels should be checked 8 to 12 hours after the first dose, two or three times weekly for the first month, and then weekly to monthly during maintenance therapy.
- Instruct the patient to maintain a fluid intake of 10 to 13 8-oz glasses (2,500 to 3,000 ml)/day to promote adequate lithium excretion.
- Teach him that the lithium may cause sodium depletion, especially during initial therapy (until he achieves consistent blood levels); instruct him not to make dietary changes that might alter his sodium intake because this might reduce lithium elimination and increase the toxicity risk.
- Inform the patient that increasing his salt intake may increase his lithium excretion, which could lead to the return of mood symptoms; stress the need to maintain adequate salt

and water intake and to eat a normal, well-balanced diet (remind him that sodium loss—which can result from diarrhea, illness, extreme sweating, or other conditions—may alter lithium levels).
- Teach the patient and family to watch for evidence of toxicity—abdominal cramps, frequent urination, diarrhea, vomiting, drowsiness, unsteadiness, muscle weakness, ataxia, and tremors; instruct him to withhold one dose and call the physician if toxic symptoms occur, but not to stop taking the drug abruptly.
- Advise the patient to take his medication with food or after meals to avoid stomach upset.
- Because lithium may impair mental and physical function, caution the patient against driving or operating dangerous equipment while on the medication.

Guidelines for patients receiving lithium

- Blood levels should be checked 8 to 12 hours after first dose, two or three times weekly for first month, then weekly to monthly during maintenance therapy.
- Instruct patient to maintain fluid intake of 10 to 13 8-oz glasses (2,500 to 3,000 ml)/day.
- Teach patient that lithium may cause sodium depletion.
- Inform patient that increasing salt intake may increase lithium excretion.
- Teach patient and family to watch for evidence of lithium toxicity.
- Advise patient to take lithium with food or after meals.
- Caution patient against driving or operating dangerous equipment.

- Anticipating possible need for high-calorie finger foods, sandwiches, and cheese and crackers to supplement diet (especially if patient can't sit still long enough to complete a meal)
    - Offering fluids frequently
- Help the patient with personal hygiene; as symptoms subside, encourage him to assume responsibility for personal care
- Involve the patient in activities that require gross motor movements, maintain a calm environment, and protect him from overstimulation (such as from large groups, loud noises, and bright colors); suggest short daytime naps to promote rest, and firmly discourage him from overexerting himself
- Provide diversionary activities suited to a short attention span
- Provide emotional support, and set realistic goals for behavior
- In a calm, clear, self-confident manner, establish limits for the patient's demanding, hyperactive, manipulative, and acting-out behaviors

Key signs and symptoms of lithium toxicity

- Abdominal cramps
- Frequent urination
- Diarrhea
- Vomiting
- Drowsiness
- Unsteadiness
- Muscle weakness
- Ataxia
- Tremors

- Avoid reinforcing socially inappropriate or suggestive comments, and tactfully divert conversations that become intimately involved with other patients or staff
- Don't leave an opening for the patient to test or argue with you
  - Includes listening to requests attentively and with a neutral attitude, but avoiding power struggles if the patient pressures for an immediate answer
  - May require explaining that you'll seriously consider the request and respond later
- Collaborate with other staff members to provide consistent responses to the patient's manipulations or acting-out behaviors
- Anticipate the need for excessive verbalization
- Watch for early signs of frustration — when the patient's anger escalates from verbal threats to hitting (an object or person); certain actions may be necessary
  - Giving him space and removing clutter from environment
  - Telling him firmly that threats and hitting are unacceptable and that he needs help to control behavior
  - Informing him that staff will assist him to a quiet area, where he'll be able to gain control over behavior so he won't hurt himself or others
- Alert the care team promptly when acting-out behavior escalates
- When an acting-out incident ends and the patient is calm and in control, discuss his feelings with him and offer suggestions to prevent recurrence
- If the patient is receiving medication for the disorder, remind him of the importance of complying with the regimen and explain the need for ongoing laboratory values

● **Nursing interventions (depressive episode)**
- Provide for the patient's physical needs; if he's too depressed to care for himself, help him with personal hygiene
- Encourage him to eat, or feed him if necessary
- If the patient is constipated, add high-fiber foods to his diet; offer small, frequent meals and fluids, and encourage physical activity
- To help the patient sleep, give back rubs or warm milk at bedtime
  - May find relaxation tapes helpful
  - May require an as-needed sleep medication for sleep deficits
- Provide continual positive reinforcement to help build self-esteem
  - Maintaining a structured routine, including activities to boost confidence and promote interaction with others (for instance, group therapy)
  - Ongoing reassurances that his depression will lift
- Assume an active role in communicating with the patient
  - By encouraging him to talk or to write down his feelings if he's having trouble expressing them
  - By listening attentively and respectfully
  - If he seems sluggish, by giving him time to formulate his thoughts
  - By recording your observations and conversations to assist in evaluating his condition
- Avoid overwhelming the patient
- Take measures to prevent the patient from self-injury or suicide

Key nursing interventions for a patient in the depressive phase of bipolar disorder

- Provide continual positive reinforcement to help build self-esteem.
- Assume an active role in communicating with patient.
- Avoid overwhelming patient.
- Take measures to prevent patient self-injury or suicide.

- Removing harmful objects (such as glass, belts, shelves, rope, and bobby pins) from the patient's environment
- Closely observing and strictly supervising medications
- Always taking suicidal thoughts, gestures, or plans seriously
- Taking suicide precautions as dictated by facility policy
• Teach the patient the importance of continuing his medication regimen, even if he doesn't feel a need for it
  - With lithium, provide appropriate instructions
  - With an antidepressant, watch for signs and symptoms of mania

CYCLOTHYMIC DISORDER

● **Defining characteristics**
  • Cyclothymic disorder is characterized by short periods of mild depression alternating with short periods of hypomania; between the depressive and manic episodes, brief periods of normal mood occur
    - Emergence of depression or hypomania within 2 months of last episode
    - In many cases, emergence of manic episodes within a few days to weeks of last episode, although onset within hours is possible
  • Both the depressive and hypomanic phases of cyclothymic disorder are shorter and less severe than those in bipolar I or II disorder
    - No delusions
    - Usually no need for hospitalization
  • In some cases, the hypomanic episodes may enhance achievement in business and artistic endeavors; however, such mood swings can have a negative impact on the patient's interpersonal and social relationships and may lead to a more severe disease state
    - May lead to an uneven work and academic history, impulsive and frequent changes of residence, repeated romantic or marital breakups, or episodic pattern of alcohol and drug abuse (many cyclothymic patients self-medicate with alcohol or illegal drugs)
    - Can progress to a more severe form of bipolar illness
    - Possibility of a full-blown manic episode or major depression, with a consequent change in diagnosis to bipolar I or II disorder (occurs in roughly one-third of patients)
  • Cyclothymic disorder affects up to 1% of the population, striking men and women equally; onset usually occurs in the teens or early 20s

● **Causes**
  • Genetic factors (most likely cause)
    - Family history of bipolar disorder, major depression, substance abuse, or suicide in many patients

● **Signs and symptoms**
  • General features
    - Odd, eccentric, or suspicious personality
    - Dramatic, erratic, or antisocial personality features
    - Inability to maintain enthusiasm for new projects
    - Pattern of pulling close and then pushing away in interpersonal relationships

Key signs and symptoms of cyclothymic disorder

Hypomanic phase
- Insomnia
- Hyperactivity and physical restlessness
- Irritability or aggressiveness
- Grandiosity or inflated self-esteem
- Increased productivity, creativity

Depressive phase
- Insomnia or hypersomnia
- Feelings of inadequacy
- Decreased productivity
- Social withdrawal
- Loss of libido or interest in pleasurable activities
- Lethargy
- Suicidal ideation

Diagnosing cyclothymic disorder

- Rule out other disorders as cause of symptoms
- Must meet *DSM-IV-TR* criteria

Key treatment options for cyclothymic disorder

- Lithium
- Carbamazepine
- Valproic acid
- Verapamil
- Various antidepressants
- Individual psychotherapy
- Couple or family therapy

Key nursing interventions for a patient with cyclothymic disorder

- Explore ways to help patient cope with frequent mood changes.
- Encourage vocational opportunities that allow flexible hours.
- Encourage patients with artistic ability to pursue their talents as a creative outlet.

– Abrupt changes in personality from cheerful, confident, and energetic to sad, blue, or mean
- Hypomanic phase
  – Insomnia
  – Hyperactivity and physical restlessness
  – Irritability or aggressiveness
  – Grandiosity or inflated self-esteem
  – Increased productivity and creativity
  – Overinvolvement in pleasurable activities, including sex
  – Rapid speech
- Depressive phase
  – Insomnia or hypersomnia
  – Feelings of inadequacy
  – Decreased productivity
  – Social withdrawal
  – Loss of libido or interest in pleasurable activities
  – Lethargy
  – Depressed speech
  – Crying
  – Suicidal ideation

Diagnosis
- Differential diagnosis (ruling out other disorders) needed for accurate diagnosis
  – Acquired immunodeficiency syndrome
  – Cushing's disease
  – Epilepsy
  – Huntington's disease
  – Hyperthyroidism
  – Premenstrual syndrome
  – Migraines
  – Multiple sclerosis
  – Neoplasm
  – Postpartum depression
  – Stroke
  – Systemic lupus erythematosus
  – Wilson's disease
  – Trauma, uremia, and vitamin deficiencies
- Must rule out other psychiatric disorders that can mimic cyclothymic disorder
  – Mood disorder caused by substance abuse or a general medical condition
  – Bipolar I or II disorder with rapid cycling
  – Borderline personality disorder
- Diagnosis confirmed if *DSM-IV-TR* criteria met

Treatment
- Pharmacologic options: lithium, carbamazepine, valproic acid, verapamil (Calan), and various antidepressants
- Other therapies (individual psychotherapy, couple or family therapy) to help the patient deal with relationship problems associated with the disorder

Nursing interventions
- Explore ways to help the patient cope with frequent mood changes

- Encourage vocational opportunities that allow flexible work hours
- Encourage patients with artistic ability to pursue their talents as a creative outlet

DYSTHYMIC DISORDER

● Defining characteristics
- Dysthymic disorder, or *dysthymia,* refers to mild depression that lasts at least 2 years in adults or 1 year in children
- The depression is relatively mild or moderate, and most patients aren't certain when they first became depressed
  - May impair functioning at home, in school, or at work
  - Hospitalization rarely needed unless suicidal intent is present
- Dysthymic disorder commonly goes unrecognized by those experiencing it as well as by their family and friends
  - Usually not seen by mental health professional unless disorder progresses to major depression (symptoms often mild and, in some cases, more physiologic than emotional)
  - Difficult to treat, even when disorder is recognized
  - Slow recovery possible if condition becomes chronic and goes untreated
- An estimated 75% of patients with dysthymic disorder have a coexisting medical disorder (such as heart disease, cancer, or diabetes) or psychiatric disorder (for instance, substance abuse or an anxiety disorder)
- Dysthymic disorder affects about 3% of the population; it's twice as common in women as it is in men, and more prevalent among the poor and unmarried

● Causes
- Below-normal serotonin levels in many patients (likely involvement of serotonin in development of disorder)
- As with many other psychiatric disorders, increased vulnerability to disorder resulting from personality problems and multiple stressors, combined with inadequate coping skills

● Signs and symptoms
- Psychological symptoms
  - Persistent sad, anxious, or empty mood
  - Loss of interest in activities previously enjoyed
  - Excessive crying
  - Increased feelings of guilt, helplessness, or hopelessness
  - Poor school or work performance
  - Social withdrawal
  - Conflicts with family and friends
  - Increased restlessness and irritability
  - Poor concentration
  - Inability to make decisions
  - Thoughts of death or suicide, or suicide attempts
- Physiologic symptoms
  - Weight or appetite changes
  - Sleep difficulties
  - Reduced energy level
  - Headache
  - Backache

Characteristics of dysthymic disorder
- Also called *dysthymia*
- Mild depression that lasts at least 2 years in adults or 1 year in children
- Twice as common in women as in men
- More prevalent among the poor and unmarried

Common causes of dysthymic disorder
- Below-normal serotonin levels
- Increased vulnerability when multiple stressors and personality problems are combined with inadequate coping skills

Key signs and symptoms of dysthymic disorder

Psychological symptoms
- Persistent sad, anxious, or empty mood
- Excessive crying
- Increased feelings of guilt, helplessness, or hopelessness

Physiologic symptoms
- Weight or appetite changes
- Sleep difficulties
- Reduced energy level

Diagnosing dysthymic disorder

- Careful psychiatric examination and medical history
- Must meet *DSM-IV-TR* criteria

Key treatment options for dysthymic disorder

- Short-term psychotherapy
- Behavioral therapy
- Group therapy
- Antidepressants, such as SSRIs or TCAs, especially for patients who exhibit pessimism

Key nursing interventions for a patient with dysthymic disorder

- Provide supportive measures, such as reassurance, warmth, availability, and acceptance.
- Teach patient about the illness.
- Encourage positive health habits.

Characteristics of major depressive disorder

- Also called *unipolar major depression*
- Syndrome of a persistently sad mood lasting 2 weeks or longer
- Incidence increases with age

Possible accompanying problems

- Feelings of guilt, helplessness, or hopelessness
- Poor concentration
- Sleep disturbances
- Lethargy
- Appetite loss or weight gain
- Anhedonia
- Loss of mood reactivity
- Thoughts of death

● **Diagnosis**
- Careful psychiatric examination and medical history by psychiatrist or other mental health professional
- Diagnosis confirmed if *DSM-IV-TR* criteria met

● **Treatment**
- Short-term psychotherapy to teach the patient more constructive ways of communicating with family, friends, and coworkers; it also allows ongoing assessment of suicidal ideation and suicide risk
- Behavioral therapy to reeducate the patient in social skills and help him make attitude changes
- Group therapy to help him change maladaptive social functioning
- Pharmacologic treatment involving antidepressants, such as selective serotonin reuptake inhibitors (SSRIs) or tricyclic antidepressants (TCAs)
- Antidepressant drugs for patients who exhibit pessimism, disinterest, and low self-esteem

● **Nursing interventions**
- Provide supportive measures, such as reassurance, warmth, availability, and acceptance—even if the patient becomes hostile
- Teach the patient about the illness and prescribed antidepressant medication
- Urge the patient to engage in activities that enhance his sense of accomplishment
- Encourage positive health habits, such as eating well-balanced meals, avoiding drugs and alcohol (which can worsen depression), and getting physical exercise (which can lift his mood)

MAJOR DEPRESSIVE DISORDER

● **Defining characteristics**
- Major depressive disorder, also called *unipolar major depression*, is a syndrome of a persistently sad mood lasting 2 weeks or longer; it may be accompanied by other problems
  - Feelings of guilt, helplessness, or hopelessness
  - Poor concentration
  - Sleep disturbances
  - Lethargy
  - Appetite loss or weight gain
  - Anhedonia (inability to feel pleasure)
  - Loss of mood reactivity (failure to feel a mood uplift in response to something positive)
  - Thoughts of death
- Feelings of sadness go beyond—and last longer than—"normal" sadness or grief; some symptoms of severe depression (such as disinterest in pleasurable activities, hopelessness, and loss of mood reactivity) rarely accompany "normal" sadness
- Major depression commonly goes undiagnosed, and those who have it typically receive inadequate treatment; it can profoundly alter a person's social, physical, family, and occupational functioning
- Suicide—the most serious complication—can occur if feelings of worthlessness, guilt, and hopelessness are so overwhelming that the person no longer considers life worth living

– Occurs in nearly 15% of patients with untreated depression
– In many cases, patient may wait 1 month after suicide ideation before seeking help from a health care provider
- At some time in their lives, about 22% of women and 16% of men in the United States experience major depressive disorder; in health care settings, an estimated 6% to 8% of patients meet the diagnostic criteria for this disorder
- The incidence of major depression increases with age
  – Onset usually in early adulthood, with recurrences throughout the patient's lifetime
  – In about 50% of patients, first episode at about age 40 (currently, more being diagnosed with first episode in their 30s)
- More than 50% of patients who have one episode go on to have at least two more
  – Recurrences possible following prolonged symptom-free period or may occur sporadically
  – In some patients, recurrences occurring in clusters; in others, recurrences growing more frequent with age
- An untreated episode can last from 1 month to 1 year—or even longer

● **Causes**
- Genetic, biochemical, physical, psychological, and social factors implicated
- Unclear relationship between psychological stress, stressful life events, and depression onset; however, the patient history commonly reveals specific personal loss or severe stress
  – One theory: Major depression provoked by stressor interacting with patient's predisposition or premorbid personality
- Two to three times more common in people with first-degree relatives with the disorder, indicating genetic vulnerability (mounting evidence of involvement of several genes, although some researchers believe a single depression gene exists)
- Biological influences pointing to neural networks of brain's prefrontal cortex and basal ganglia as possible primary defect sites
  – May involve serotonin, neuroendocrine, and hypothalamic-pituitary-adrenal regulation systems
  – May be affected by differences in biological rhythms, as seen by changes in circadian rhythms and various neurochemical and neurohormonal factors
  – May be associated with abnormal cortisol levels (in dexamethasone suppression test, about 50% of patients with depression fail to suppress cortisol levels)
- Must be distinguished from secondary depression, which may be caused by specific event or can result from wide range of recognizable organic conditions
  – Metabolic disturbances, such as hypoxia and hypercalcemia
  – Endocrine disorders, such as diabetes and Cushing's disease
  – Neurologic diseases, such as Parkinson's disease and Alzheimer's disease
  – Cancer (especially of the pancreas)
  – Viral and bacterial infections, such as influenza and pneumonia
  – Cardiovascular disorders such as heart failure
  – Pulmonary disorders such as chronic obstructive lung disease

Common causes of major depressive disorder

- Genetic, biochemical, physical, psychological, and social factors implicated
- Biological influences pointing to neural networks of brain's prefrontal cortex and basal ganglia as possible primary defect sites
- Possible involvement of serotonin, neuroendocrine, and hypothalamic-pituitary-adrenal regulation systems
- Possibly, drugs prescribed for certain medical and psychiatric conditions, such as antihypertensives, psychotropics, antiparkinsonian drugs, opioid and nonopioid analgesics, and steroids

– Musculoskeletal disorders such as degenerative arthritis
– GI disorders such as irritable bowel syndrome
– Genitourinary problems such as incontinence
– Collagen vascular diseases such as systemic lupus erythematosus
– Anemias
- May be caused by drugs prescribed for certain medical and psychiatric conditions
    – Antihypertensives
    – Psychotropics
    – Antiparkinsonian drugs
    – Opioid and nonopioid analgesics
    – Numerous cardiovascular medications
    – Oral antidiabetics
    – Antimicrobials
    – Steroids
    – Chemotherapeutic agents
    – Cimetidine (Tagamet)
- Alcohol and illicit drug abuse (may contribute)

Signs and symptoms

- May seem unhappy or apathetic in assessment interviews
- May report range of signs and symptoms
    – Feeling "down in the dumps"
    – Increased or decreased appetite
    – Sleep disturbances (for example, insomnia or early awakening)
    – Disinterest in sex
    – Difficulty concentrating or thinking clearly
    – Easy distractibility
    – Indecisiveness
    – Low self-esteem
    – Poor coping
    – Constipation or diarrhea
    – Suicidal thoughts
- Possible worsening of symptoms in morning (patient report)
- Possible agitation (such as hand-wringing or restlessness) or psychomotor retardation (slow movements) on physical examination
- In severe depression, possible delusions of persecution or guilt, which can have an immobilizing effect
- Possible life problems or losses that may explain or contribute to depression (psychosocial history)
- Physical disorder or use of a prescription drug or other substance that can cause depression (medical history)
- Clues related to suicidal thoughts, a preoccupation with death, or previous suicide attempts
    – Requires use of direct questioning because many patients are reluctant to verbalize suicidal thoughts unless prompted
    – May require referral to mental health specialist or immediate hospitalization if patient has specific suicide plan or significant risk factors — history of a suicide attempt, profound hopelessness, concurrent medical illness, substance abuse, or social isolation

---

Key signs and symptoms of major depressive disorder

- Feeling "down in the dumps"
- Increased or decreased appetite
- Sleep
- Disinterest in sex
- Difficulty concentrating or thinking clearly
- Easy distractibility
- Indecisiveness
- Low self-esteem
- Poor coping
- Constipation or diarrhea
- Suicidal thoughts
- Possible worsening of symptoms in morning (patient report)
- Clues related to suicidal thoughts, a preoccupation with death, or previous suicide attempts

● Diagnosis

- Psychological tests, such as the Beck Depression Inventory, to determine symptom onset, severity, duration, and progression
- Dexamethasone suppression test showing failure to suppress cortisol secretion in depressed patients (although test has high false-negative rate)
- Toxicology screening suggesting drug-induced depression
- Diagnosis confirmed if *DSM-IV-TR* criteria met

● Treatment

- Antidepressant medication to achieve remission and prevent relapse; classified according to class
    - SSRIs
    - Serotonin/norepinephrine reuptake inhibitors (SNRIs)
    - Atypical antidepressants
    - TCAs
    - Monoamine oxidase (MAO) inhibitors
- Generally work by modifying the activity of relevant neurotransmitter pathways (see *Pharmacologic therapy for mood disorders,* pages 132 to 135)
- No ideal antidepressant for all patients; several factors should be considered when choosing an appropriate antidepressant
    - Patient's metabolism
    - Possible adverse effects
    - Agents that have been effective with other family members
    - Potential for toxicity (especially if suicidal overdose is a concern)
    - Patient's cultural and religious background (some patients may fear addiction or believe that medication is too strong for the body)
- Response needs reevaluating after the first 2 weeks of drug therapy, then at approximately 6 weeks, and then every 3 months
    - May require dosage changes at any time during treatment
    - Requires frequent assessment and monitoring for side effects or adverse reactions
- After remission, drug therapy continues for at least 6 to 9 months
    - As preventive measure for patient with history of recurrent depression, may be maintained on a low dose of antidepressant drug after acute episode resolves
- SSRIs: first-line treatment for patients with depression
    - Include citalopram (Celexa), escitalopram (Lexapro), fluoxetine (Prozac), fluvoxamine (Luvox), paroxetine (Paxil), and sertraline (Zoloft)
    - Inhibit serotonin reuptake and may inhibit reuptake of other neurotransmitters
    - Lack most of disturbing adverse effects associated with TCAs and MAO inhibitors
- SNRIs, such as venlafaxine (Effexor), inhibit norepinephrine uptake
    - Generally used as second-line agents for patients with major depressive disorder
- Atypical antidepressants, including bupropion (Wellbutrin), nefazodone (Serzone), trazodone (Desyrel), and mirtazapine (Remeron): second-line agents; their mechanism of action isn't well understood
    - Bupropion: thought to inhibit reuptake of serotonin, norepinephrine, and dopamine to varying degrees

(Text continues on page 134.)

Diagnosing major depressive disorder

- Psychological tests, such as the Beck Depression Inventory
- Dexamethasone suppression test showing failure to suppress cortisol secretion in depressed patients (although test has high false-negative rate)
- Toxicology screening suggesting drug-induced depression

Key treatment options for major depressive disorder

Basic treatment options
- ECT
- Antidepressants

SSRIs
- First-line treatment
- Inhibit serotonin reuptake; may inhibit reuptake of other neurotransmitters

SNRIs
- Example: Venlafaxine
- Used as second-line agents
- Inhibit norepinephrine uptake

TCAs
- Older class of antidepressants
- Inhibit reuptake of norepinephrine, serotonin, and dopamine
- Cause gradual decline in beta-adrenergic receptors
- Cause intolerable adverse effects; not used first-line

MAO inhibitors
- Examples: Phenelzine, tranylcypromine
- Increase norepinephrine, serotonin, and dopamine levels by inhibiting MAO
- May have actions that contribute to antidepressant effect
- Rarely used today because of high risk of adverse reactions and dangerous interactions
- Conservative doses may be combined with a TCA

Pharmacologic options for treating mood disorders

- MAO inhibitor: isocarboxazid
- TCAs: amitriptyline, imipramine
- SSRI: fluoxetine
- Anticonvulsant: valproic acid
- Antimanic: lithium

Pharmacologic therapy for mood disorders

This chart highlights several of the drugs used to treat mood disorders.

DRUG	ADVERSE EFFECTS	CONTRAINDICATIONS
Monoamine oxidase (MAO) inhibitor		
Isocarboxazid (Marplan)	• Blurred vision • Constipation • Dry mouth • Drowsiness or insomnia • Fatigue • Hepatic dysfunction (jaundice, malaise, right-upper-abdominal-quadrant pain, change in stool color or consistency) • Hypertensive crisis • Hypomania • Muscle twitching • Orthostatic hypotension • Skin rash • Vertigo • Weakness • Weight gain	• Cardiovascular or cerebrovascular disease • Confusion, uncooperativeness • Advanced age or debilitation • Glaucoma • Heart failure • History of severe headaches • Impaired renal function • Liver disease • Paranoid schizophrenia • Pregnancy
Tricyclic antidepressant		
Amitriptyline (Elavil) Imipramine (Tofranil)	• Agranulocytosis • Arrhythmias • Blurred vision • Bone marrow depression • Constipation • Dry mouth • Esophageal reflux • Galactorrhea • Hallucinations • Heart failure • Increased or decreased libido • Jaundice and fatigue • Mania • Myocardial infarction (MI) • Orthostatic hypotension or hypertension • Palpitations • Shock • Slowed intracardiac conduction • Urinary hesitancy • Weight gain	• Concomitant use of MAO inhibitors • Recent MI • Renal or hepatic disease
Selective serotonin reuptake inhibitor		
Fluoxetine (Prozac)	• Dry mouth • Insomnia • Nausea • Nervousness • Rash • Vertigo • Weight loss	• MAO-inhibitor use (avoid using within 14 days of taking an MAO inhibitor)

NURSING CONSIDERATIONS

- Monitor patient's blood pressure every 2 to 4 hours during initial therapy; instruct him to change positions slowly.
- Assess for signs and symptoms of hypertensive crisis.
- Monitor fluid intake and output.
- Monitor the patient for suicide risk.
- Caution the patient not to ingest foods and beverages containing tyramine, caffeine, or tryptophan (warn him that tyramine can cause a hypertensive crisis); provide a list of foods and beverages that contain such substances.
- Instruct the patient to avoid meperidine (Demerol), epinephrine, local anesthetics, decongestants, cough medicines, diet pills, and most over-the-counter agents.
- Teach the patient to wear medical identification jewelry.
- Advise the patient to go to the emergency department immediately if hypertensive crisis develops.

- Supervise drug ingestion.
- Monitor blood pressure and pulse for signs of orthostatic hypotension; instruct the patient to change positions slowly.
- Monitor liver function and complete blood counts.
- Institute suicide precautions as needed.
- Be aware that special monitoring is required if the patient poses a suicide risk or has a history of angle-closure glaucoma or seizure disorder.
- Tell the patient to avoid driving or operating hazardous machinery if drowsiness occurs.
- Instruct the patient to avoid alcohol and over-the-counter agents unless the physician approves.
- Inform the patient that the drug may take up to 4 weeks to become effective.

- Administer drug in the morning, with or without food.
- Monitor for weight loss if nausea occurs.
- Advise the patient to wait 5 weeks after stopping fluoxetine before starting an MAO inhibitor.
- Tell the patient to avoid alcoholic beverages.
- Instruct the patient to report adverse effects to the physician, especially rash or itching.

(continued)

Nursing considerations for treating mood disorders

- Monitor blood pressure every 2 to 4 hours during initial therapy with an MAO inhibitor.
- Assess patient taking an MAO inhibitor for hypertensive crisis.
- Monitor liver function and CBC when patient is taking a tricyclic antidepressant.
- Administer SSRIs in the morning with or without food.
- Advise patient taking an SSRI to avoid alcohol.
- Monitor serum drug levels of lithium.
- Advise patients taking lithium to maintain adequate sodium intake.

Pharmacologic therapy for mood disorders *(continued)*

DRUG	ADVERSE EFFECTS	CONTRAINDICATIONS
Anticonvulsant (for treatment of bipolar disorder)		
Valproic acid (Depakote)	• Abdominal cramps • Diarrhea or constipation • Double vision or seeing "spots" • Increased urination • Indigestion • Nausea • Prolonged bleeding time • Sedation • Skin rashes • Vomiting	• Liver disease
Antimanic		
Lithium (Eskalith)	• Below 1.5 mEq/L: fine hand tremors, dry mouth, increased thirst, increased urination, nausea • 1.5 to 2 mEq/L: vomiting, diarrhea, muscle weakness, ataxia, dizziness, confusion, slurred speech • 2 to 2.5 mEq/L: persistent nausea and vomiting, blurred vision, muscle twitching, hyperactive deep tendon reflexes • 2.5 to 3 mEq/L: myoclonic twitches or movements of an entire limb, choreoathetoid movements, urinary and fecal incontinence • Above 3 mEq/L: seizures, cardiac arrhythmias, hypotension, peripheral vascular collapse, death	• Early pregnancy

- Nefazodone and trazodone: inhibit serotonin and norepinephrine reuptake
- Mirtazapine: thought to inhibit serotonin and norepinephrine reuptake while blocking two specific serotonin receptors
- TCAs, an older class of antidepressants: inhibit the reuptake of norepinephrine, serotonin, and dopamine, and cause a gradual decline in beta-adrenergic receptors
  - Include amitriptyline (Elavil), amoxapine (Asendin), clomipramine (Anafranil), desipramine (Norpramin), doxepin (Sinequan), imipramine (Tofranil), nortriptyline (Pamelor), and trimipramine (Surmontil)
  - Can be effective but may cause intolerable adverse effects and generally aren't used as first-line agents
- MAO inhibitors, such as phenelzine (Nardil) and tranylcypromine (Parnate): increase norepinephrine, serotonin, and dopamine levels by inhibiting MAO, an enzyme that inactivates them; they may have additional actions that contribute to their antidepressant effect

NURSING CONSIDERATIONS

- Monitor liver function tests and platelet counts.
- Instruct the patient to take drug with meals if stomach upset occurs.
- Urge the patient to report excessive bruising or unexplained bleeding.
- Caution the patient not to discontinue the drug abruptly.
- Instruct the patient not to crush tablets.
- Caution the patient to avoid alcohol while taking this drug.

- Monitor serum drug levels.
- Instruct the patient to swallow (not to chew) extended-release preparations whole.
- Supervise administration to ensure that the medication is swallowed.
- To relieve dry mouth or increased thirst, instruct the patient to increase fluids or eat sugarless gum or hard candy.
- If the patient has increased urination, suggest limiting fluids after 8 p.m.; evaluate for diabetes insipidus, dilute urine, or low specific gravity.
- For nausea, suggest taking the drug with food.
- Instruct the patient to maintain adequate sodium intake.
- Inform the patient that metallic taste may occur while taking this drug.
- Teach the patient to take the drug even when feeling better, and not to stop it abruptly.
- Instruct the patient to monitor weight weekly.
- Caution the patient not to take the drug with alcohol.
- Instruct the patient to notify the physician if severe vomiting or diarrhea occurs.
- Instruct female patients to use a reliable form of birth control while taking this drug.
- Stress the need for the physician's approval before taking any new medications.
- Instruct the patient not to stop taking the drug without discussing it with the physician.

- – May be prescribed for patients with atypical depression (for example, depression marked by increased appetite and sleep, rather than anorexia and insomnia) or for patients who don't respond to TCAs
- – Although commonly effective, are rarely used today because of high risk of adverse reactions, causing hypertensive crisis and dangerous interactions with various foods and medications; conservative doses may be combined with a TCA for depression refractory to either type of drug alone
- Medication combined with psychotherapy (which can improve the treatment outcome by helping the patient cope with low self-esteem and self-demoralization), and electroconvulsive therapy (ECT) (which is sometimes used to treat severe depression)
- Short-term psychotherapy to aid in relieving major depression; many psychiatrists believe the best results are achieved by combining individual, family, or group psychotherapy with medication

Key facts about ECT

- Controversial
- Used to treat severe depression in certain cases
- Psychotherapy and medication aren't effective
- Its use poses a lower risk than other treatments
- A patient is at immediate risk for suicide

Key nursing interventions for a patient with major depressive disorder

- Provide for patient's physical needs.
- Plan activities for times when patient's energy level peaks.
- Assume active role in initiating communication.
- Avoid feigned cheerfulness.
- Ask patient whether he thinks about death or suicide.
- Know that suicidal thoughts signal immediate need for consultation and assessment.
- Be aware that there's a higher risk of suicide with lifting of depressed mood.

- Although controversial, ECT to treat severe depression when psychotherapy and medication aren't effective, when its use poses a lower risk than other treatments, or when a patient is at immediate risk for suicide (produces faster results than antidepressant medication does)
  - One-second electrical current passed through the brain using electrodes placed above temples; current produces brief seizure (lasts 30 to 60 seconds)
  - Insertion of bite block prevents tongue biting during seizure
  - Atropine or glycopyrrolate (to reduce secretions, prevent aspiration, and reduce the risk of bradycardia) as well as short-acting general anesthesia, muscle relaxant, and oxygen
  - Brain waves, heart rhythm, and arterial oxygen saturation monitored during treatment
  - Patient must fast for 6 to 8 hours before treatment; immediately before session, patient asked to void, and dentures, glasses, hearing aids, contact lenses, and hairpins removed
  - Total of 6 to 12 treatments in typical course for major depression; 2 or 3 per week (typically, every other day)
  - Requires informed consent, including a full explanation of the procedure and its potential benefits and risks
  - Contraindications: recent myocardial infarction, history of stroke, and intracranial lesions
  - Potential adverse effects: headache, short-term memory loss, and muscle aches

● **Nursing interventions**
- Provide for the patient's physical needs
  - Assisting with self-care and personal hygiene (patient may be too depressed to do this alone)
  - Encouraging him to eat (may need to feed him)
  - If constipated, providing high-fiber foods; offering small, frequent meals; and encouraging physical activity and fluid intake
  - Giving warm milk or back rubs at bedtime to improve sleep
- Record all observations and conversations with the patient (these are valuable in evaluating his response to treatment)
- Plan activities for times when the patient's energy level peaks
- Assume an active role in initiating communication
  - By sharing observations of patient's behavior
  - By speaking slowly and allowing ample time for him to respond (may think and react sluggishly)
  - By encouraging him to talk about and write down feelings
  - By listening attentively and respectfully (to show him he's important)
  - By avoiding interruptions and remaining nonjudgmental
  - By providing a structured routine; may include noncompetitive activities (to build self-confidence and promote interaction with others) and urging him to socialize and join group activities
- Avoid feigned cheerfulness, but don't hesitate to laugh with him and point out the value of humor
- Try to spend some time with the patient each day so he doesn't become isolated; avoid long periods of silence, which tend to increase anxiety

- Reassure the patient that he can help ease depression by expressing his feelings, engaging in pleasurable activities, and improving his grooming and hygiene
- Teach the patient about depression; emphasize that effective methods are available to relieve symptoms
- Help the patient recognize distorted perceptions and link them to his depression; when he learns to recognize depressive thought patterns, he can consciously begin to substitute self-affirming thoughts
- Ask the patient whether he thinks about death or suicide
  - Signals an immediate need for consultation and assessment (early detection of suicidal thoughts may thwart suicide attempt)
  - Higher risk of suicide with lifting of depressed mood (see *Recognizing suicide potential in patients with major depression*)
- If the patient is taking an antidepressant, stress the need for compliance and review adverse reactions
  - For patients taking drugs that produce strong anticholinergic effects (such as amitriptyline and amoxapine), suggest using sugarless gum or hard candy to relieve dry mouth

---

Recognizing suicide potential in patients with major depression

A patient with major depression is already at increased risk for suicide. However, as his mood begins to elevate and depressive feelings lift, he's considered at an even higher risk. Stay alert for these signs:

- overwhelming anxiety (the most common trigger for a suicide attempt)
- withdrawal and social isolation
- saying farewell to friends and family
- putting affairs in order
- giving away prized possessions
- sending covert suicide messages and death wishes
- expressing obvious suicidal thoughts ("I'd be better off dead")
- describing a suicide plan
- hoarding medications
- talking about death and a feeling of futility
- behavior changes, especially as his depression begins to subside.

TAKING ACTION
If you think your patient is at risk for suicide, take these steps:
- Keep communication lines open. Maintaining personal contact may help the suicidal patient feel he isn't alone or without resources or hope. Continuity of care and consistency of primary nurses also can help him maintain emotional ties to others — the ultimate technique for preventing suicide.
- To ensure a safe environment, check for dangerous conditions, such as exposed pipes, windows without safety glass, and access to the roof or open balconies.
- Remove belts and sharp objects, such as razors, knives, nail files and clippers, suspenders, light cords, and glass, from the patient's room.
- Make sure an acutely suicidal patient is observed around the clock. Stay alert when he uses a sharp object (as when shaving), takes medications, or uses the bathroom (to prevent hanging or other injury). Assign him a room near the nurses' station and with another patient.

Key nursing interventions for a patient with major depressive disorder

- For patient taking an antidepressant, stress need for compliance and review adverse reactions.
- For patients taking drugs that produce strong anticholinergic effects, suggest using sugarless gum or hard candy to relieve dry mouth.
- Caution patient taking a sedating antidepressant to avoid activities that require alertness.
- Caution patient taking a TCA or an SSRI to avoid alcoholic beverages or other central nervous system depressants.
- For patient taking an MAO inhibitor, tell him he must avoid foods that contain tyramine, caffeine, or tryptophan; give him a list of specific foods and beverages to avoid.

Key signs and symptoms of suicide potential

- Overwhelming anxiety
- Withdrawal and social isolation
- Saying farewell to friends and family
- Putting affairs in order
- Sending covert suicide messages
- Expressing obvious suicidal thoughts
- Describing a suicide plan
- Hoarding medications
- Talking about death
- Behavior changes

TIME-OUT FOR TEACHING

Foods to avoid with MAO inhibitors

If your patient is taking a monoamine oxidase (MAO) inhibitor, instruct him to avoid these food items, which can cause a hypertensive reaction:

- Aged cheeses
- Avocados
- Bananas
- Beer
- Canned figs
- Chianti
- Chocolate
- Coffee
- Colas
- Fava beans
- Liver
- Meat tenderizers
- Pickled herring
- Raisins
- Sherry
- Sour cream
- Soy sauce
- Yeast extracts
- Yogurt

  - Caution the patient taking a sedating antidepressant (such as amitriptyline or trazodone) to avoid activities that require alertness, including driving and operating mechanical equipment
- Monitor the patient for seizures because some antidepressants lower the seizure threshold
- Inform the patient that antidepressants, especially bupropion, may take several weeks to produce the desired effect
- Caution the patient taking a TCA or an SSRI to avoid drinking alcoholic beverages or taking other central nervous system depressants during therapy
- If the patient is taking an MAO inhibitor, emphasize that he must avoid foods that contain tyramine (can produce hypertensive crisis), caffeine, or tryptophan; give him a list of specific foods and beverages to avoid (see *Foods to avoid with MAO inhibitors*)

NCLEX CHECKS

It's never too soon to begin your NCLEX preparation. Now that you've reviewed this chapter, carefully read each of the following questions and choose the best answer. Then compare your responses to the correct answers.

1. Assessment of a patient reveals severe pathologic mood swings, from hyperactivity and euphoria to sadness and depression. Which diagnosis should the nurse suspect?
- ☐ **1.** Dysthymic disorder
- ☐ **2.** Cyclothymic disorder
- ☐ **3.** Bipolar disorder
- ☐ **4.** Depressive disorder

2. When caring for a patient who's predisposed to bipolar disorder, the nurse should be aware that a bipolar episode may be triggered by:

☐ **1.** hypothyroidism.
☐ **2.** hyperparathyroidism.
☐ **3.** antimanic drugs.
☐ **4.** anticonvulsant drugs.

3. What frequency of depressive episodes would the nurse interpret as indicative of rapid-cycling bipolar disorder?

☐ **1.** No episodes of depression
☐ **2.** One or more episodes of depression or mania in 1 year
☐ **3.** Two or more episodes of depression or mania in 1 year
☐ **4.** Four or more episodes of depression or mania in 1 year

4. Which patient would the nurse expect to prepare for ECT?

☐ **1.** A female patient with dysthymic disorder
☐ **2.** An elderly male with major depressive disorder and a history of stroke
☐ **3.** A female patient with depression and hypomania due to a cyclothymic disorder
☐ **4.** A middle-age, female patient with major depression and an immediate risk of suicide

5. Which instructions would the nurse include in a teaching plan for a patient who has been prescribed lithium?

☐ **1.** Limit fluids to 33 oz (1,000 ml) daily
☐ **2.** Maintain a fluid intake of 10 to 13 8-oz glasses (2,500 to 3,000 ml) daily
☐ **3.** Restrict sodium intake
☐ **4.** Exercise outside in hot weather

6. When planning care for a patient with bipolar disorder who's experiencing a manic episode, which nursing actions are most appropriate? Select all that apply:

☐ **1.** Having the patient participate in gross motor physical activities
☐ **2.** Providing high-calorie finger foods for the patient
☐ **3.** Encouraging the patient to continue activities until exhausted
☐ **4.** Urging the patient to participate in large group functions
☐ **5.** Allowing the patient to continue to engage in hyperactive behavior

7. The physician has prescribed lithium 600 mg t.i.d. in syrup form for a patient who has difficulty swallowing capsules. The label on the drug reads *Lithium 300 mg/ 5 ml.* How many milliliters should the nurse administer for each dose?

_____

8. A patient is scheduled for ECT at 10 a.m. Which action would be most appropriate?

☐ **1.** Giving the patient a clear liquid breakfast
☐ **2.** Catheterizing the patient for a morning urine sample
☐ **3.** Administering prescribed medications to reduce secretions
☐ **4.** Allowing the patient to keep his dentures in his mouth

TOP 10

Items to study for your next test on mood disorders

1. Abnormalities in affect
2. Four types of mood disorders
3. Possible causes of mood disorders
4. Classification of bipolar disorders
5. Signs and symptoms of manic and depressive phases
6. Nursing interventions for patients with bipolar disorder during manic and depressive phases
7. Characteristics of major depressive disorder
8. Signs and symptoms of depression
9. Major medications for the treatment of depression
10. Nursing interventions for patients with depression

9. A patient receiving lithium has a serum drug level of 2.3 mEq/L. What would the nurse most likely assess given this serum drug level?

- ☐ **1.** Urinary incontinence
- ☐ **2.** Seizures
- ☐ **3.** Muscle weakness
- ☐ **4.** Hyperactive deep tendon reflexes

10. Which instruction would the nurse most likely include in the teaching plan for a patient receiving amitriptyline?

- ☐ **1.** Avoid foods containing caffeine.
- ☐ **2.** Change positions slowly.
- ☐ **3.** Maintain adequate fluid and sodium intake.
- ☐ **4.** Report excessive bruising or bleeding.

ANSWERS AND RATIONALES

1. CORRECT ANSWER: 3
Severe pathologic mood swings occur in bipolar disorder. Dysthymic disorder involves a depressed mood with no evidence of mania. In cyclothymic disorder, the patient's mood swings would be much milder than those described for this scenario. Depressive disorder involves a depressed mood or loss of interest in previously pleasurable activities, and no manic symptoms.

2. CORRECT ANSWER: 1
In a patient who's predisposed to bipolar disorder, hypothyroidism may trigger a disease episode. Other possible triggers include stressful life events (such as a serious loss, chronic illness, or financial problems), use of antidepressants to treat depression, and sleep deprivation. Hyperparathyroidism, antimanic drugs, and anticonvulsant drugs aren't triggers for this disorder.

3. CORRECT ANSWER: 4
Rapid cycling is a variant form of bipolar disorder in which four or more episodes of depression and mania occur within a 12-month period.

4. CORRECT ANSWER: 4
ECT may be used to treat major depression as well as certain psychotic disorders, particularly in situations of severe depression when psychotherapy and medications have been ineffective, when ECT poses a lower risk than other treatments do, or when the patient is at an immediate risk for suicide. ECT isn't used for dysthymic disorder or cyclothymic disorder, and it's contraindicated in patients with recent myocardial infarction, a history of stroke, and intracranial lesions.

5. CORRECT ANSWER: 2
A patient taking lithium must maintain a fluid intake of 10 to 13 8-oz glasses (2,500 to 3,000 ml) per day to promote adequate excretion of the drug. Sodium depletion can occur during initial therapy until consistent blood levels are achieved; therefore, consistent intake is necessary. Exercising outside in hot weather would lead to excess sodium depletion, which would alter serum lithium levels.

6. CORRECT ANSWER: 1, 2

During a manic episode, the patient should engage in activities that require gross motor movement. Because of the patient's hyperactivity, the nurse should provide high-calorie finger foods to supplement his diet. Allowing the patient to overextend himself or continue activities until exhausted is inappropriate. The patient needs a calm environment and should be protected from overstimulation, including exposure to large groups. The nurse needs to set firm, consistent limits for the patient's demanding, hyperactive, manipulative, and acting-out behavior.

7. CORRECT ANSWER: 10

Using the formula D/H × V, set up the problem as follows:

$$\frac{600}{300} \times 5 \text{ milliliters}$$

Then solve:

$$2 \times 5 \text{ milliliters} = 10 \text{ milliliters}$$

8. CORRECT ANSWER: 3

In this situation, the nurse should administer the prescribed medication (such as atropine or glycopyrrolate) to reduce secretions, prevent aspiration, and reduce the risk of bradycardia. The patient needs to fast for 6 to 8 hours before the ECT, so giving the patient a clear-liquid breakfast would be inappropriate. The patient should void and remove dentures, glasses, hearing aids, contact lenses, and hairpins before the procedure begins. A catheterized urine specimen isn't necessary.

9. CORRECT ANSWER: 4

With a serum drug level between 2 and 2.5 mEq/L, assessment findings include hyperactive deep tendon reflexes, persistent nausea and vomiting, blurred vision, and muscle twitching. Urinary incontinence is associated with drug levels of 2.5 to 3 mEq/L. Seizures are associated with drug levels above 3 mEq/L. Muscle weakness is seen with drug levels ranging from 1.5 to 2 mEq/L.

10. CORRECT ANSWER: 2

Amitriptyline is a tricyclic antidepressant that can cause orthostatic hypotension. Therefore, the nurse would instruct the patient to change positions slowly. Avoiding foods containing caffeine, tyramine, or tryptophan would be appropriate for patients receiving MAO inhibitors. Maintaining an adequate sodium and fluid intake is important when lithium is the prescribed drug. Excessive bruising or bleeding is an adverse reaction associated with valproic acid, which is sometimes used to treat bipolar disorder.

6

Anxiety disorders

LEARNING OBJECTIVES

After studying this chapter, you should be able to:

- Identify positive and negative effects of anxiety.
- Describe how anxiety disorders impair functioning.
- Identify the proposed causes of anxiety disorders.
- List the most common anxiety disorders.
- Explain how to distinguish acute stress disorder from posttraumatic stress disorder.
- Identify the drugs commonly used to treat anxiety disorders.
- Discuss assessment and intervention for patients with anxiety disorders.

CHAPTER OVERVIEW

Anxiety disorders are a group of conditions marked by extreme or pathologic anxiety or dread. Sufferers experience disturbances of thinking, mood, behavior, and physiologic activity. Many with such disorders are anxious most of the time, with no apparent cause.

The anxiety may be so uncomfortable that the individual stops doing certain everyday activities to avoid the feeling of dread. Some people have terrifying bouts of intense anxiety that immobilize them. The overwhelming feelings of anxiety, impending catastrophe, guilt, shame, helplessness, or worthlessness cause sufferers to cling to maladaptive behaviors, ultimately worsening their symptoms.

UNDERSTANDING ANXIETY DISORDERS

General information

- Anxiety is a universal feeling—everyone experiences some degree of worry, uncertainty, or apprehension
- At mild or moderate levels, anxiety rarely threatens one's coping ability, and can even motivate a person to try new things and take risks (such as interviewing for a new job)
- The degree of anxiety a person experiences, along with his ability to perceive it accurately and channel it appropriately, determines whether the anxiety will help or hinder his level of functioning
  - When perceived as mild or moderate, may feel uneasy or fearful but still able to function
  - When perceived as severe, will feel threatened and either avoid the anxiety or become overwhelmed by it
- Anxiety disorders are the most common type of psychiatric disorder
- Anxiety disorders are highly treatable; however, only about one-third of sufferers receive treatment
  - Left untreated, these disorders can become chronic and can progressively worsen, increasing the risk of suicide and other serious complications
- Anxiety may be mild, moderate, or severe (panic level), and is classified according to signs and symptoms and diagnostic criteria
  - Acute stress disorder
  - Agoraphobia
  - Generalized anxiety disorder (GAD)
  - Obsessive-compulsive disorder (OCD)
  - Panic disorder
  - Phobia, social and specific
  - Posttraumatic stress disorder (PTSD)
- In the United States, anxiety disorders affect more than 19 million adults ages 18 to 54 (about 13% of the total population) and account for nearly one-third of the $148 billion mental health bill
- Those with anxiety disorders are three to five times more likely than the general population to visit a physician, and six times more likely to be hospitalized for a psychiatric disorder
- Anxiety disorders can occur at any age, and they affect twice as many women as men
- Anxiety disorders are commonly accompanied by other psychiatric illnesses, especially mood disorders and substance abuse—as well as various physiologic disorders

CAUSES

Genetic factors

- Some anxiety disorders (panic disorder, OCD, GAD, and major phobias) are inherited
- Researching specific genetic factors that might explain or contribute to an inherited risk

Key facts about anxiety

- A universal feeling
- Degree of anxiety, along with the ability to perceive it accurately and channel it appropriately, determines whether a person's anxiety will help or hinder his level of functioning
- May be mild, moderate, or severe (panic level)
- Classified according to signs and symptoms and diagnostic criteria

Classifying anxiety disorders

- Acute stress disorder
- Agoraphobia
- GAD
- OCD
- Panic disorder
- Phobia, social and specific
- PTSD

- Studies focusing on the possibility that the genes that regulate specific neuro-transmitters, such as serotonin and dopamine, are defective

Common causes of anxiety disorders

- Biochemical factors
- Brain atrophy
- Underdeveloped frontal and temporal lobes
- Abnormalities involving the amygdala and hippocampus

● **Biochemical factors**
  - Some experts believe in a biological vulnerability to stress; increases susceptibility to environmental stimuli
  - Neurotransmitter imbalances and breathing abnormalities: also contribute
  - Studies suggesting hypersensitivity to the effects of carbon dioxide
    - Hypersensitivity: may be aggravated in crowded spaces, such as airplanes or elevators
    - Hypersensitive people: exposure to carbon dioxide aggravates anxiety symptoms; over time, may develop pattern of impaired breathing and sense of panic that evolves into full-fledged anxiety disorder

● **Neuroanatomic factors**
  - Scientists using magnetic resonance imaging (MRI) and other neuroimaging techniques to locate the brain areas or abnormalities associated with anxiety responses
  - Identification of brain atrophy, underdeveloped frontal and temporal lobes, and abnormalities involving the amygdala (which regulates fear, memory, and emotion) and the hippocampus (which plays a role in emotion and memory storage)

● **Psychological factors**
  - Some theories suggesting that certain anxiety disorders arise when unconscious defense mechanisms become overwhelmed and dysfunctional
  - Several studies showing a strong correlation between parents' fears and those of their children (in other words, a child "learns" fears by observing a parent's fearful reaction to an object or situation)

● **Other factors**
  - Traumatic events triggering anxiety disorders
    - PTSD most obvious example
    - Include trauma following separation and loss (as in panic disorders)
    - May trigger psychological, genetic, or biochemical factors in those vulnerable to the disorder
    - May trigger biological propensity leading to phobia, even after a single exposure (as in fear of snakes)
  - Some associated with particular medical conditions; however, no causal relationship established
  - Gender playing a role in disorder development; women are at higher risk than men are
  - Additional risk factors for anxiety disorders
    - Marital separation or divorce
    - History of childhood physical or sexual abuse
    - Low socioeconomic status

Characteristics of acute stress disorder

- May begin as early as 2 days after the trauma
- Unlike PTSD, acute stress disorder resolves within 4 weeks
- Acute stress disorder may be rediagnosed as PTSD if symptoms last longer

ACUTE STRESS DISORDER

● **Defining characteristics**
  - Acute stress disorder is a syndrome of anxiety and behavioral disturbances that occurs within 4 weeks of an extreme trauma (possibly involving serious

physical or emotional injury or threats to the patient's life, including combat, rape, or a near-death experience in an accident)
- Generally, symptoms start during or shortly after the trauma
    - Feelings of numbness
    - Dissociation
    - Lack of reality surrounding the event
- Symptoms generally impair functioning in at least one key area (such as social or occupational settings, or relationships)
- Acute stress disorder may begin as early as 2 days after the trauma
- Unlike PTSD, acute stress disorder resolves within 4 weeks; the condition may be rediagnosed as PTSD if symptoms last longer
- Prognosis depends on such factors as severity and duration of the trauma, and the patient's level of functioning
    - More rapid recovery possible with immediate psychological care and much social support
    - If untreated, may progress to PTSD, substance abuse, or major depression

Causes
- Exposure to trauma (major precipitant)
- See "Posttraumatic stress disorder," page 166, for other possible causes

Signs and symptoms
- Generalized anxiety
- Hyperarousal
- Avoidance of reminders of the traumatic event
- Persistent, intrusive recollections of the traumatic event in flashbacks, dreams, or recurrent thoughts or visual images
- Irritability
- Physical restlessness
- Sleep disturbances
- Exaggerated startle reflex
- Poor concentration
- Hallmark is dissociation (defense mechanism in which patient separates anxiety-provoking thoughts and emotions from rest of psyche)
    - Characterized by the world seeming dreamlike or unreal
    - Feelings of observing self from a distance or that a body part has somehow changed
    - May be accompanied by poor memory of traumatic event or even complete event-related amnesia

Diagnosis
- Although initially based on recent history of trauma, physical examination to help rule out organic causes of signs and symptoms
- Diagnosis confirmed if *Diagnostic and Statistical Manual of Mental Disorders, Fourth Edition, Text Revision (DSM-IV-TR)* criteria met

Treatment
- Social supports, psychotherapy, cognitive or behavioral therapy, and pharmacotherapy; those experiencing hyperarousal may also benefit from relaxation techniques such as deep-breathing exercises
- Supportive counseling or short-term psychotherapy helps the patient examine the trauma in a supportive environment, strengthen previously helpful coping mechanisms, and learn new coping strategies

Common causes of acute stress disorder
- Exposure to trauma: major precipitant

Key signs and symptoms of acute stress disorder
- Hyperarousal
- Avoidance of reminders of traumatic event
- Persistent, intrusive recollections of traumatic event in flashbacks, dreams, or recurrent thoughts or visual images
- Exaggerated startle reflex
- Dissociation (hallmark of disorder)

Diagnosing acute stress disorder
- Recent history of trauma
- Physical examination to rule out organic causes of signs and symptoms
- Must meet *DSM-IV-TR* criteria

Key treatment options for acute distress disorder
- Psychotherapy
- Cognitive or behavioral therapy
- Pharmacotherapy
- Supportive counseling

- Cognitive or behavioral therapy may involve trauma education, cognitive restructuring of the traumatic event to help the patient see it from a different perspective, and gradual reexposure with less avoidance
- Drugs may be used if nonpharmacologic methods aren't effective; antianxiety agents, beta-adrenergic blockers (such as clonidine [Catapres] or propranolol [Inderal]), or antidepressants may be prescribed

● **Nursing interventions**
- Encourage the patient to discuss the stressful event and identify it as traumatic (to help validate that the situation was beyond her personal control)
- Urge her to talk about her anxiety and her other feelings about the trauma to help her cope with the reality of the event
- Encourage the patient to identify any feelings of survivor guilt, inadequacy, or blame; expressing these feelings can help her understand that her survival may have been due to chance, rather than being related to any personal action or inaction
- Teach the patient relaxation techniques, such as progressive muscle relaxation and deep breathing
- Administer antianxiety medications as ordered

AGORAPHOBIA

● **Defining characteristics**
- Agoraphobia is the intense fear or avoidance of situations or places that may be difficult or embarrassing to leave or in which help might not be available
  - Worry about inability to get somewhere safe, and fear of ensuing panic attack or panic symptoms (such as dizziness, vomiting, loss of control, or difficulty breathing)
  - Eventually, avoidance of potentially uncomfortable situations
- Agoraphobia usually occurs in patients with a history of panic disorder
- Without treatment, agoraphobia may worsen
  - In extreme cases, patient literally becomes prisoner in own home; too fearful to leave "safe" zone
  - In less severe cases, may be able to engage in activities or travel if a trusted companion goes along
- Many experts view agoraphobia as an adverse behavioral outcome of repeated panic attacks and the subsequent worry, preoccupation, and avoidance
- Some of the most common fears among agoraphobic patients include crowds, large public spaces (such as parks, malls, theaters, and supermarkets), and places where the person feels trapped (such as airplanes, inside a car in rush-hour traffic, or on a bridge)
- Most patients can verbalize what they fear and where they fear it, although some know only that they have a sense of dread
- Nearly 6% of adults develop agoraphobia at some point in their lives
  - In a given year, occurs in about 2.2% of adults ages 18 to 54
  - Twice as common in women as it is in men
  - Age of onset usually in 20s or 30s
- Agoraphobic patients have higher depression and suicide rates than those of the general population and may be prone to alcohol and sedative abuse

Causes
- Exact cause unknown; theories include biochemical imbalances (especially related to neurotransmitters) and environmental factors
  - Panic attack in given situation or place (such as a shopping mall) may lead to association of panic with specific situation or place, and avoidance
- May run in families, suggesting genetic basis

Signs and symptoms
- Overriding fear of open or public spaces (primary symptom)
  - Deep concern that help might not be available in such places
  - Avoidance of public places and confinement to home
- When accompanied by panic disorder, fear that having panic attack in public will lead to embarrassment or inability to escape (for symptoms of a panic attack, see "Panic disorder," page 154)

Diagnosis
- Based on evidence of signs and symptoms
- When present without panic disorder, diagnosis confirmed when *DSM-IV-TR* criteria met

Treatment
- Medication and behavioral therapy
- Pharmacologic therapy, including a tricyclic antidepressant (TCA), such as amitriptyline (Elavil), or a selective serotonin-reuptake inhibitor (SSRI) such as paroxetine (Paxil)
  - A benzodiazepine, such as alprazolam (Xanax), may be used to treat a panic attack in progress
- Desensitization, which gradually exposes the patient to the situation that triggers fear and avoidance (mainstay of treatment)
  - Helps patient learn to cope with the situation and break the mental connection between the situation and anxiety
  - May include antianxiety medications to reduce anxiety during desensitization sessions
- Relaxation techniques as well as psychotherapy, in which patients discuss underlying emotional conflicts with a therapist or support group

Nursing interventions
- Encourage the patient to discuss the feared object or situation
- Collaborate with the patient and multidisciplinary team to develop and implement a systematic desensitization program that gradually exposes the patient to the feared situation in a controlled environment
- Provide training in assertiveness skills to reduce submissive and fearful responses; such strategies allow the patient to experiment with new coping skills and encourage her to discard ineffective ones
- Administer antianxiety or antidepressant medications as ordered

GENERALIZED ANXIETY DISORDER

Defining characteristics
- GAD is characterized by anxiety that's persistent, overwhelming, uncontrollable, and out of proportion to the stimulus
- Usually, GAD emerges slowly and tends to be chronic

Common causes of agoraphobia
- Exact cause unknown
- May have genetic basis or biochemical influence

Key signs and symptoms of agoraphobia
- Overriding fear of open or public spaces (primary symptom)
- Deep concern that help might not be available in such places
- Avoidance of public places and confinement to home

Diagnosing agoraphobia
- Evidence of signs and symptoms
- Must meet *DSM-IV-TR* criteria when present without panic disorder

Key treatment options for agoraphobia
- Medication and behavioral therapy
- Pharmacologic therapy
- A benzodiazepine to treat a panic attack in progress
- Desensitization (mainstay of treatment)
- Relaxation techniques
- Psychotherapy

Key nursing interventions for a patient with agoraphobia
- Encourage patient to discuss the feared object or situation.
- Collaborate with patient and multidisciplinary team to develop and implement a systematic desensitization program.
- Provide training in assertiveness skills.
- Administer antianxiety or antidepressant medications as ordered.

Characteristics of GAD

- Anxiety that's persistent, overwhelming, uncontrollable, and out of proportion to the stimulus
- Usually emerges slowly and tends to be chronic
- Effects range from mild to severe and incapacitating
- Affects an estimated 3% of general population
- Up to 25% of patients with GAD develop panic disorder

Common causes of GAD

- Genetic predisposition
- Imbalances in serotonin and GABA
- Possible predisposition in children of anxious parents
- Stress (may be trigger)

Key signs and symptoms of GAD

Evidence of excessive physiologic arousal
- Shortness of breath
- Tachycardia or palpitations
- Dry mouth
- Sweating
- Nausea or diarrhea
- Frequent urination
- Inability to relax
- Muscle tension, aches, and spasms
- Irritability
- Trembling
- Cold, clammy hands

- – Occasionally triggered by a stressful event
- – Marked by periods of exacerbation and remission
- Effects of GAD range from mild to severe and incapacitating
  - – May involve self-medication with alcohol and antianxiety drugs to relieve anxiety
  - – Untreated, can cause constant, unremitting tension that ultimately results in immunosuppression, leaving the patient more susceptible to physical illnesses
- GAD affects an estimated 3% of the general population, occurring more commonly in women than in men
  - – Usual onset, early 20s
  - – Affects all age-groups, including children and elderly people
- Up to 25% of patients with GAD develop panic disorder; many also have other psychiatric disorders, such as social phobia, specific phobia, depression, or dysthymic disorder

Causes

- Exact cause unknown; certain genetic, biochemical, psychosocial, and other factors suspected
- Genetic predisposition (vulnerability to increased anxiety): may contribute
- Imbalances in serotonin and gamma-aminobutyric acid (GABA), an amino acid: may play key role in susceptibility
  - – Serotonin vital to feelings of well-being
  - – GABA helpful in preventing nerve cells from overfiring
- Children of anxious parents may be predisposed; learn to see world as dangerous and uncontrollable
- Stress may merely be trigger for (not cause of) GAD; increased stress (death of a loved one, an illness, job loss, or divorce) can trigger anxiety attacks

Risk factors

- Unresolved conflicts
- Tendency to misinterpret events
- Shyness and avoidance of new situations

Signs and symptoms

- Manifestations of excessive physiologic arousal
  - – Shortness of breath
  - – Tachycardia or palpitations
  - – Dry mouth
  - – Sweating
  - – Nausea or diarrhea
  - – Frequent urination
  - – Inability to relax
  - – Muscle tension, aches, and spasms
  - – Irritability
  - – Fatigue
  - – Restlessness
  - – Trembling
  - – Headache
  - – Cold, clammy hands
  - – Insomnia

- Evidence of distorted cognitive processes
  - Poor concentration
  - Unrealistic assessment of problems
  - Excessive anxiety and worry over minor matters
  - Fears of grave misfortune or death
- Evidence of poor coping
  - Avoidance
  - Procrastination
  - Poor problem-solving skills

Diagnosis
- Psychiatric evaluation to rule out phobias, OCD, depression, and acute schizophrenia (anxiety is central feature of many mental disorders)
- Diagnosis confirmed if *DSM-IV-TR* criteria met

Treatment
- For mild anxiety, nonpharmacologic methods tried first
  - Relaxation techniques and biofeedback to decrease arousal
  - Psychotherapy to help the patient identify and deal with the cause of anxiety, anticipate her reactions, and plan effective responses to anxiety
- Cognitive therapy to reduce cognitive distortions by teaching the patient how to restructure her thoughts and view her worries more realistically
  - In one cognitive therapy approach, patient taught to record worries and list evidence that justifies or contradicts each one
  - Learns that "worrying about worry" maintains anxiety; avoidance and procrastination are ineffective problem-solving techniques
- Biofeedback training to ease physical symptoms of anxiety by teaching the patient how to become aware of—and then consciously control—various body functions (including blood pressure, heart and respiratory rates, skin temperature, and perspiration)
  - Using biofeedback device, patient learns when changes in these functions occur
  - With adequate training, can repeat response at will, even when not hooked up to device
- Pharmacologic therapy if anxiety significantly impairs the patient's daily functioning
  - Antianxiety agents, including such benzodiazepines as diazepam (Valium); benzodiazepines reduce anxiety by decreasing vigilance, easing somatic symptoms (for instance, muscle tension)
    - Generally given for several weeks to patients with acute anxiety and those with chronic anxiety who experience a new stressor
    - Should begin at the lowest possible dose and be increased slowly
    - Shouldn't be taken for more than 6 weeks (to reduce potential for tolerance and abuse)
  - SSRIs
  - TCAs, such as imipramine (Tofranil), or the anxiolytic drug buspirone (BuSpar) for patients with chronic anxiety and those who relapse after benzodiazepine therapy
    - Buspirone considered initial drug of choice for anxious patients with history of substance abuse; causes less sedation and rarely leads to physical dependence or tolerance

Key signs and symptoms of GAD

Evidence of distorted cognitive processes
- Poor concentration
- Unrealistic assessment of problems
- Excessive anxiety and worry over minor matters
- Fears of grave misfortune or death

Evidence of poor coping
- Avoidance
- Procrastination
- Poor problem-solving skills

Diagnosing GAD
- Psychiatric evaluation to rule out phobias, OCD, depression, and acute schizophrenia

Key treatment options for GAD
- Cognitive therapy
- Biofeedback training
- Pharmacologic therapy (antianxiety agents, SSRIs, and TCAs)

Pharmacologic options for treating GAD

Antianxiety agents
- Benzodiazepines such as diazepam
- Reduce anxiety by decreasing vigilance, easing somatic symptoms

TCAs
- Imipramine
- Buspirone: Initial drug of choice for anxious patients with history of substance abuse

Strategies for easing anxiety

- Progressive muscle relaxation
- Guided imagery
- Deep breathing
- Time-management skills
- List making
- Realistic goal setting
- Group tasking in small increments

Key nursing interventions for a patient with GAD

- Stay with patient when she's anxious, and encourage her to discuss her feelings.
- Remain calm and nonjudgmental.
- Suggest activities that distract from anxiety.
- Reduce environmental stimuli.

TIME-OUT FOR TEACHING

Easing anxiety

Various techniques can help ease anxiety. Such methods reduce the risk of hyperventilation, help the patient focus on something other than anxiety, and interrupt the flow of negative or stressful thoughts. Appropriate techniques for patients with generalized anxiety may include:

- progressive muscle relaxation
- guided imagery
- deep breathing.
  Other relaxation techniques help manage anxiety, including:
- time-management skills
- list making
- realistic goal setting
- group tasking in small increments.

- As effective as benzodiazepines (which treat somatic symptoms); also treats worry associated with GAD
- Delayed onset of action (several weeks)

Nursing interventions

- Stay with the patient when she's anxious, and encourage her to discuss her feelings
  - Remain calm, nonjudgmental
  - Suggest activities that distract from anxiety
  - Reduce environmental stimuli
- When the patient is more receptive, teach her appropriate ways to ease and manage anxiety (see *Easing anxiety*)
- Provide nutritional counseling to reduce stress (such as advising the patient to avoid caffeine and alcohol)
- Make appropriate referrals to a mental health professional
- Dissuade the patient from visiting the hospital emergency department for symptom relief because of the frantic atmosphere
- Administer prescribed antianxiety medications as ordered
- Inform the patient and her family that these drugs may cause adverse reactions (drowsiness, fatigue, ataxia, blurred vision, slurred speech, tremors, and hypotension), which should be reported to the prescribing physician
- Advise the patient beginning treatment with buspirone that the drug has a delayed onset of action; tell her to expect a delay in symptom relief (several weeks)
- Advise the patient not to discontinue medications except with the physician's approval; abrupt withdrawal could cause severe symptoms

OBSESSIVE-COMPULSIVE DISORDER

Defining characteristics

- OCD is characterized by unwanted, recurrent, intrusive thoughts or images (obsessions) that the person tries to alleviate through repetitive behaviors or mental acts (compulsions)
  - Obsessions: produce anxiety
  - Compulsions: meant to reduce the anxiety or prevent some dreaded event from happening (typically include overt behaviors, such as

hand washing and checking, and mental acts, such as praying and counting)

- Obsessive-compulsive behaviors may be simple, or complex and ritualized
  - Complex: tend to take up more than 1 hour per day
  - Extreme ritualistic behaviors: can take hours to complete, becoming the patient's major life activity
- OCD can cause significant distress and may severely impair occupational and social functioning; it can even endanger the patient's health and safety (for example, severe dermatitis or a skin infection may result from compulsive hand washing)
- In most cases, the patient is aware that his obsessions are excessive or irrational and that they interfere with daily activities; the patient may be embarrassed and may attempt to hide the symptoms
- OCD affects about 2% of the general population, striking men and women equally
  - In males, typically begins in adolescence to young adulthood; in females, in young adulthood
  - In about one-third of adults, symptomatic during childhood
  - Onset usually gradual—over months or years
  - In most cases, takes a fluctuating course, with exacerbations linked to stressful events; in some cases, psychosocial functioning steadily deteriorates
- Many OCD sufferers also have major depressive disorder, panic disorder, social phobia, specific phobia, eating disorders, substance abuse, or personality disorders

● **Causes**
- Possible involvement of genetic, biological, and psychological factors (see *The strep connection*)
- Apparent association with Tourette syndrome
  - In clinical samples, approximately 20% to 30% reporting past history of tics, suggesting neurobehavioral connection (as in Tourette syndrome)
  - About one-quarter meeting full criteria for Tourette syndrome
  - Up to 50% of people with Tourette syndrome developing OCD

The strep connection

Researchers have found an association between obsessive-compulsive disorder (OCD) and beta-hemolytic streptococci infection. Specifically, studies of children have linked the sudden appearance of obsessions, compulsions, and motor or vocal tics with streptococcal throat infection.

Possibly, an autoimmune response to the infection occurs, in which antibodies attack both healthy and infected cells. This onslaught could cause inflammation of the basal ganglia, a brain region involved in movement and motor control.

Sad syndrome, called *pediatric autoimmune neuropsychiatric disorders associated with streptococcal infections (PANDAS)*, typically affects children ages 5 to 11, and has a dramatic, sudden onset. In some of these children, OCD symptoms respond to prompt antibiotic treatment.

Characteristics of OCD

- Unwanted, recurrent, intrusive thoughts or images (obsessions) that the person tries to alleviate through repetitive behaviors or mental acts (compulsions)
- Obsessions: produce anxiety
- Compulsions: meant to reduce anxiety or prevent some dreaded event from happening
- Obsessive-compulsive behaviors may be simple, or complex and ritualized
- Complex: tend to take up more than 1 hour per day
- Extreme ritualistic behaviors: can take hours to complete, becoming the patient's major life activity
- Affects about 2% of general population
- Many OCD sufferers also have major depressive disorder, panic disorder, social phobia, specific phobia, eating disorders, substance abuse, or personality disorders

Common causes of OCD

- Apparent association with Tourette syndrome
- Anatomic-physiologic disturbances in brain areas

Freudian psychoanalytical theory
- Result of conflict between ego and id
- Impulses repugnant to ego controlled by unconscious defense mechanisms

Behavioral theory
- Conditioned response to anxiety-provoking events
- Obsession caused by linking anxiety with neutral object or event
- Compulsive behavior also learned and reinforced

Key signs and symptoms of OCD

- Repetitive thoughts that cause stress
- Repetitive behaviors, such as hand washing, counting, or checking and rechecking whether a door is locked
- Engagement in culturally prescribed ritual behavior that exceeds cultural norms; occurs at times and places that others in culture would judge inappropriate and interferes with social role functioning

Diagnosing OCD

- Demonstration of ritualistic behavior that's irrational or excessive
- Enlarged basal ganglia in some patients
- Increased glucose metabolism in part of the basal ganglia

Key treatment options for OCD

- Exposure and response prevention (primary behavioral technique used)
- Relaxation techniques
- Support groups

  - Tends to run in families; risk higher among first-degree relatives with Tourette syndrome
- Possible involvement of anatomic-physiologic disturbances in brain areas involved in learning or acquiring and maintaining habits and skills
- Freudian psychoanalytical theory
  - Result of conflict between ego and id (unconscious part of psyche that gives rise to instinctual impulses)
  - Impulses repugnant to ego controlled by unconscious defense mechanisms
- Behavioral theory
  - Conditioned response to anxiety-provoking events
  - Obsession caused by linking anxiety with neutral object or event
  - Compulsive behavior also learned and reinforced
  - Patient continues practicing compulsive behaviors that initially helped control the anxiety, even though behaviors no longer helpful
- Increased risk from sociological factors, such as being young, divorced, separated, or unemployed (reasons not fully understood)

Signs and symptoms

- Manifestations
  - Repetitive thoughts that cause stress
  - Repetitive behaviors, such as hand washing, counting, or checking and rechecking whether a door is locked
  - Engagement in culturally prescribed ritual behavior that exceeds cultural norms; occurs at times and places that others in culture would judge inappropriate and interferes with social role functioning
- Degree of social impairment caused by preoccupation with obsessions and compulsions
- Perceived need to achieve perfection

Diagnosis

- Suggested by demonstration of ritualistic behavior that's irrational or excessive
- Enlarged basal ganglia in some patients (MRI and computed tomography)
- Increased glucose metabolism in part of the basal ganglia (positron-emission tomography scanning)
- Diagnosis confirmed if *DSM-IV-TR* criteria met

Treatment

- Exposure and response prevention (the primary behavioral technique used) proven effective in about 80% of cases; involves exposing the patient to the object or situation that triggers his obsessions, then asking him to refrain from engaging in his usual compulsive response
  - Includes having patient write down what happens as a result of the behavioral restraint; shows him that not performing the ritual doesn't result in distressing outcomes
  - Helps patient to manage his intense anxiety until it subsides
  - Based on its success, has led to use in telephone-access therapy (patients call in and receive computer-generated response-prevention therapy)
- Relaxation techniques, including deep breathing, progressive muscle relaxation, meditation, imagery, and music
- Support groups to help decrease the patient's isolation

- Partial hospitalization and day treatment programs when a patient's phobias prevent him from carrying out activities of daily living
- Pharmacologic treatments, including benzodiazepines, monoamine oxidase (MAO) inhibitors, SSRIs, and TCAs

Nursing interventions

- Assess the patient's physical needs, noting such cues as chafed or reddened hands, or hair loss (due to compulsive pulling; be aware that compulsive hand washing can cause skin breakdown)
- Provide for basic needs, such as rest, nutrition, and grooming, if the patient becomes involved in ritualistic thoughts and behaviors to the point of self-neglect; be alert for inadequate food and fluid intake and exhaustion due to rituals or preoccupations
- Let the patient know you're aware of his behavior, and help him to explore the feelings associated with that behavior
  - Approaching the patient unhurriedly
  - Listening attentively
  - Offering feedback
  - Discussing patterns leading to the behavior or recurring problems
  - Identifying disturbing topics of conversation that reflect the patient's underlying anxiety or terror
  - Maintaining an accepting attitude
  - Avoiding displays of shock, amusement, or criticism of the ritualistic behavior
- Give the patient time to carry out the ritualistic behavior (unless it's dangerous) until he can be distracted by some other activity because blocking such behavior could increase his anxiety to an intolerable level
- Establish reasonable demands and limits on the patient's behaviors, and make their purpose clear
- Avoid situations that increase the patient's frustration and provoke his anger, which may interfere with treatment
- Encourage the use of active diversions (whistling or humming a tune) to divert his attention from the unwanted thoughts and promote a pleasurable experience
- Help the patient decrease his compulsive behavior and find new ways of coping and solving problems
  - Limiting number of times per day he may indulge in compulsive behavior, then gradually shortening time allowed
  - Refocusing time and attention on other feelings or problems
  - Explaining how to channel emotional energy to relieve stress (for example, through creative endeavors)
  - Engaging him in activities that produce positive accomplishments and boost confidence and self-esteem
- Evaluate the patient's insight, and look for signs of improved behavior (reduced compulsive behavior and fewer obsessive thoughts); note when interventions don't work, and recommend alternative strategies as needed
- Help the patient identify progress and set realistic expectations; encourage the use of appropriate coping mechanisms to relieve loneliness and isolation
- Monitor the patient for suicidal behaviors and thoughts; he may develop feelings of overwhelming hopelessness and helplessness as he realizes the absurdity of his behavior but feels powerless to control it
- Monitor for desired and adverse effects of prescribed drugs

Key nursing interventions for a patient with OCD

- Give patient time to carry out the ritualistic behavior (unless it's dangerous) until he can be distracted by some other activity.
- Establish reasonable demands and limits on the patient's behaviors, and make their purpose clear.
- Encourage use of active diversions to divert his attention from the unwanted thoughts and promote a pleasurable experience.
- Limit number of times per day he may indulge in compulsive behavior; then gradually shorten time allowed.
- Refocus time and attention on other feelings or problems.
- Explain how to channel emotional energy to relieve stress.
- Engage him in activities that produce positive accomplishments and boost confidence and self-esteem.

PANIC DISORDER

● **Defining characteristics**
- Panic disorder represents anxiety in its most severe form
  - Characterized by recurrent, unexpected panic attacks that cause intense apprehension and feelings of impending doom
  - Between attacks, marked by persistent worrying that another attack may occur; may change patient's behavior
- Roughly 2% to 4% of the general population experiences panic disorder at some time in their lives
  - Affects about twice as many women as it does men
  - Most common age of onset is from late adolescence to mid-adulthood; rarely begins after age 50
  - With earlier onset, a greater risk of coexisting illnesses, chronicity, and impairment
- The frequency of panic attacks and the high level of anxiety they cause may lead to functional impairments
- Panic is an extreme level of anxiety and is different from fear (response to external stimuli) and anxiety (response to internal conflict)
- Panic attacks occur suddenly, with no warning
  - Usually build to peak intensity within 10 to 15 minutes and rarely last longer than 30 minutes
  - May continue to recur for hours
- During the attack, the patient may fear he's dying, going crazy, or losing control of his emotions or behavior
  - Feels strong urge to escape or flee the place where the attack began
  - If chest pain or shortness of breath occurs, may go to a hospital emergency department or seek some other type of urgent assistance
- The frequency and severity of panic attacks vary from one person to the next; they may arise once per week or in clusters separated by months
- Because of the spontaneous occurrence of panic attacks (without exposure to a known anxiety-producing situation), constant worry over when the next attacks will occur may restrict the affected person's lifestyle in an attempt to avoid them
- At some point, about 50% of those with panic disorder develop severe avoidance, warranting a separate diagnosis of panic disorder with agoraphobia (see "Agoraphobia," page 146)
  - Person with panic disorder and agoraphobia may be unable to carry out normal daily activities; may grow so fearful that becomes unable to leave home
- For many sufferers, panic disorder is complicated by major depressive disorder (50% to 65% lifetime comorbidity)
- The tendency to self-medicate with alcohol or antianxiety drugs may result in alcoholism and substance abuse disorders (20% to 30% comorbidity)
- Many patients with panic disorder have additional anxiety disorders
  - Social phobia (up to 30% comorbidity)
  - GAD (up to 25% comorbidity)
  - Specific phobia (up to 20% comorbidity)
  - OCD (up to 10% comorbidity)

Characteristics of panic disorder

- Anxiety in its most severe form
- Recurrent, unexpected panic attacks that cause intense apprehension and feelings of impending doom
- Between attacks, marked by persistent worrying that another attack may occur; may change patient's behavior
- Panic attacks occur suddenly, with no warning
- Usually build to peak intensity within 10 to 15 minutes and rarely last longer than 30 minutes
- May continue to recur for hours
- During attack, patient may fear he's dying, going crazy, or losing control of his emotions or behavior
- Patient feels strong urge to escape or flee place where attack began
- If chest pain or shortness of breath occurs, may go to hospital emergency department or seek other type of urgent assistance

Causes

- May be triggered by intense stress or sudden loss; however, underlying cause probably involves combination of genetic, biochemical, and other factors
- Tends to run in families
  - In first-degree relatives of up to 17% of patients
  - To a much higher degree in identical twins, supporting theory of genetic basis
- Higher norepinephrine levels found in patients with panic attacks, suggesting defect in catecholamine system
- Affected people may have heightened sensitivity to somatic (physical) symptoms
  - May, in turn, trigger the autonomic system
  - Triggers series of events that leads to panic attack
- Learning theory proposes that person misinterprets symptoms; may explain some cases
  - Produces fear that mild anxiety symptoms are the start of a major physical illness
  - Results in exaggeration of fear, leading to panic attack
- May result from failure to resolve early childhood conflict of dependence versus independence
- Has been linked to medical conditions (first experience of condition may be so frightening that thinking about it can lead to a panic attack)
  - Migraine
  - Obstructive sleep apnea
  - Cardiovascular disease, including mitral valve prolapse
  - GI disorders, including irritable bowel syndrome
  - Chronic fatigue syndrome
  - Premenstrual syndrome
  - Asthma

Signs and symptoms

- Can mimic heart attack
  - Palpitations and rapid heart beat
  - Sweating
  - Generalized weakness or trembling
  - Shortness of breath or rapid, shallow breathing
  - Sensations of choking, smothering, or a lump in the throat
  - Chest pain or pressure
  - Abdominal pain, nausea, heartburn, diarrhea, or other GI distress
  - Dizziness, tingling sensations, or light-headedness
  - Chills, pallor, or flushing
- Diminished ability to focus or think clearly, even with direction
- Fidgeting or pacing
- Rapid speech
- Exaggerated startle reaction

Diagnosis

- Tests to rule out organic or pharmacologic basis for symptoms (some physical conditions and drug effects can mimic panic disorder)
  - Serum glucose measurements (to rule out hypoglycemia)
  - Urine catecholamine and vanillylmandelic acid tests (can exclude pheochromocytoma)

Common causes of panic disorder

- Possible trigger: intense stress or sudden loss
- Family predisposition
- High norepinephrine levels, suggesting defect in catecholamine system
- Heightened sensitivity to somatic symptoms
- Misinterpretation of symptoms
- Medical conditions

Key signs and symptoms of panic disorder

- Can mimic heart attack
- Diminished ability to focus or think clearly, even with direction
- Fidgeting or pacing
- Rapid speech
- Exaggerated startle reaction

Diagnosing panic disorder

- Must rule out organic cause for signs and symptoms
- Must meet *DSM-IV-TR* criteria

- Thyroid function tests (can eliminate hyperthyroidism)
- Urine and serum toxicology tests (can rule out presence of psychoactive substances—such as barbiturates, caffeine, and amphetamines—capable of triggering panic attacks)
- Diagnosis confirmed if *DSM-IV-TR* criteria met

Treatment

- Highly treatable; responds well to a combination of patient teaching, cognitive or behavioral therapies, and relaxation techniques; however, some patients also require medication.
- Teaching the patient about the disorder and its physiologic effects to help her overcome it; many patients experience some relief simply by understanding exactly what panic disorder is and that many others suffer from it
- Cognitive therapy using cognitive restructuring for patients who worry that their panic attacks mean they're going crazy or they're about to have a heart attack
  - Teaches the patient to replace negative thoughts with more realistic, positive ways of viewing the attacks
  - Helps the patient to identify and evaluate the thoughts that precede anxiety, then restructure them to gain a more realistic perception
  - Helps the patient identify possible triggers for the panic attacks, such as a particular thought or situation or even a slight change in heartbeat
  - Helps the patient understand that panic attack is separate and independent of the trigger; diminishes trigger's hold on the patient and its ability to induce attack
  - Using interoceptive exposure technique, therapist guides the patient through repeated exposure to sensations she experiences during a panic attack (such as palpitations or dizziness)
    - Involves evoking feared sensations by using such methods as controlled hyperventilation or physical exertion (such as running up a flight of stairs to cause tachycardia)
    - Teaches patient that sensations need not progress to full-blown attack
- Behavioral therapy involving desensitization, which resembles interoceptive exposure but lacks the cognitive component
  - Involves helping the patient break down a fearful situation into small, manageable steps
  - Allows the patient to perform the steps one at a time until she can master the most difficult step
  - Also can help the patient deal with situational avoidance
- Relaxation techniques to help the patient cope with a panic attack by easing physical symptoms and directing her attention elsewhere
  - Deep-breathing exercises, which also reduce the risk of hyperventilation (a contributing factor for anxiety)
  - Progressive relaxation, which involves conscious tightening and relaxation of the skeletal muscles in a sequential fashion
  - Positive visualization or guided imagery, in which the patient elicits peaceful mental images or some other purposeful thought or action, promoting feelings of relaxation, renewed hope, and a sense of being in control of a stressful situation
  - Listening to calming music

Key treatment options for panic disorder

- Cognitive therapy using cognitive restructuring
- Behavioral therapy involving desensitization
- Relaxation techniques to help patient cope with a panic attack

• Pharmacologic therapy with antianxiety drugs (especially benzodiazepines) or antidepressants
  – Rapid stabilization of panic symptoms promoted by combining antianxiety drug with antidepressant
  – Beta-adrenergic blockers (control irregular heartbeats) of benefit to some patients

● **Nursing interventions**
  • During a panic attack
    – Stay with the patient until the attack subsides (if left alone, she may grow even more anxious)
    – Avoid touching the patient until you've established rapport (she may be too stimulated or frightened to find touch reassuring)
    – If the patient loses control, guide her to a smaller, quieter area
    – Avoid insincere expressions of reassurance
    – Maintain a calm, serene approach
    – Speak in short, simple sentences, and slowly give the patient one direction at a time; avoid giving lengthy explanations and asking too many questions
    – Reduce external stimuli, including exposure to groups of people
    – Provide a safe environment, and prevent harm to the patient and others
    – Keep in mind that the patient's perceptual field may be narrowed; therefore, avoid exposure to excessive stimuli (which may be overwhelming) and dim bright lights as necessary
    – Encourage the patient to express her feelings and to cry, if necessary
    – Allow her to pace around the room
  • Between panic attacks
    – Encourage the patient to discuss her fears; help her to identify situations or events that trigger the attacks
    – Discuss alternative coping mechanisms
    – Monitor therapeutic and adverse effects of prescribed medications
    – Teach the patient how to recognize adverse reactions
    – Instruct the patient to notify the physician before discontinuing medication because abrupt withdrawal could cause severe symptoms

PHOBIA, SOCIAL

● **Defining characteristics**
  • Social phobia (sometimes called *social anxiety disorder*) refers to marked, persistent fear or anxiety in social or performance situations, which causes the sufferer to avoid these situations whenever possible (usually out of fear that she'll be embarrassed or ridiculed)
    – Commonly involves anxieties about speaking or eating in public and using a public restroom
    – Associated with deep concern that others will see the patient's anxiety symptoms (such as sweating or blushing) or will judge her as weak, stupid, or crazy; in some cases, fear of fainting, losing bowel or bladder control, or going mentally blank

---

Key nursing interventions for a patient with a panic attack

• Stay with patient until attack subsides.
• Avoid touching patient until you've established rapport.
• Maintain a calm, serene approach.
• Speak in short, simple sentences, and slowly give patient one direction at a time; avoid giving lengthy explanations and asking too many questions.
• Reduce external stimuli, including exposure to groups of people.
• Provide a safe environment, and prevent harm to patient and others.
• Keep in mind that patient's perceptual field may be narrowed; therefore, avoid exposing her to excessive stimuli and dim bright lights as necessary.

Characteristics of social phobia

• Sometimes called *social anxiety disorder*
• Marked, persistent fear or anxiety in social or performance situations
• Sufferer avoids these situations whenever possible
• More common in women
• Rarely develops after age 25

Common causes of social phobia

- Family predisposition
- Possible role of biological and environmental factors
- Environmental influences

Key signs and symptoms of social phobia

- Fear or avoidance of eating, writing, or speaking in public; being stared at; or meeting strangers
- Pronounced sensitivity to criticism
- Low self-esteem
- Scholastic underachievement because of test anxiety
- Blushing
- Profuse sweating
- Trembling
- Nausea or stomach upset
- Difficulty talking

Diagnosing social phobia

- No specific diagnostic test for social phobia
- Must meet *DSM-IV-TR* criteria

- – Even when around familiar people, may feel overwhelmed, fearing that others are watching her every move and making negative judgments about her
  - – Linked with shyness and social inhibition
- An estimated 2% to 7% of people in the United States suffer from social phobia
  - – More common in women
  - – Typically starts in childhood or adolescence
  - – Rarely develops after age 25
- The person with social phobias generally has anticipatory anxiety for days or weeks before the dreaded event, further handicapping her performance and heightening embarrassment
- Social phobia may be limited to one specific situation, such as speaking in public; however, in its most severe form, it's generalized to the point that the patient has symptoms almost any time she's near other people
- Severity of symptoms and impairments typically fluctuates with job or academic demands and the stability of the patient's social relationships; the disorder can be quite debilitating
  - – Can prevent the patient from going to work or school on some days
  - – Can cause loss of a job or job promotion out of fear of speaking in public
  - – Can result in continual inconvenience (for instance, from fear of using a public lavatory)
  - – May cause other health problems (high rates of alcohol abuse and other psychiatric conditions, such as depression and eating disorders)
- After the disorder is established, complete remission is unlikely without treatment

Causes

- May run in families (suggested by preliminary studies)
- Possible role of biological and environmental factors
  - – Possible physiologic or hormonal basis for increased sensitivity to disapproval
  - – May involve the amygdala (brain structure that controls fear responses)
- Theories about environmental factors focus on social modeling or observational learning, proposing that a person acquires fear from observing the behavior and consequences of others

Signs and symptoms

- Fear or avoidance of eating, writing, or speaking in public; being stared at; or meeting strangers
- Pronounced sensitivity to criticism
- Low self-esteem
- Scholastic underachievement because of test anxiety
- Blushing
- Profuse sweating
- Trembling
- Nausea or stomach upset
- Difficulty talking

Diagnosis

- No specific diagnostic test
- Diagnosis confirmed if *DSM-IV-TR* criteria met

Treatment

- Desensitization therapy to gradually reintroduce the feared situation while coaching the patient on relaxation techniques (progressive muscle relaxation, deep-breathing exercises, listening to calming music)
- Role-playing in guided imagery to allow the patient to rehearse ways to relax while confronting a feared object or situation
- Assertiveness training to help the patient become assertive in her interpersonal interactions
- Modeling behavior
  - Patient observes someone modeling, or demonstrating, appropriate behavior when confronted with the feared situation
- A behavioral technique called negative thought stopping to reduce the frequency and duration of disturbing thoughts by interrupting them and substituting competing thoughts
  - Teaches patient to recognize negative thoughts
  - Involves using an intense distracting stimulus (such as snapping a rubber band around the wrist) to stop the thought
  - With practice, allows patient to control thoughts without using distracting stimulus
- Drugs, such as benzodiazepines, SSRIs, MAO inhibitors, TCAs, and beta-adrenergic blockers; however, relapse rates are high when medication is used as a sole treatment
  - Beta-adrenergic blockers (such as propranolol [Inderal]) to slow heart rate, lower blood pressure, and reduce nervous tension, sweating, panic, and shakiness

Nursing interventions

- No matter how illogical the patient's phobia seems, avoid the urge to trivialize her fears; remember that the patient fears criticism and that her behavior represents an essential coping mechanism
  - Should focus on encouraging the patient to interact with others; provide continuous support, positive reinforcement
  - Should avoid pep talks, ridicule (may alienate the patient or worsen already low self-esteem)
- Teach the patient progressive muscle relaxation, guided imagery, or thought-stopping techniques as appropriate
- Ask the patient how she normally copes with her fear; when she's able to face the fear, encourage her to explore and verbalize her personal strengths and resources with you
- Suggest ways to channel energy and relieve stress, such as running and creative activities
- Don't let the patient withdraw completely; if she's being treated as an outpatient, suggest small steps to overcome her fears (such as planning a brief shopping trip with a supportive family member or friend)
- To increase self-esteem and reduce anxiety, explain to the patient that her phobia is a way of coping with anxiety, especially if she perceives her behavior as silly or unreasonable
- If the patient is taking an antidepressant or antianxiety agent, stress the importance of complying with the prescribed therapy, and the need to report adverse reactions

Key treatment options for social phobia

- Desensitization therapy
- Role-playing in guided imagery
- Assertiveness training
- Modeling behavior
- Negative thought stopping

Key nursing interventions for a patient with social phobia

- Avoid urge to trivialize patient's fears.
- Teach patient progressive muscle relaxation, guided imagery, or thought-stopping techniques as appropriate.
- Suggest ways to channel energy and relieve stress.
- Don't let the patient withdraw completely.

Characteristics of specific phobia

- Onset in childhood to early adulthood
- More persistence seen in adult phobias

Classifying specific phobia

- Natural environment
- Animal
- Blood-injection-injury
- Situational
- Other

Common causes of specific phobia

- Unknown cause but may have some genetic influence
- Predisposing factors (observing or experiencing a trauma) may contribute
- Usually not caused by a single traumatic event
- May adopt phobias of other family members

PHOBIA, SPECIFIC

- ● **Defining characteristics**
  - The person with specific phobia (also called *simple phobia*) experiences intense, irrational anxiety when anticipating a specific feared entity (such as a snake) or situation (such as being in an enclosed space)
    - Involves real-life exposure or exposure through images from movies, television, photographs, or imagination
    - In many cases, leads to avoidance or disabling behavior that interferes with activities or even confines person to the home
    - May reach panic-level anxiety, especially if no apparent escape from the feared entity or situation
  - Specific phobias are classified as five main types
    - Natural environment
    - Animal
    - Blood-injection-injury
    - Situational
    - Other
  - A wide range of specific phobias has been identified
    - Enclosed spaces
    - Insects, bugs, other animals
    - Heights
    - Elevators and escalators
    - Tunnels
    - Water
    - Storms
    - Blood or injections
    - Driving on freeways
    - Flying on airplanes
  - Many people have multiple specific phobias (see *Types of phobias*)
  - Although adults with specific phobias realize their fears are irrational and out of proportion to any actual danger, they still experience severe anxiety or panic attacks when facing (or perhaps even thinking about) the source of their fear
    - May try avoiding the stimulus; when impossible, may try to endure exposure with great difficulty
    - May make important career or personal decisions to avoid exposure
  - Specific phobias affect about 10% of the population, occurring in more women than men
    - Onset in childhood to early adulthood (usually mid-20s)
    - In most cases, persist for years or even decades; only about 20% remit spontaneously without treatment
    - More persistence seen in adult phobias; childhood phobias usually disappear over time (some continue into adulthood)

- ● **Causes**
  - Cause unknown; seem to run in families (especially those involving blood or injury), so genetic predisposition may play role

Types of phobias

There are a wide range of phobias that patients can suffer from. Some of these phobias are listed below.

A

Ablutophobia: Fear of washing
Acarophobia: Fear of itching or insects that cause itching
Acerophobia: Fear of sourness
Aerophobia: Fear of drafts
Achluophobia: Fear of darkness
Ailurophobia: Fear of cats
Antlophobia: Fear of floods
Apiphobia: Fear of bees
Arachnophobia: Fear of spiders
Astrapophobia: Fear of lightning

B

Bacteriophobia: Fear of bacteria
Bathmophobia: Fear of stairs or steep slopes
Bathophobia: Fear of depth
Blennophobia: Fear of slime
Bogyphobia: Fear of the bogeyman
Botanophobia: Fear of plants
Bromidrosiphobia or bromidrophobia: Fear of body smells

C

Cacophobia: Fear of ugliness
Cancerophobia: Fear of cancer
Carnophobia: Fear of meat
Catagelophobia: Fear of being ridiculed
Catapedaphobia: Fear of jumping from high or low places
Cathisophobia: Fear of sitting
Chaetophobia: Fear of hair
Coprastasophobia: Fear of constipation

D

Demophobia: Fear of crowds
Didaskaleinophobia: Fear of going to school
Dikephobia: Fear of justice
Dishabiliophobia: Fear of undressing in front of someone
Domatophobia or oikophobia: Fear of houses

Dysmorphophobia: Fear of deformity
Dystychiphobia: Fear of accidents

E

Ecclesiophobia: Fear of church
Ecophobia: Fear of home
Eisoptrophobia: Fear of mirrors or seeing oneself in a mirror
Emetophobia: Fear of vomiting
Enochlophobia: Fear of crowds

F

Febriphobia: Fear of fever
Frigophobia: Fear of cold or cold things

G

Gamophobia: Fear of marriage
Gerascophobia: Fear of growing old
Geumaphobia or geumophobia: Fear of taste
Glossophobia: Fear of speaking in public
Gynephobia or gynophobia: Fear of women

H

Heliophobia: Fear of the sun
Herpetophobia: Fear of reptiles or creepy, crawly things
Heterophobia: Fear of the opposite sex
Hierophobia: Fear of religious or sacred things
Hippophobia: Fear of horses
Hypsiphobia: Fear of height

I

Iatrophobia: Fear of doctors
Ichthyophobia: Fear of fish
Ideophobia: Fear of ideas
Illyngophobia: Fear of vertigo or feeling dizzy when looking down
Iophobia: Fear of poison
Insectophobia: Fear of insects
Isolophobia: Fear of solitude

Common phobias

- Arachnophobia: Fear of spiders
- Dysmorphophobia: Fear of deformity
- Ecophobia: Fear of home
- Enochlophobia: Fear of crowds
- Heliophobia: Fear of the sun
- Heterophobia: Fear of the opposite sex
- Insectophobia: Fear of insects
- Macrophobia: Fear of long waits
- Menophobia: Fear of menstruation
- Noctiphobia: Fear of the night
- Photophobia: Fear of light
- Scotophobia: Fear of darkness
- Xenophobia: Fear of strangers of foreigners
- Zoophobia: Fear of animals

(continued)

Key signs and symptoms of specific phobia

- Severe anxiety with exposure or even threat of exposure
- Low self-esteem
- Depression
- Feelings of weakness, cowardice, or ineffectiveness

Diagnosing specific phobia

- History of anxiety when exposed to specific entity or situation
- Must meet *DSM-IV-TR* criteria

Types of phobias *(continued)*

K
Kainophobia: Fear of anything new, novel
Kakorrhaphiophobia: Fear of failure or defeat
Katagelophobia: Fear of ridicule
Kathisophobia: Fear of sitting down
Kopophobia: Fear of fatigue

L
Levophobia: Fear of objects to the left
Ligyrophobia: Fear of loud noises
Lilapsophobia: Fear of tornadoes and hurricanes
Logophobia: Fear of words

M
Macrophobia: Fear of long waits
Mageirocophobia: Fear of cooking
Maieusiophobia: Fear of childbirth
Medomalacuphobia: Fear of losing an erection
Menophobia: Fear of menstruation
Metallophobia: Fear of metal
Microbiophobia: Fear of microbes
Myctophobia: Fear of darkness
Myrmecophobia: Fear of ants

N
Neopharmaphobia: Fear of new drugs

Neophobia: Fear of new scenes; aversion to all that's unknown or not understood
Nephophobia: Fear of clouds
Noctiphobia: Fear of the night
Nostophobia: Fear of returning home
Novercaphobia: Fear of one's stepmother

O
Ochlophobia: Fear of crowds or mobs
Ochophobia: Fear of vehicles
Oenophobia: Fear of wines
Olfactophobia: Fear of smells
Ombrophobia: Fear of rain
Optophobia: Fear of opening one's eyes
Ornithophobia: Fear of birds

P
Pagophobia: Fear of ice or frost
Panphobia: Fear of everything
Panthophobia: Fear of suffering and disease
Pediculophobia: Fear of lice
Pedophobia: Fear of children
Phalacrophobia: Fear of becoming bald
Photophobia: Fear of light
Pogonophobia: Fear of beards
Potamophobia: Fear of rivers
Prosophobia: Fear of progress

- Predisposing factors
  - Experiencing or observing a trauma
  - Repeated warnings of danger about the feared entity or situation
- Generally not caused by single traumatic event (such as being bitten by a dog); instead, patient may learn to adopt phobias of other family members
- Apparent role of spontaneous, unexpected panic attacks in development of specific phobia

● **Signs and symptoms**
- Severe anxiety with exposure or even threat of exposure (most common)
- Low self-esteem
- Depression
- Feelings of weakness, cowardice, or ineffectiveness due to routine avoidance of object of the phobia

● **Diagnosis**
- History of anxiety when exposed to or anticipating specific entity or situation
- Diagnosis confirmed if *DSM-IV-TR* criteria met

Psellismophobia: Fear of stuttering
Pyrophobia: Fear of fire

R
Ranidaphobia: Fear of frogs
Rhypophobia: Fear of defecation
Rhytiphobia: Fear of getting wrinkles
Rupophobia: Fear of dirt

S
Sciophobia: Fear of shadows
Scoleciphobia: Fear of worms
Scolionophobia: Fear of school
Scotophobia: Fear of darkness
Scriptophobia: Fear of writing in public
Selachophobia: Fear of sharks
Selaphobia: Fear of light flashes
Siderodromophobia: Fear of trains
Syngenesophobia: Fear of relatives

T
Thaasophobia: Fear of sitting
Thanatophobia; Fear of death
Thalassophobia: Fear of the sea
Thermophobia: Fear of heat
Tocophobia: Fear of pregnancy or child-
    birth
Triskaidekaphobia: Fear of the num-
    ber 13
Trypanophobia: Fear of injections

U
Uranophobia: Fear of heaven
Urophobia: Fear of urine or urinating

V
Vaccinophobia: Fear of inoculations
Verbophobia: Fear of words
Verminophobia: Fear of germs
Vestiphobia: Fear of clothing

W
Wiccaphobia: Fear of witches and
    witchcraft

X
Xanthophobia: Fear of the color yellow
    or the word *yellow*
Xenophobia: Fear of strangers or for-
    eigners
Xerophobia: Fear of dryness
Xylophobia: Fear of wooden objects;
    fear of forests
Xyrophobia: Fear of razors

Z
Zelophobia: Fear of jealousy
Zoophobia: Fear of animals

● **Treatment**
- Systematic desensitization or exposure therapy; in a controlled environ-
  ment, a mental health professional or a trusted companion gradually ex-
  poses the patient to what frightens her until the fear begins to fade
  - Extremely beneficial for about 75% of patients
  - Especially helpful for phobias involving driving, flying, heights, bridges,
    and elevators
- Relaxation, breathing exercises, and thought stopping (can help reduce anxi-
  ety symptoms)
- Role-playing in guided imagery (teaches patient to relax while confronting
  source of fear)
- Hypnosis
- No proven drug treatment; benzodiazepines, beta-adrenergic blockers, and
  SSRIs to help reduce symptoms
  - Situational use of medications to reduce anxiety symptoms in advance of
    a phobic situation such as flying in an airplane
  - Antianxiety drugs to manage short-term anxiety (not useful as long-term
    treatment) (see *Pharmacologic therapy for anxiety disorders,* pages 164 to
    167)
    (*Text continues on page 166.*)

**Key treatment options
for specific phobia**
- Systematic desensitization or
  exposure therapy
- Relaxation techniques
- Breathing exercises
- Thought stopping
- Role-playing in guided imagery
- Hypnosis
- No proven drug treatment

Pharmacologic options for treating anxiety disorders

- Benzodiazepines: alprazolam and diazepam
- Beta-adrenergic blocker: propranolol
- MAO inhibitors: phenelzine sulfate and tranylcypromine sulfate
- SSRIs: fluoxetine and paroxetine
- TCAs: amitriptyline and imipramine
- Other antianxiety agent: buspirone

Pharmacologic therapy for anxiety disorders

This chart highlights several drugs used to treat anxiety disorders.

DRUG	ADVERSE EFFECTS	CONTRAINDICATIONS
Benzodiazepines		
Alprazolam (Xanax) Diazepam (Valium)	• Ataxia • Confusion • Constipation • Double or blurred vision • Dry mouth • Sedation • Skin reactions (rash, urticaria, photosensitivity) • Vertigo • Weight change	• Acute alcohol intoxication • Acute angle-closure glaucoma or untreated open-angle glaucoma • Coma • Depression or psychosis without anxiety • Pregnancy or breast-feeding • Shock • Concomitant MAO inhibitor use (within 14 days of taking)
Beta-adrenergic blockers		
Propranolol (Inderal)	• Bradycardia • Dizziness • Emotional lability • Fatigue • Fever • GI disturbances • Heart block • Impaired concentration • Impotence and decreased libido • Mental depression • Skin rash • Shortness of breath • Sore throat • Worsening of angina	• Concomitant use of reserpine, MAO inhibitors, digoxin, calcium channel blockers, theophylline, norepinephrine, or dopamine • Compromised cardiac function • Diabetes • Respiratory disease
Monoamine oxidase (MAO) inhibitors		
Phenelzine sulfate (Nardil) Tranylcypromine sulfate (Parnate)	• Blurred vision • Constipation • Drowsiness or insomnia • Dry mouth • Fatigue • Hepatic dysfunction (jaundice, malaise, right-upper-abdominal-quadrant pain, change in stool color or consistency) • Hypertensive crisis • Hypomania • Muscle twitching • Orthostatic hypotension • Skin rash • Vertigo • Weakness • Weight gain	• Cardiovascular or cerebrovascular disease • Confusion or uncooperativeness • Advanced age or debilitation • Glaucoma • Heart failure • History of severe headache • Impaired renal function • Liver disease • Pregnancy • Paranoid schizophrenia
Selective serotonin reuptake inhibitors (SSRIs)		
Fluoxetine (Prozac) Paroxetine (Paxil)	• Insomnia • Nausea • Nervousness • Vertigo	• Concomitant MAO inhibitor use (within 14 days of taking)

NURSING CONSIDERATIONS

- Monitor closely after giving each dose because of a possible disinhibitory effect (excitement) rather than calming effect.
- Administer cautiously in elderly patients and in patients with epilepsy, myasthenia gravis, impaired hepatic or renal function, history of substance abuse, or other central nervous system depressant use.
- Assess for unexplained bleeding.
- Monitor liver function and blood counts.
- Instruct patient to avoid alcohol, antidepressants, and anticonvulsants.
- Caution patient not to drive or operate hazardous machinery until drowsiness subsides.
- Stress the importance of avoiding abrupt drug withdrawal.

- Take patient's apical pulse for 1 full minute after giving dose.
- Monitor cardiac function (fluid intake and output, daily weight, serum electrolytes).
- Assess for signs and symptoms of depression.
- Advise patient not to change dose or stop drug without physician's approval.
- Instruct patient to report weight gain of more than 2 lb (0.9 kg) per week.
- Inform diabetic patients that drug may mask hypoglycemia symptoms.
- Instruct patient to take drug with food to minimize GI disturbance.
- Teach patient which adverse effects to report.

- Use with caution in elderly patients.
- Monitor patient's blood pressure every 2 to 4 hours during initial therapy; instruct patient to change positions slowly.
- Assess for signs and symptoms of hypertensive crisis.
- Monitor fluid intake and output.
- Monitor for suicide risk.
- Caution patient not to ingest foods and beverages containing tyramine, caffeine, or tryptophan; warn him that tyramine can cause a hypertensive crisis (provide a list of foods and beverages that contain such substances).
- Instruct patient to avoid meperidine (Demerol), epinephrine, local anesthetics, decongestants, cough medicines, diet pills, and most over-the-counter (OTC) agents.
- Advise patient to go to the emergency department if hypertensive crisis develops.
- Instruct patient to wear medical identification jewelry.

- Give in morning with or without food.
- Monitor for weight loss if nausea occurs.
- Instruct patient to avoid alcoholic beverages.
- Tell patient to report adverse effects, especially rash or itching.

(continued)

Pharmacologic therapy for anxiety disorders *(continued)*

DRUG	ADVERSE EFFECTS	CONTRAINDICATIONS
Tricyclic antidepressants (TCAs)		
Amitriptyline (Elavil) Imipramine (Tofranil)	• Agranulocytosis • Arrhythmias • Blurred vision • Bone marrow depression • Constipation • Dry mouth • Esophageal reflux • Galactorrhea • Hallucinations • Heart failure • Increased or decreased libido • Jaundice and fatigue • Mania • Myocardial infarction (MI) • Orthostatic hypotension or hypertension • Palpitations • Shock • Slowing of intracardiac conduction • Urinary hesitancy • Weight gain	• Concomitant use of MAO inhibitors • Recent MI • Renal or hepatic disease
Other antianxiety agent		
Buspirone (BuSpar)	• Dizziness • Excitement • Headache • Light-headedness • Nausea • Nervousness	• Concomitant MAO inhibitor therapy • Renal or hepatic impairment

● Nursing interventions

- Encourage the patient to discuss the feared entity or situation
- Collaborate with the patient and the multidisciplinary team to develop and implement a systematic desensitization program
- Teach assertiveness skills to help reduce submissive, fearful responses (enables the patient to experiment with new coping skills and discard those that haven't worked in the past)
- Instruct the patient in relaxation and thought-stopping techniques as appropriate
- Administer medications as ordered (to calm the patient and possibly help her change her behavior by reducing anxiety during desensitization sessions)

POSTTRAUMATIC STRESS DISORDER

● Defining characteristics

- PTSD is characterized by persistent, recurrent images and memories of a serious traumatic event that the person has either experienced or witnessed, impairing her ability to function

NURSING CONSIDERATIONS

- Monitor blood pressure and pulse for signs of orthostatic hypotension.
- Monitor patient for suicidal thoughts and behaviors.
- Supervise drug ingestion.
- Know that special monitoring is required if patient has a history of angle-closure glaucoma or seizure disorder.
- Monitor for adverse effects.
- Monitor liver function and complete blood counts.
- Tell patient to change positions slowly.
- Instruct patient to avoid driving or hazardous machinery if drowsiness occurs.
- Teach patient to avoid alcohol and OTC agents unless the physician approves.
- Inform patient that desired drug effects may take up to 4 weeks to appear.

- Assist with ambulation if needed.
- Instruct patient to inform all health care providers of all prescription, OTC, and recreational drug use.
- Caution patient against driving or operating machinery until drowsiness subsides.
- Instruct patient to report adverse effects.
- Inform the patient that improvement may take 3 to 4 weeks.
- Advise patient to have liver and kidney tests periodically.

   - Includes such traumatic events as wartime combat, natural disasters, rapes, accidents, and acts of violence
   - May involve flashbacks, reliving event, nightmares about event—along with avoidance of reminders
- Impairments caused by PTSD can range from mild to severe, affecting nearly every aspect of the person's life
   - Often described as irritable, anxious, fatigued, forgetful, socially withdrawn
   - May have survivor guilt (survived a catastrophe that took another life or lives [possibly many])
   - May become hypervigilant, easily aroused, and easily startled (to avoid stimuli that trigger memories of traumatic event)
- PTSD can be acute or chronic
   - Acute PTSD diagnosed if symptoms appear within 6 months of trauma
   - Delayed or chronic PTSD diagnosed if symptoms begin later than 6 months after incident
   - Remission within 6 months in about 50% of cases
- An estimated 5% to 10% of people in the United States experience PTSD at some time in their lives, with women more likely to be affected than men are

Characteristics of PTSD

- Persistent, recurrent images and memories of a serious traumatic event that the person has either experienced or witnessed, impairing her ability to function
- Includes such traumatic events as wartime combat, natural disasters, rapes, accidents, and acts of violence
- May involve flashbacks, reliving event, nightmares about event—along with avoidance of reminders

Common causes of PTSD

- Triggering traumatic event
- Some may be biochemically predisposed

Key signs and symptoms of PTSD

- Anger
- Poor impulse control
- Chronic anxiety and tension
- Avoidance of people, places, and things associated with the traumatic experience
- Emotional detachment or numbness
- Social withdrawal
- Decreased self-esteem

Diagnosing PTSD

Key assessment findings
- Inability to recall specific aspects of the traumatizing event
- Recurring dreams, flashbacks, or thoughts of the traumatic event
- Feeling or acting as one did when event originally occurred
- Intense distress when faced with cues reminiscent of event

- Patients with PTSD are at increased risk for developing other anxiety, mood, and substance-related disorders—especially alcohol abuse
- Signs and symptoms may occur up to several years after the traumatic event

● **Causes**
- Triggering traumatic event
- Some may be biochemically predisposed
  - May involve impairment of the alpha$_2$-adrenergic receptor response, which inhibits stress-induced release of norepinephrine in PTSD patients
  - Results in progressive behavioral sensitization and generalization to stimulus cues from the original trauma, with responses of increased sympathetic activity

● **Risk factors**
- Limited social supports
- High anxiety levels
- Low self-esteem
- Neurotic and extroverted characteristics
- Family history of PTSD or depression
- History of substance abuse
- Previous diagnosis of an acute stress disorder that failed to resolve within 1 month
- Although preexisting psychopathology may predispose to PTSD, can develop in anyone, especially if stressor is extreme
- Genetic factors

● **Signs and symptoms**
- Anger
- Poor impulse control
- Chronic anxiety and tension
- Avoidance of people, places, and things associated with the traumatic experience
- Emotional detachment or numbness
- Depersonalization (sense of loss of identity as a person)
- Difficulty concentrating
- Difficulty falling or staying asleep
- Hyperalertness, hyperarousal, and exaggerated startle reflex
- Inability to recall details of the traumatic event
- Labile affect (rapid, easily changing affective expression)
- Social withdrawal
- Decreased self-esteem
- Loss of sustained beliefs about people or society
- Self-destructive behavior
- Hopelessness
- Relationship problems
- Survivor's guilt

● **Diagnosis**
- Key assessment findings
  - Inability to recall specific aspects of the traumatizing event
  - Recurring dreams, flashbacks, or thoughts of the traumatic event
  - Feeling or acting as one did when event originally occurred

– Intense distress when faced with cues reminiscent of event
* Diagnosis confirmed if *DSM-IV-TR* criteria met

Treatment

* Nonpharmacologic treatment options: interoceptive exposure, desensitization, relaxation techniques, and psychotherapy
* Individual psychotherapy: gives the patient a chance to talk through the traumatic experience with a nonthreatening person and thus gain some perspective
    – Encouraging patient to confront feelings of loss, grief, and anxiety to help resolve emotional numbness
* Group therapy: helps the patient realize she isn't alone; a skilled group therapist can assist group members in confronting stressful feelings in a supportive environment
* When indicated, alcohol or drug rehabilitation
* Exploration and practice of more positive coping strategies
* Drugs
    – SSRIs (first-line drug for PTSD to treat depression)
    – Benzodiazepines (to reduce symptoms of acute stress and anxiety)
    – Beta-adrenergic blockers (thought to reduce anxiety by preventing functional activity of adrenaline and noradrenaline)
    – TCAs (to reduce insomnia and dream disturbance, anxiety, guilt, flashbacks, and depression)
    – MAO inhibitors (used rarely but may reduce depression, nightmares and night terrors, flashbacks, violent outbursts, and startle reactions)

Nursing interventions

* Establish trust by accepting the patient's current level of functioning and assuming a positive, consistent, honest, and nonjudgmental attitude
* Encourage the patient to express her grief, complete the mourning process, and gain coping skills to relieve anxiety and desensitize her to memories of the traumatic event
* Use crisis intervention techniques as needed
* Deal constructively with the patient's displays of anger
    – Encourage the patient to assess angry outbursts by identifying how anger escalates
    – Assist in regaining control over angry impulses; help to identify situations in which she lost control, to talk about past and precipitating events
    – Use displacement (such as pounding and throwing clay or destroying selected items) as means of dealing with violent urges (from self or others); provide safe, staff-monitored room
    – Encourage move from physical to verbal expressions of anger
* Help the patient relieve shame and guilt precipitated by real actions (such as killing or mutilation) that violated a consciously held moral code
    – Put behavior into perspective, recognize isolation and self-destructive behavior as forms of atonement, accept forgiveness from herself and others
* Carefully review the healing process with the patient; remind her not to equate setbacks with treatment failure
* Administer prescribed medications as ordered

Key treatment options for PTSD

* SSRIs (first-line drugs to treat depression)
* Benzodiazepines
* Beta-adrenergic blockers
* TCAs
* MAO inhibitors

Key nursing interventions for a patient with PTSD

* Deal constructively with patient's displays of anger.
* Encourage patient to assess angry outbursts by identifying how anger escalates.
* Assist in regaining control over angry impulses; help to identify situations in which patient lost control, to talk about past and precipitating events.
* Use displacement as means of dealing with violent urges (from self or others); provide safe, staff-monitored room.
* Encourage move from physical to verbal expressions of anger.

- Teach the patient about prescribed medications and adverse effects, and advise her not to discontinue medication without first consulting her physician
- Evaluate her response to the prescribed drug regimen; be aware that, although benzodiazepines are fast-acting, they may lose their effectiveness with prolonged use
- Provide referrals to clergy, community resources, and group therapy with other victims (for peer support and forgiveness)

NCLEX CHECKS

It's never too soon to begin your NCLEX preparation. Now that you've reviewed this chapter, carefully read each of the following questions and choose the best answer. Then compare your responses to the correct answers.

1. When assessing a patient for acute stress disorder, the nurse is aware that signs and symptoms may occur:

- ☐ **1.** immediately after a trauma.
- ☐ **2.** as soon as 2 days after a trauma.
- ☐ **3.** about 1 month after a trauma.
- ☐ **4.** within 6 months after a trauma.

2. The nurse interprets a patient's fear of being in situations or places that may be difficult or embarrassing to leave as evidence of:

- ☐ **1.** social phobia.
- ☐ **2.** panic disorder.
- ☐ **3.** agoraphobia.
- ☐ **4.** GAD.

3. The nurse identifies unresolved conflicts, a tendency to misinterpret events, and avoidance of new situations as potential risk factors for:

- ☐ **1.** panic disorder.
- ☐ **2.** GAD.
- ☐ **3.** social phobia.
- ☐ **4.** cacophonia.

4. The fear of losing one's mind or having a heart attack is most likely to occur in:

- ☐ **1.** panic disorder.
- ☐ **2.** social phobia.
- ☐ **3.** GAD.
- ☐ **4.** myctophobia.

5. The nurse is assessing a patient who describes flashbacks of an extremely terrifying and painful experience in which she saw hundreds of people die in an airline crash. The nurse notes that the patient is also easily startled and appears hypervigilant. Which disorder should the nurse suspect in this situation?

- ☐ **1.** OCD
- ☐ **2.** Panic disorder
- ☐ **3.** Agoraphobia
- ☐ **4.** PTSD

TOP 10

Items to study for your next test on anxiety disorders

1. Seven classifications of anxiety disorders
2. Factors contributing to the development of anxiety disorders
3. Characteristics differentiating acute stress disorder and PTSD
4. Signs and symptoms of agoraphobia
5. Manifestations and treatment of OCD
6. Nursing interventions for a patient with OCD
7. Nursing interventions for a patient with panic disorder during an acute attack
8. Five main types of specific phobias
9. Four key assessment findings related to PTSD
10. Pharmacologic therapy for anxiety disorders

6. A patient states, "I'm so afraid of embarrassing myself in public. My face gets so red and I start to perspire. Then the words just won't come out." The nurse interprets these statements as possibly indicating:

☐ **1.** GAD.
☐ **2.** panic disorder.
☐ **3.** specific phobia.
☐ **4.** social phobia.

7. A patient with a history of panic attacks reports feeling "trapped" after having an attack. The nurse interprets this as indicating that the patient fears a loss of:

☐ **1.** maturity.
☐ **2.** control.
☐ **3.** memory.
☐ **4.** identity.

8. Which signs and symptoms would the nurse expect to assess in a patient with GAD? Select all that apply:

☐ **1.** Depersonalization
☐ **2.** Fear of dying
☐ **3.** Poor concentration
☐ **4.** Shortness of breath
☐ **5.** Heightened problem solving
☐ **6.** Realistic assessment of the situation

9. When teaching the family of a patient with GAD about her buspirone prescription, which information should the nurse include?

☐ **1.** The drug is a major first-line agent for treating GAD.
☐ **2.** The risk of sedation is increased with this drug.
☐ **3.** It effectively treats the worry associated with GAD.
☐ **4.** The drug begins to work in about 1 week.

10. The physician orders 2.5 mg diazepam I.M. stat for a client with acute anxiety. The vial label reads *Diazepam 5 mg/ml.* How many milliliters should the nurse administer?

_____

ANSWERS AND RATIONALES

1. CORRECT ANSWER: 2
Acute distress disorder may cause symptoms as soon as 2 days after a trauma and typically within 4 weeks of the traumatic event. Symptoms of acute PTSD typically manifest within 6 months of the trauma.

2. CORRECT ANSWER: 3
Agoraphobia is the fear and avoidance of being in situations or places that may be too difficult or embarrassing to leave, or in which help may not be available. Social phobia involves marked, persistent fear or anxiety in social or performance situations. Panic disorder involves recurrent and unexpected severe anxiety (panic) that causes intense apprehension and feelings of impending doom. GAD involves anxiety that's persistent, overwhelming, uncontrollable, and out of proportion to the stimulus.

3. CORRECT ANSWER: 2

The risk of GAD is higher in persons with unresolved conflicts, and a tendency to misinterpret events and avoid new situations. Panic disorder, social phobia, and cacophobia (fear of ugliness) share some, but not all, of these risk factors.

4. CORRECT ANSWER: 1

Anxiety severe enough to cause the patient to fear she's losing her mind or having a heart attack occurs with panic disorder. Social phobia, GAD, and myctophobia (fear of darkness) may have a panic component, but the anxiety is less severe.

5. CORRECT ANSWER: 4

Flashbacks of a trauma along with hypervigilance and being easily startled are characteristics of PTSD. They aren't major components of panic disorder, agoraphobia, or OCD.

6. CORRECT ANSWER: 4

Social phobia is characterized by a dread of being scrutinized and, subsequently, embarrassed in public. Generalized anxiety disorder involves anxiety that's persistent, overwhelming, uncontrollable, and out of proportion to the stimulus. Panic disorder involves recurrent and unexpected severe anxiety (panic) that causes intense apprehension and feelings of impending doom. Specific phobia involves intense, irrational anxiety when exposed to anticipating a specific feared object or situation.

7. CORRECT ANSWER: 2

People who fear loss of control during a panic attack commonly make statements about feeling trapped, getting hurt, or having little or no personal control over their situation. Loss of maturity would be indicated by a regression to a previous developmental level. Loss of memory would be suggested by forgetfulness or confusion. Loss of identity would be indicated by statements involving dissociation.

8. CORRECT ANSWER: 2, 3, 4

The patient with GAD may exhibit fear of grave misfortune or death, poor concentration, shortness of breath, poor (not heightened) problem solving, and unrealistic (not realistic) assessment of the situation. Depersonalization is seen with panic disorder.

9. CORRECT ANSWER: 3

Buspirone is used to treat the worry associated with GAD; it doesn't treat the somatic symptoms associated with the disorder. It may be prescribed for patients with chronic anxiety and for those who relapse after benzodiazepine therapy. The initial drug of choice for GAD patients with a history of substance abuse, buspirone causes less sedation and rarely leads to physical dependence or tolerance. The drug's onset of action takes several weeks.

10. CORRECT ANSWER: 0.5

Using the formula D/H × V, set up the problem as follows:

$$\frac{2.5 \text{ milligrams}}{5 \text{ milligrams}} \times 1 \text{ milliliter}$$

Then solve:

$$\frac{1}{2} \times 1 \text{ milliliter} = 0.5 \text{ milliliter}$$

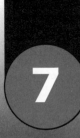

7

Somatoform disorders

LEARNING OBJECTIVES

After studying this chapter, you should be able to:

- Explain how stress can be converted to physical symptoms.
- Name the most common somatoform disorders.
- Identify the differences between conversion disorder and factitious disorders.
- State the proposed causes of somatization and somatoform disorders.
- Describe the treatments commonly used for somatoform disorders.
- List the signs and symptoms of somatoform disorders.
- Discuss the assessment and interventions for patients with somatoform disorders.

CHAPTER OVERVIEW

Somatoform disorders are a group of psychiatric disorders in which the patient has persistent somatic (physical) complaints that can't be explained by a physical disorder, substance use, or another mental disorder. Instead, the symptoms are linked to psychological factors. Distress and preoccupation with the symptoms can lead to occupational, academic, social, and other impairments.

Formerly called *psychosomatic disorders,* somatoform disorders account for about 5% of primary care patient visits.

Defining somatization

- Conversion of emotional or mental states into bodily symptoms
- Internalization of anxiety, stress, and frustration
- Feelings expressed through physical symptoms instead of direct confrontation

Characteristics of somatoform disorders

- Patients don't feign their symptoms (as in malingering, or conscious "faking")
- Patients believe their symptoms indicate a real physical disorder
- Patients have difficulty accepting that symptoms have a psychological origin

Classifying somatoform disorders

- BDD
- Conversion disorder
- Factitious disorders
- Hypochondriasis
- Pain disorder
- Somatization disorder

UNDERSTANDING SOMATOFORM DISORDERS

● **General information**
  - *Somatization* refers to the conversion of emotional or mental states into body symptoms
    – Internalization of anxiety, stress, and frustration
    – Feelings expressed through physical symptoms instead of direct confrontation
  - Although relatively few patients have a disorder that meets the criteria for a true somatoform disorder, psychosomatic symptoms are extremely common
    – More females than males
    – Common among elderly people
  - Patients with somatoform disorders don't feign their symptoms (as in malingering, or conscious "faking")
    – Believe their symptoms indicate a real physical disorder
    – Have difficulty accepting that symptoms have a psychological origin, primarily because they don't produce the symptoms intentionally or feel a sense of control over them
  - Failure to recognize somatization and to manage it appropriately can have frustrating, costly, and potentially dangerous consequences
    – May go from physician to physician in search of a diagnosis and treatment
    – Leads to numerous tests that fail to identify organic disease, and treatments (if prescribed) that don't ease the patient's suffering
    – May lead to misdiagnosis of organic conditions and complications from diagnostic, medical, or surgical procedures
  - Somatoform disorders are classified according to type
    – Body dysmorphic disorder (BDD)
    – Conversion disorder
    – Factitious disorders
    – Hypochondriasis
    – Pain disorder
    – Somatization disorder

● **Coexisting disorders**
  - Many patients with somatoform disorders also have personality disorders— probably because of the inherent relationship between physical illness and certain personality traits or types of character structure
  - Some patients also have coexisting depressive or anxiety disorders
    – Panic attacks or agoraphobia (common with somatization disorder)
    – Depression (common with pain disorder)
    – Obsessive-compulsive disorder (OCD) (common with BDD)

● **Cultural and ethnic factors**
  - Culture and ethnicity may affect the prevalence of psychosomatic symptoms and somatoform disorders; may have different views when compared with Western (American) cultures
    – Asians and Africans: more likely to experience certain types of physical sensations, such as burning hands or feet and sensation of ants crawling under the skin

– Greek and Puerto Rican men: higher rates of somatization disorder than in American men
- Culture and ethnicity also can affect the types of treatment a patient will consider
  – May be suspicious of alternative medicine
  – May prefer using alternative techniques but are reluctant to disclose this information because of previous experiences with skeptical health care professionals

CAUSES

Psychodynamic theories
- Somatoform disorders result from repression of emotions such as after a traumatic event
- The symptoms are physical manifestations of the patient's repressed emotions

Stress
- Among children and adolescents, family stress is thought to be a common cause of somatoform disorders

Learned responses
- Behavioral theorists view psychosomatic symptoms as responses that the patient has consciously learned
- The patient subsequently maintains these responses because they bring some type of reward; for example, the symptoms may allow the patient to do certain things
  – Gain concern or sympathy
  – Avoid unpleasant tasks
  – Explain or justify failures
- In hypochondriasis and somatization disorder, a child may unconsciously reflect or imitate a parent's behavior — especially if the parent reaped considerable secondary gain (such as attention) from the symptoms (see *Primary and secondary gain,* page 176)

Psychobiological mechanisms
- Some experts describe four independent psychobiological mechanisms at work in somatization (an individual may have a single mechanism or a combination)
  – Heightened body sensations
  – Increased autonomic arousal
  – Identification of the "patient" within a family
  – Perceived need to be sick
- Somatoform disorders may be linked to a heightened awareness of normal body sensations; paired with a cognitive bias, this awareness may predispose the patient to interpret any physical symptom as a sign of physical illness
  – May cause the patient (who's already worried about physical disease) to focus attention on common variations in bodily sensations — to the point that these sensations become disturbing and unpleasant
  – Makes patient think the sensations confirm the suspected presence of physical disease
  – Leads to exacerbation of concern, further increasing anxiety and amplifying the sensations

Common causes of somatoform disorders
- Psychodynamic factors
- Stress
- Learned responses
- Psychobiological mechanisms

Psychobiological mechanisms causing somatoform disorders
- Heightened body sensations: may predispose patient to interpret any physical symptom as sign of physical illness
- Increased autonomic arousal
- Identification of the "patient" within a family: identifying one family member as the "patient" may provide a focus that relieves anxiety
- Perceived need to be sick

Primary and secondary gain

Primary gain
- Refers to relief of the unconscious psychological conflict, wish, or need that's causing the physical symptom

Secondary gain
- Refers to the benefit, resources, or advantages that come from having the symptom

Primary and secondary gain

Primary gain refers to relief of the unconscious psychological conflict, wish, or need that's causing the physical symptom. As the patient's anxiety increases and threatens to emerge into consciousness, she "converts" it to physical symptoms. This relieves the pressure to deal with it directly.

Secondary gain, in contrast, refers to the benefit, resources, or advantages that come from having the symptom — such as avoiding difficult situations or getting emotional support or sympathy that the patient might otherwise not receive.

- Some patients with somatoform disorders may have heightened autonomic arousal
  - May be associated with effects of body chemicals that cause norepinephrine release, resulting in such symptoms as tachycardia or gastric hypermotility
  - May also cause pain and muscle tension associated with muscular hyperactivity, as in muscle-tension headache
- In a family under stress, identifying one member as the "patient" may provide a focus that relieves anxiety
  - Causes dysfunctional family patterns, with a single member taking on the "sick" role
  - May be reinforced by health care providers, who focus medical attention on the "sick" family member's disability and illness
- Patients with somatoform disorders may seek the "sick" role because it provides relief from stressful interpersonal expectations and, in most societies, offers attention and caring

EVALUATION AND TREATMENT

Diagnosis
- Accurate diagnosis of somatoform disorders can prevent unnecessary laboratory tests, surgery, and other procedures
- The patient should undergo a thorough physical workup to rule out medical and neurologic conditions and, in patients with pain, to assess pain severity
- Other psychiatric disorders that resemble somatoform disorder must also be ruled out

Treatment considerations
- A patient with a somatoform disorder should develop a long-term relationship with a single, trusted primary health care provider to help guard against unnecessary tests and treatments
- Specialist referrals should be minimized to ensure continuity of care and effective patient monitoring — and to avoid the perception that the health care provider is "abandoning" the patient
- Referrals to mental health professionals should be handled with great sensitivity

Treatment considerations in somatoform disorders

- Long-term relationship should be established with a single, trusted primary health care provider.
- Specialist referrals should be minimized.
- Referrals to mental health professionals should be handled with great sensitivity.

Patient's role in treatment

- The patient should take an active role in treatment and be willing to take responsibility for moving forward with the treatment plan (such as by keeping a diary of symptoms and activities)
- The patient should be encouraged to get regular exercise because self-initiated physical activity fosters responsibility and a sense of control
- Periodic conferences should be scheduled with the patient and family to provide a forum for communication and education
- Teaching the patient about signs and symptoms of disorders linked to anxiety or depression may decrease stress and ease symptoms
- Many patients improve just by learning about the mind-body connection (the effects of the mind and emotions on physical symptoms and disease)
- Parents and child-care providers need to be taught about the symptoms of stress in children, which can manifest as physical disorders (see *Stress-related disorders in children*)

Stress-related disorders in children

Stress can produce certain disorders in children. These disorders include stuttering, sleepwalking and sleep terrors, functional enuresis, and functional encopresis.

STUTTERING

In *stuttering,* speech rhythms are abnormal, with repetitions and hesitations at the beginning of words. Sometimes, these abnormalities are accompanied by movements of the face, shoulders, and respiratory muscles.

Stuttering is most common in children of average or superior intelligence who fear they can't meet the expectations of socially striving, success-oriented families. Sometimes, however, it's associated with mental dullness, poor social background, and a history of birth trauma. Stuttering can lower a child's self-esteem and cause anxiety, humiliation, and withdrawal from social situations.

About 80% of stutterers recover after age 16. Evaluation and treatment by a speech pathologist teaches the stutterer to place equal weight on each syllable in a sentence, to breathe properly, and to control anxiety.

SLEEPWALKING AND SLEEP TERRORS

In *sleepwalking,* the child calmly rises from bed in an altered state of consciousness and walks about, with no subsequent recollection of dream content.

In *sleep terrors,* he awakens terrified, in a state of clouded consciousness and is typically unable to recognize his parents and familiar surroundings. Visual hallucinations may also occur.

Sleep terrors are a normal developmental occurrence in children ages 2 and 3 years. They most commonly occur within 30 minutes to 3½ hours after the child falls asleep. Associated signs include tachycardia, tachypnea, diaphoresis, dilated pupils, and piloerection. Usually, sleep terrors are self-limiting and subside within a few weeks.

(continued)

Patient's role in treatment of somatoform disorders

- Patient should take active role in treatment.
- Patient should be encouraged to get regular exercise.
- Periodic conferences should be scheduled with patient and family.
- Teaching patient about signs and symptoms of disorders linked to anxiety or depression may decrease stress and ease symptoms.
- Many patients improve just by learning about mind-body connection.
- Parents and care providers need to be taught about symptoms of stress in children.

Stress-related disorders in children

Stuttering
- Abnormal speech rhythms
- Repetitions and hesitations at beginning of words

Sleepwalking
- Child calmly rises from bed in an altered state of consciousness
- No subsequent recollection of dream content

Sleep terrors
- Child awakens terrified in a state of clouded consciousness
- Normal development occurrence in children ages 2 and 3
- Most commonly occur within 30 minutes to 3½ hours after child falls asleep

Stress-related disorders in children

Functional enuresis
- Bed-wetting
- Normal occurrence up to ages 3 and 4
- May be linked to stress
- Imipramine may help
- Dry-bed therapy

Functional encopresis
- Evacuation of stool into child's clothes or inappropriate receptacles
- Predisposing factor: psychosocial stress

Key treatment options for somatoform disorders
- Cognitive and behavioral therapies
- Psychoanalysis
- Family therapy
- Alternative therapies

Alternative therapies for treatment of somatoform disorders
- Acupuncture
- Hydrotherapy
- Therapeutic massage
- Meditation
- Botanical medicine
- Homeopathic treatments

Stress-related disorders in children *(continued)*

FUNCTIONAL ENURESIS

Functional enuresis (bed-wetting) is characterized by intentional or involuntary voiding of urine, usually at night. Considered normal in children up to ages 3 and 4, functional enuresis persists in 10% of children up to age 5, in 5% to age 10, and in 1% of males up to age 18.

This condition may be linked to stress, as from the birth of a sibling, a move to a new home, parental divorce or separation, hospitalization, faulty toilet training, or unrealistic (age-inappropriate) responsibilities. Associated problems include low self-esteem; social withdrawal from peers because of ostracism, ridicule, and embarrassment; and anger, rejection, and punishment by caregivers.

If enuresis persists into late childhood, treatment with imipramine (Tofranil) may help. However, this drug can cause schizophrenia-like symptoms in young children. *Dry-bed therapy* may include the use of an alarm apparatus (wet bell pad), social motivation, self-correction of accidents, and positive reinforcement.

FUNCTIONAL ENCOPRESIS

Functional encopresis is the evacuation of stool into the child's clothes or inappropriate receptacles. It's associated with low intelligence, cerebral dysfunction, or other developmental symptoms such as a lag in language development.

Predisposing factors may include psychosocial stress and inadequate or inconsistent toilet training. Related problems include repressed anger, withdrawal from peers, and low self-esteem.

The child should undergo a medical examination to rule out physical disorders. Child, adult, and family therapy may be needed to reduce anger and disappointment over the child's development and to improve parenting techniques.

Therapeutic approaches
- The most effective treatments for somatoform disorders are cognitive and behavioral therapies and similar approaches that aim to reduce symptoms and stabilize the personality
- Psychoanalysis and other forms of insight-oriented psychotherapy are less effective, although some patients may benefit from group therapy or support groups
- Family therapy may be recommended for children or adolescents with somatoform disorders, particularly if the parents seem to be using the child to divert attention from other difficulties
- For patients with pain disorder, family therapy can help avoid reinforcement of dependency among family members
- Alternative therapies may relieve stress, pain, and other symptoms, not just on a physical level but also on a mental, emotional, and spiritual level
  - Acupuncture
  - Hydrotherapy
  - Therapeutic massage
  - Meditation
  - Botanical medicine
  - Homeopathic treatments

BODY DYSMORPHIC DISORDER

● **Defining characteristics**
- BDD is characterized by preoccupation with an imagined or slight defect in physical appearance that causes the patient much distress or impairment in social or occupational functioning; in extreme cases, it results in psychiatric hospitalization, suicidal ideation, or suicide attempts
- A patient with BDD views himself as hideous or grotesque, even though others offer reassurances that his appearance is fine
  - Can't be convinced that the flaw is minimal or, in many cases, nonexistent
  - Thinks about the perceived defect for at least 1 hour each day
- Most patients perceive a flaw of the face or head — especially the skin, nose, hair, or ears
  - May worry about having acne or scarring
  - May think nose is too big or facial features are asymmetrical
- In some cases, patients focus on the shape or size of a particular body part (breasts, genitals, muscles, or buttocks) or are preoccupied with several body parts; for instance, young male patients may believe they're "puny," and obsessively try to gain weight and add muscle
- To confirm or avoid the perceived defect, patients typically engage in ritualistic, compulsive behaviors that they believe will reduce their anxiety; however, these behaviors actually intensify the anxiety
  - May frequently check appearance in mirrors (or, conversely, avoid mirrors)
  - May compare perceived defect with others' defects
  - May engage in excessive grooming (combing hair, applying makeup, or picking skin)
  - Usually seeks constant reassurance from others that defect is "not that bad"
- Many patients consult cosmetic specialists, such as plastic surgeons and dermatologists; some even stay in hiding, convinced that they're hideous
- In the United States, BDD occurs in 1% to 2% of the general population, affecting males and females equally (prevalence may be underestimated because BDD frequently goes undiagnosed)
  - Among those seeking cosmetic surgery, ranges from 2% to 7%
  - Among psychiatric patients, about 12%
- Many sufferers are too embarrassed to reveal their distress to others (including health care professionals); some downplay the problem or don't even realize they need help
  - May be trivialized by family members who don't realize that BDD is an extreme distortion that the sufferer can't simply "get over" or "grow out of"
  - May go unreported by some health care professionals who are unaware that BDD is a known psychiatric disorder that responds to appropriate treatment
- Usually begins during late teens (average age of onset is 17 years)
- The disorder may come on gradually or abruptly; usually follows a fluctuating but chronic course
  - With appropriate treatment, has a good prognosis

Characteristics of BDD

- Preoccupation with imagined or slight defect in physical appearance that causes patient much distress or impairment in social or occupational functioning
- In extreme cases, results in psychiatric hospitalization, suicidal ideation, or suicide attempts
- Usually begins during late teens (average age of onset: 17 years)
- May come on gradually or abruptly; usually follows fluctuating but chronic course
- May predispose patient to major depressive disorder

Common causes of BDD

- Biological explanation: possible genetic predisposition to psychiatric disorders
- Psychological explanation: low self-esteem and tendency to judge oneself almost exclusively by appearance

Key signs and symptoms of BDD

Related to perceived flaw

- Frequent checking of reflection in mirror, or avoidance of mirrors
- Frequently comparing appearance with that of others, or scrutiny of others' appearance
- Attempting to cover perceived defect
- Seeking corrective treatment to eradicate perceived defect
- Touching perceived problem area frequently

Related to behavior

- Feelings of acute distress over appearance
- Avoidance of social situations where perceived defect may be exposed

- Without treatment, may cause delusions or increasingly depressed—even suicidal—behavior
- Many patients with BDD have additional psychiatric disorders
  - Depression
  - OCD
  - Eating disorders
  - Anxiety disorders
  - Agoraphobia
  - Trichotillomania (hair-pulling)
- BDD may predispose the patient to major depressive disorder
  - In clinical settings, occurs in about 60% of patients (lifetime risk in about 80%)
  - Puts patient at high risk for suicide (especially females with perceived facial defects)

Causes

- Exact cause unknown; one biological and one psychological explanation proposed (both may be correct)
- Proposed biological explanation: Some may have genetic predisposition to psychiatric disorders, increasing risk of developing BDD
  - Onset possibly precipitated by certain stresses or life events, especially during adolescence
  - Possibly also associated with imbalance of serotonin or other brain chemicals
- Proposed psychological explanation: Low self-esteem and tendency to judge oneself almost exclusively by appearance may contribute
  - May be perfectionistic, striving for an impossible ideal and not being satisfied with appearance
  - Can lead to excessive scrutiny and heightened perception of self-appearance by increasingly focusing on every imperfection or slight abnormality
  - May begin avoiding certain situations or using maladaptive behavior in attempt to escape scrutiny or judgment by others, which only intensifies excessive attention on self
- Societal values (largely based on Western culture in the United States) playing large role; adolescents particularly vulnerable to this type of pressure
  - Based on idealized—in some cases, unrealistic—standards of beauty
  - Comparisons made to so-called "beautiful" celebrities, such as actors and models
  - Reinforced through media (television, movies, magazines, ads) and by peers

Signs and symptoms

- Variable symptom severity (patient to patient)
  - Some patients capable of managing distress, functioning on a day-to-day basis (although not to full potential)
  - Others with severe functional impairment; in extreme cases, so embarrassed by appearance that they become reclusive
- Common signs and symptoms focusing on perceived flaw
  - Frequent checking of reflection in mirror, or avoidance of mirrors
  - Frequently comparing appearance with that of others, or scrutiny of others' appearance

- Attempting to cover perceived defect with clothing, makeup, or hat, or by changing posture or hairstyle
- Seeking corrective treatment, such as surgery or dermatologic therapy, to eradicate perceived defect (even though physicians, family, and friends think such measures aren't necessary)
- Seeking constant reassurance from others about the perceived flaw or, conversely, attempting to convince others of its repulsiveness
- Performing long grooming rituals, such as repeatedly combing or cutting hair or applying makeup or cover-up products
- Picking skin or squeezing pimples or blackheads for hours
- Touching the perceived problem area frequently
- Measuring body part that's perceived as repulsive
- Distress and avoidant behavior
  - Anxiety and self-consciousness around peers
  - Feelings of acute distress over appearance, causing functional impairment
  - Avoidance of social situations where the perceived defect may be exposed
  - Difficulty maintaining relationships with peers, family, spouses or partners
  - Poor school or work performance or frequent use of sick days
  - Low self-esteem
  - Suicidal thoughts or behaviors

Diagnosis

- Requires careful diagnostic analysis because may be misdiagnosed as anorexia nervosa, social phobia, agoraphobia, panic disorder, trichotillomania, depression, or OCD (closely linked to OCD, in particular)
  - Shared features of obsessive and compulsive behaviors
  - BDD considered a "spectrum" disorder of OCD (has same core symptoms but focuses on just one aspect of appearance)
- Diagnostic instruments used to assess severity
  - Yale-Brown Obsessive-Compulsive Scale modified for BDD
  - National Institutes of Health Body Dysmorphic Disorder Scale
  - Psychiatric Status Rating Scale for BDD
  - Global Assessment of Functioning Scale
  - Schneier Disability Profile
  - Fixity of Beliefs Questionnaire
  - Hamilton Depression Rating Scale
- Diagnosis confirmed if *Diagnostic and Statistical Manual of Mental Disorders, Fourth Edition, Text Revision (DSM-IV-TR)* criteria met

Treatment

- Treatment goals
  - Enhance self-esteem
  - Reduce preoccupation with perceived flaw and decrease time spent on compulsive behavior
  - Eliminate harmful effects of compulsive behaviors
  - Improve functional abilities
  - Encourage patient to express—and cope with—feelings of anxiety as they arise without resorting to excessive behaviors
- Group therapy to reduce the patient's sense of helplessness and help him to directly communicate his thoughts, feelings, and desires

Diagnosing BDD

Possible misdiagnoses
- Anorexia nervosa
- Social phobia
- Agoraphobia
- Panic disorder
- Trichotillomania
- Depression
- OCD

Diagnostic tests
- Yale-Brown Obsessive-Compulsive Scale modified for BDD
- National Institutes of Health Body Dysmorphic Disorder Scale
- Psychiatric Status Rating Scale for BDD
- Global Assessment of Functioning Scale
- Schneier Disability Profile
- Fixity of Beliefs Questionnaire
- Hamilton Depression Rating Scale

Key treatment options for BDD

- Group therapy
- Behavior therapy
- SSRIs
- TCAs

Treatment goals in BDD

- Enhance self-esteem
- Reduce preoccupation with perceived flaw and decrease time spent on compulsive behavior
- Eliminate harmful effects of compulsive behaviors
- Improve functional abilities
- Encourage patient to express—and cope with—feelings of anxiety as they arise without resorting to excessive behaviors

- Cognitive-behavioral therapy
  - Forbidding the patient from performing behaviors that heighten discomfort and worsen the disorder
  - Teaching to resist compulsive behaviors
  - Decreasing the time spent on obsessive thoughts and compulsive behavior
  - Helping the patient to face the situations that have been avoided
- Various behavior therapy techniques
  - Aversion therapy: involves applying a painful stimulus to the patient to create an aversion to his obsession with the perceived defect
  - Thought stopping: breaks the habit of thinking disturbing thoughts by interrupting them and substituting competing ones; uses an intense distracting stimulus (such as snapping a rubber band around the wrist) to stop the offending thought while the patient focuses on achieving calmness and muscle relaxation
  - Thought replacement (thought switching): teaches the patient to strengthen positive thoughts to the point that they eventually replace obsessive (negative) ones
  - Response prevention: aims to prevent compulsive behavior through distraction, persuasion, or redirection of activity; hospitalization or family involvement may be necessary
  - Flooding (implosion therapy): exposes the patient to images of perceived flaw for prolonged periods until it no longer causes distress; involves gradually increasing exposure and requires strong interpersonal support or antianxiety medication
- Selective serotonin reuptake inhibitors (SSRIs), including fluvoxamine (Luvox), to diminish preoccupation, distress, depression, and anxiety
- Tricyclic antidepressant (TCA): clomipramine (Anafranil)
- Certain drugs—lithium, neuroleptics, trazodone (Desyrel), and benzodiazepines—usually ineffective and may even exacerbate symptoms of BDD

● **Nursing interventions**
- Approach the patient unhurriedly
- Promote an accepting, nonjudgmental atmosphere; avoid expressions of shock, amusement, or criticism of the patient's behavior
- Address the patient's physical needs
  - Observing for evidence of infection (caused by skin breakdown from constantly picking at the skin)
  - Possible interventions to promote rest, nutrition, and grooming (may be needed if patient becomes involved in ritualistic thoughts and behaviors to the point of self-neglect)
- Allow the patient time to carry out compulsive or ritualistic behavior (unless it's dangerous) until some distraction or other activity can be implemented
  - Don't block ritualistic behavior; could raise patient's anxiety to intolerable level
  - Set reasonable limits, constraints on obsessive behaviors (clearly explain why needed)
  - Avoid creating situations that increase frustration, provoke anger (may interfere with treatment)
- Let the patient know you're aware of the behavior, and help him explore feelings associated with it

---

Behavior therapy techniques

- Aversion therapy
- Thought stopping
- Thought replacement
- Response prevention
- Flooding

Key nursing interventions for a patient with BDD

- Promote an accepting, nonjudgmental atmosphere; avoid expressions of shock, amusement, or criticism of patient's behavior.
- Address patient's physical needs.
- Allow patient time to carry out compulsive or ritualistic behavior (unless dangerous) until some distraction or other activity can be implemented.
- Let patient know you're aware of the behavior, and help him explore feelings associated with it.

– Identifying disturbing topics of conversation that reflect underlying anxiety or terror

– Listening attentively and offering feedback

• Work with the patient to decrease the time spent on obsessive thoughts and maladaptive behaviors and to find better ways of coping with problems

– Gradually shortening the time allowed for engaging in the behavior (and helping the patient focus on other feelings) or problems for the remainder of the time

– Suggesting active diversions, such as whistling or humming, to divert the patient's attention away from unwanted thoughts

– Engaging patient in activities that create positive accomplishments and raise self-esteem and confidence

– Encouraging use of appropriate techniques to relieve stress, loneliness, and isolation

• Monitor the patient for evidence of developing insight and improved behavior, such as fewer obsessive thoughts and reduced time spent on ritualistic behavior

• Evaluate behavioral changes, noting which interventions work and recommending alternative strategies when needed

• Monitor for desired and adverse effects of drug therapy as appropriate

HYPOCHONDRIASIS

● **Defining characteristics**

• Hypochondriasis is marked by the persistent conviction that one has or is likely to get a serious disease—despite medical evidence and reassurance to the contrary

• The patient with this disorder typically bases his conviction on bodily sensations or symptoms that have been misinterpreted

– Doesn't consciously cause symptoms and isn't consciously aware of the benefits they bring (such as increased attention)

– Doesn't suffer from delusions

• It can lead to significant psychological distress or impairment in social and occupational functioning

– May have a long history of previously unfounded complaints, which contributes to overlooking of serious organic diseases

– May be at risk for complications from multiple evaluations, tests, and invasive procedures

• In general medical clinic populations, it's found in about 6% of all patients; it accounts for about 5% of all psychiatric patients

• The disorder affects as many men as it does women

– Most common between ages 20 and 30

– Seen increasingly in children and adolescents

– May also develop in elderly people with no previous history of health-related fears (see *Assessing elderly patients for somatoform disorders,* page 184)

• The condition may persist for years but usually occurs as a series of episodes rather than continual treatment-seeking

– Flare-ups typically following stressful events

Characteristics of hypochondriasis

● Marked by persistent conviction that one has or is likely to get a serious disease—despite medical evidence and reassurance to the contrary

● Patient's conviction based on bodily sensations or symptoms that have been misinterpreted

● Patient doesn't consciously cause symptoms and isn't consciously aware of benefits they bring

● Patient doesn't suffer from delusions

● Affects as many men as women

Assessment data for somatoform disorders in elderly patients

- Past level of functioning
- Extent of current disabilities
- Cognitive deficits
- Psychosocial status

Assessing elderly patients for somatoform disorders

Elderly patients may perceive themselves to be in poor health even if they have no significant physical impairments. Their tendency to present with somatoform complaints poses a challenge to assessment and management.

As a first step, the patient should undergo a comprehensive medical evaluation (and laboratory tests as needed) to check for a physical basis for complaints. Cognitive and psychiatric examinations may also be warranted.

ESSENTIAL ASSESSMENT DATA
When assessing an elderly patient for a somatoform disorder, always gather a complete history.
- Past level of functioning
- Extent of current disabilities
- Cognitive deficits
- Manifestations of emotional distress
  Also assess the patient's psychosocial status.
- Living situation
- Social supports
- Role within the family
- Key support people outside the family

To verify the patient's information, obtain a collaborative history from family members, if possible.

FAMILY STRESS AND ABUSE
Be aware that the family may respond to the patient's somatoform symptoms by giving him more time and attention. In some cases, however, family members become angry and frustrated as conflicts arise and escalate. The patient may even suffer neglect and abuse. If you suspect such treatment, make sure it's reported to the proper authorities.

- Permanent recovery in only about 5% of patients
- In those with overlapping depression, usually a poor prognosis for recovery from depression

● **Causes**
- Exact cause unknown; may involve biologically based hypersensitivity to internal stimuli
- More common in people who have had an organic disease
  - Found in nearly 8% of first-degree relatives of patients with hypochondriasis
  - Have high rate of other somatoform disorders as well as anxiety and depressive disorders
- Psychological factors (probable role)
  - In adults, may reflect self-centeredness or wish to be taken care of; enables patient to take on dependent, sick role, thereby escaping responsibilities or postponing unwelcome challenges
  - Emotionally, may be linked to — or may be expression of — anger or guilt
  - May also be linked to anxiety and depression
  - In elderly patients, may be associated with depression or grief
- Contributing factors
  - Death of loved one
  - Serious illness in family member or friend
  - History of serious illness

Common causes of hypochondriasis

- More common in people who have had an organic disease
- Psychological factors (probable role)
- May reflect self-centeredness or wish to be taken care of
- May be linked to — or may be expression of — anger or guilt
- May be linked to anxiety and depression

Signs and symptoms

- Range from specific to general complaints
- Characteristically involve a single body system
- Complaints rarely follow recognizable pattern of organic disease
    - Usually reflect preoccupation with normal body functions (not supported by abnormal physical findings)
- In many cases, patient asked about complaint provides detailed description of each symptom, including location, quality, and duration; complaints may change as evaluation proceeds
- Typically, concerns not relieved by examination and physician's reassurance; patient tends to believe physician has failed to find real cause
- Certain physical sensations and symptoms commonly misinterpreted as signs of organic disease
    - Borborygmi (rumbling sounds caused by gas and fluids moving through the intestines)
    - Abdominal bloating
    - Crampy discomfort
    - Cardiac awareness (feeling the heart beating)
    - Sweating
- Common sensory complaints
    - Anesthesia
    - Paresthesia
    - Deafness
    - Blindness
    - Tunnel vision
- Common motor complaints
    - Abnormal movements
    - Gait disturbances
    - Weakness
    - Paralysis
    - Tremors
    - Tics
    - Jerks
- In some patients, neurologic complaints, including seizurelike symptoms and symptoms that mimic those of degenerative neurologic disorders
- Other assessment findings
    - Abnormal focus on bodily functions and sensations
    - Anger, frustration, and depression
    - Frequent visits to a health care provider despite assurance of good health
    - Intensified symptoms when around sympathetic people
    - Rejection of notion that symptoms are stress-related
    - Use of symptoms to avoid difficult situations

Diagnosis

- Projective psychological tests (such as inkblot interpretation and sentence completion tests) showing a preoccupation with somatic concerns
- Complete patient history with emphasis on current psychological stressors
- Tests to rule out underlying organic disease, although invasive procedures should be minimized; typically, test results inconsistent with complaints and physical findings

---

Key signs and symptoms of hypochondriasis

- Characteristically involves a single body system
- Complaints rarely follow recognizable pattern of organic disease
- Typically, concerns not relieved by examination and physician's reassurance

Misinterpreted physical signs and symptoms
- Borborygmi
- Abdominal bloating
- Crampy discomfort
- Cardiac awareness
- Sweating

Common sensory complaints
- Anesthesia
- Paresthesia
- Deafness
- Blindness
- Tunnel vision

Common motor complaints
- Abnormal movements
- Gait disturbances
- Weakness
- Paralysis
- Tremors
- Tics
- Jerks

Diagnosing hypochondriasis

- Projective psychological tests
- Complete patient history
- Tests to rule out underlying organic disease

- Diagnosis possibly suggested by history and physical findings; however, diagnosis confirmed only if *DSM-IV-TR* criteria met

Treatment

- Goal: Help the patient lead a productive life despite distressing symptoms and fears
- Appropriate teaching and a supportive relationship with one competent, trusted health care professional crucial
- After medical evaluation is complete, telling the patient he doesn't have a serious disease but that continued medical follow-up will help control his symptoms
  - May not make hypochondriasis disappear, but may ease some of the patient's anxiety
  - May also be therapeutic to link the diagnosis to psychological stressors; conversely, telling the patient that symptoms are imaginary could be counterproductive
- Regular outpatient follow-up to help detect organic illness and help the patient deal with symptoms
  - Later development of organic disease in up to 30% of patients with hypochondriasis
  - Psychological influence on symptoms not acknowledged by most patients with hypochondriasis; most resist psychiatric treatment
- Psychotherapy: individual, group, or family therapy, as needed
  - Individual psychotherapy: uses psychodynamic principles to help patient understand unconscious conflicts
  - Group therapy: provides support to help patient learn to cope with symptoms and improve social skills
  - Family therapy: focuses on improving family members' awareness of their interaction patterns and on enhancing their communication with one another
- Behavior modification (provides incentives, motivation, and rewards to control symptoms)
- Medication for patients with overlapping psychiatric conditions, such as depression and anxiety disorders
  - Benzodiazepines, such as lorazepam (Ativan) or alprazolam (Xanax)
  - SSRIs
  - TCAs, such as amitriptyline (Elavil) or imipramine (Tofranil)

Nursing interventions

- Help the patient deal with ineffective individual coping and altered health maintenance
- Assess the patient's knowledge about the effects that emotions and stress can have on physiologic functioning; provide appropriate teaching
- Encourage the patient to express feelings rather than repress them, which can have physical consequences
- Respond to the patient's symptoms in a matter-of-fact way to reduce the secondary gain obtained from talking about them
- Engage the patient in conversations that focus on something other than physical maladies
- Create a supportive relationship that helps the patient feel cared for and understood

---

Key treatment options for hypochondriasis

- Goal: help patient lead productive life despite distressing symptoms and fears
- Appropriate teaching and supportive relationship with one competent, trusted health care professional crucial
- Psychotherapy
- Behavior modification

Key nursing interventions for a patient with hypochondriasis

- Encourage patient to express feelings rather than repress them.
- Help patient learn nonpharmacologic strategies to reduce distress, including imagery, relaxation, hypnosis, biofeedback, and massage.
- Teach assertiveness techniques, if appropriate.

TIME-OUT FOR TEACHING

Relaxation techniques

If your patient has symptoms related to stress or anxiety, relaxation techniques may help. Simple relaxation techniques include:

- Deep breathing, in which the patient takes a series of slow, deep breaths and releases each breath slowly
- Meditation, in which the patient either clears his mind or focuses on a single soothing thought, image, or sound.

DEEP BREATHING

Provide your patient with these instructions to teach him how to perform deep breathing:

- Instruct him to sit in a comfortable position with his eyes closed.
- Tell him to focus on a peaceful sound or image and then to breathe in through his nose to a count of 4.
- Have him hold his breath for a count of 2.
- Instruct him to breathe out through his mouth for a count of 6. He should repeat this cycle for 30 seconds to 5 minutes.

MEDITATION

Meditation may offset some of the negative physiologic effects of stress through a mechanism called the *relaxation response*. Meditating takes about 20 minutes and can be done anywhere, at any time — or it may be done as a scheduled activity. Tell the patient that learning to meditate takes some practice — ideally, he should practice it daily.

Techniques include concentrative and mindful meditation. For *concentrative* meditation, instruct the patient to focus on a peaceful image, thought, or sound, or his own breathing.

For *mindful* meditation, instruct him to remain aware of all sensations, feelings, images, thoughts, sounds, and smells that pass through his mind — without actually thinking about them.

Whichever technique the patient uses, encourage him to make a conscious effort to relax his muscles and maintain a comfortable posture as he meditates. Closing his eyes can help him focus on inner peace.

Relaxation techniques

Deep breathing

- Instruct patient to sit in comfortable position with eyes closed.
- Tell him to focus on peaceful sound or image and then breathe in through his nose to a count of 4.
- Have him hold his breath for a count of 2.
- Instruct him to breathe out through his mouth for a count of 6.
- Patient should repeat this cycle for 30 seconds to 5 minutes.

Meditation

- Takes about 20 minutes; it can be done anywhere, at any time.
- Concentrative meditation: Instruct patient to focus on peaceful image, thought, or sound, or his own breathing.
- Mindful meditation: Instruct patient to remain aware of all sensations, feelings, images, thoughts, sounds, and smells that pass through his mind — without actually thinking about them.

- Keep in mind that the patient with hypochondriasis feels real pain and distress, so denying his symptoms or challenging his behavior is never appropriate; instead, help him find new ways to deal with stress other than developing physical symptoms
- Recognize that the patient will probably never be symptom-free, and don't get angry when he continues to complain about the symptoms; such anger can drive him away to yet another unnecessary medical evaluation
- Help the patient learn nonpharmacologic strategies to reduce distress, including imagery, relaxation, hypnosis, biofeedback, and massage (see *Relaxation techniques*)
- Teach assertiveness techniques, if appropriate
- If the patient is willing to try psychotherapy, make the necessary referral for individual, group, or family therapy, as needed

Characteristics of pain disorder

- Complaints of persistent pain
- Psychological factors play key role in pain's onset, severity, or maintenance
- Predominant feature is the pain itself
- Remissions and exacerbations may occur

Complications

- Psychoactive substance dependence
- Multiple surgical interventions
- Complications of extensive diagnostic evaluations

Common causes of pain disorder

- No specific cause
- Stress or conflict may underlie the problem
- One theory equates patient's unconscious conversion of conflicts to pain
- Behavioral theory: pain behaviors reinforced when rewarded and inhibited when punished

PAIN DISORDER

● Defining characteristics

- In pain disorder, the patient complains of persistent pain, which results predominantly or exclusively from psychological factors yet isn't feigned or intentionally produced
- The pain is severe enough to warrant medical attention and becomes the patient's main focus of attention
  - Causes the patient significant distress
  - May be acute or chronic
  - Impairs the patient's social, occupational, or other important areas of functioning
- In some cases, the patient has an underlying physical disorder that explains the pain—but not its severity or duration or the resulting disability
  - May have sought treatment for the underlying disorder and been treated for pain as well
  - May have familiarity with medications used to treat pain, including their dosages and routes of administration
- As with many psychiatric conditions (especially anxiety and mood disorders), psychological factors play a key role in the pain's onset, severity, and maintenance; however, with pain disorder, the predominant feature is the pain itself
- The prevalence of pain disorder is unknown; however, roughly 10% to 15% of adults in the United States have some form of work disability because of back pain alone
  - More common among blue-collar workers (possibly a result of increased risk of job-related injuries)
  - Twice as many males as females experience chronic headache
  - Peak age of onset is 30s or 40s
- Remissions and exacerbations may occur; the disorder may result in complications
  - Psychoactive substance dependence
  - Multiple surgical interventions
  - Complications of extensive diagnostic evaluations
- Concomitant disorders may include substance dependence, anxiety, and depression

● Causes

- No specific cause; stress or conflict may underlie the problem
  - Can result from chronic anxiety and depression, which predispose a patient to pain disorder by decreasing the pain threshold
  - May be associated with a recent traumatic, stressful, or humiliating experience
- For some, the pain may have special significance; may serve as way to get attention, sympathy, or relief from responsibilities; or may be used to manipulate others and gain advantage in interpersonal relationships
- One psychological theory: patient converts unconscious conflicts to pain symptoms or expresses intrapsychic conflict through pain
- Behavioral theory: pain behaviors reinforced when rewarded, and inhibited when ignored or punished

Signs and symptoms

- Pain involving part of body; most commonly back, head, abdomen, or chest
- If contributing medical condition, physical findings consistent with that condition
- May relate long history of medical evaluations and procedures in multiple settings, without much noticeable pain relief
- Key assessment findings
  - Acute or chronic pain not explained by a physiologic cause
  - Pain severity, duration, or resulting disability not explained by underlying physical disorder
  - Insomnia
  - Anger, frustration, and depression
  - Anger directed at health care professionals (because they have failed to relieve pain)
  - Drug-seeking behavior in an attempt to relieve pain
  - Frequent visits to multiple health care providers to seek pain relief

Diagnosis

- Challenging to diagnosis (perception of pain is subjective)
- Tests to rule out physical and neurologic conditions, as well as other psychiatric disorders (especially other somatoform disorders and malingering); any ordered diagnostic test will fail to reveal organic cause of pain (or severity or duration)
- Diagnosis confirmed if *DSM-IV-TR* criteria met

Treatment

- Easing the patient's pain and helping him live with it
- Attending a comprehensive pain center and receiving treatment for any coexisting psychiatric disorders
- A continuing, supportive relationship with an understanding health care professional and regularly scheduled follow-up appointments
- Several supportive measures
  - Hot or cold packs
  - Physical therapy
  - Distraction techniques
  - Hypnotherapy
  - Cutaneous stimulation with massage
  - Transcutaneous electrical nerve stimulation
  - Anxiety-reducing measures
- Alternative therapies for relief (see *Common alternative therapies,* page 190)
- Psychotherapy
  - May gain insight by emphatically pointing out the link between pain and an obvious psychosocial stressor
  - Not for all patients; some are unable or unwilling to associate their problem with a psychosocial stressor and will reject any form of psychotherapy
- Analgesics; regularly scheduled doses are usually more effective than those given as needed (can help reduce the patient's anxiety about asking for pain medication, and eliminate unnecessary confrontations)
- Other medications

Common alternative therapies

- Nutritional therapy
- Herbal therapy
- Homeopathic remedies
- Acupuncture or acupressure
- Hydrotherapy
- Naturopathic manipulative therapy
- Aromatherapy

Common alternative therapies

A patient with pain disorder or other somatoform disorders may consider trying one of these alternative therapies.

- *Nutritional therapy* – Uses whole foods, nutritional supplements (if needed), and controlled fasting to treat disease and maintain health.
- *Herbal therapy* – May be taken internally or applied externally to treat the internal conditions that manifest as disease. For example, capsaicin, ginger, sarapin, bromelain, arnica, or hypericum (usually in the form of a tea) may be used for complaints of chronic pain.

  If the patient experiences abdominal pain, a combination of herbs, such as chamomile, cinnamon, fennel, ginger, lemon balm, and peppermint, can be used as a tea. Meadowsweet has been shown to have pain-relieving properties, and ginger has been identified as an anti-inflammatory herb.
- *Homeopathic remedies* – Dilute preparations of natural substances that, in large amounts, cause certain symptoms but in small amounts may relieve them.
- *Acupuncture or acupressure* – Commonly used to relieve pain; involves the insertion of very fine needles into or application of pressure onto designated points on the skin to stimulate the body's vital energy flow.

  For example, light sensitive pressure applied to the temples with the fingertips can help relieve headache pain. Additional acupressure sites for head-

ache pain are in the forehead (above the right eyebrow), the inside aspect between the thumb and index finger of the left hand, and the area at the base of the great toe on the left foot. Abdominal pain can be relieved by acupressure at the epigastric area, just below the ribs at the midline.
- *Hydrotherapy* – Involves the use of special baths and other water-based treatments to cure disorders and maintain health.
- *Naturopathic manipulative therapy* – Uses physical treatments that may include manipulation of the bones and spine (in a manner similar to chiropractic) as well as massage, heat, cold, touch, electricity and sound, ultrasound, diathermy, and therapeutic exercises.

  For example, massage with oil applied to the thigh using slow rhythmic strokes toward the heart can help relieve upper leg pain.
- *Aromatherapy* – Involves the inhalation of application of essential oils distilled from various plants.

  For example, a patient with a somatoform disorder involving nausea may drink a glass of honey water with peppermint. Headache pain may be relieved with such oils as eucalyptus, black pepper, lavender, marjoram, peppermint, rosemary, or rose, which can be inhaled or used in baths or massages to the scalp or face.

  – Anxiolytics (benzodiazepines), such as lorazepam (Ativan) and alprazolam (Xanax)
  – TCAs, such as amitriptyline (Elavil), imipramine (Tofranil), or doxepin (Sinequan) — rarely used as first-choice drugs
- Placebos never used in an effort to "prove" to the patient that his pain is psychogenic; discovery of the deceit can lead to anger and distrust by the patient

Nursing interventions

- Assess and record characteristics of the patient's pain, including its severity, duration, precipitating or alleviating factors, and any resulting disabilities
- Provide assistance in relieving the patient's pain and reducing his anxiety
- Ensure a safe, accepting environment to promote therapeutic communication
  - A caring atmosphere in which the patient's complaints are taken seriously and every effort is made to provide relief
  - Acknowledgement of the patient's pain (eliminates his need to try to convince you it's real); remember, never tell the patient his pain is imaginary or make him wait longer for medication that's due
- Help the patient understand what's contributing to his pain, and encourage him to recognize situations that precipitate his pain
- Offer attention at times other than when the patient complains of pain, to weaken the link to secondary gain (and to strengthen notion that pain isn't need to receive positive attention)
- Provide nonpharmacologic comfort measures, such as repositioning, back massage, or heat application, whenever possible
- Teach the patient coping strategies to help him deal with the pain — for example, progressive muscle relaxation or deep-breathing exercises
- Encourage him to remain independent despite his pain
- Consider psychiatric referrals — but realize that the patient may resist such intervention

CONVERSION DISORDER

Defining characteristics

- Conversion disorder is marked by the loss of or change in voluntary motor or sensory functioning (for instance, blindness, paralysis, or anesthesia) that suggests a physical illness but has no demonstrable physiologic basis
- The specific symptom or deficit has a psychological basis
  - Exacerbation during times of emotional stress
  - Relief of stress or inner conflict provided by the symptom
  - Attention, support, or avoidance of responsibilities provided by the symptom
- The conversion symptom itself isn't life-threatening and usually has a short duration
  - Considered clinically significant and distressing enough to disrupt social, occupational, or other important areas of functioning
  - Not under the patient's voluntary control (symptom isn't feigned or intentionally produced, as in factitious disorders or malingering) (see *Facts about factitious disorders,* pages 192 and 193)
  - May be associated with unconscious motives of primary or secondary gain
- Conversion symptoms can severely impede the patient's normal activities
  - With prolonged loss of function, may lead to serious complications, such as contractures, disuse atrophy, and pressure ulcers (although rare)
  - May be at increased risk for complications from unnecessary diagnostic or therapeutic medical procedures

Key nursing interventions for a patient with pain disorder

- Help patient understand what's contributing to his pain; encourage him to recognize situations that precipitate his pain.
- Offer attention at times other than when patient complains of pain, to weaken the link to secondary gain.
- Provide nonpharmacologic comfort measures whenever possible.
- Teach patient coping strategies to help him deal with the pain.

Characteristics of conversion disorder

- Marked by loss of or change in voluntary motor or sensory functioning that suggests a physical illness but has no demonstrable physiologic basis
- Specific symptom or deficit has psychological basis
- Exacerbation during times of emotional stress
- Relief of stress or inner conflict provided by the symptom
- Attention, support, or avoidance of responsibilities provided by the symptom
- Rare
- Most common somatoform disorder in children and adolescents
- Rarely chronic
- About one-third of patients also have somatization disorder

Key facts about factitious disorders

- Conditions in which patient deliberately produces or exaggerates symptoms of a physical or mental illness to assume the role of a sick person
- Main types: Factitious disorders with physical symptoms (Munchausen syndrome); factitious disorders with psychological symptoms

Munchausen syndrome
Symptoms are:
- fabricated
- self-inflicted
- an exacerbation or exaggeration of preexisting disorder
- a combination of above

Factitious disorders with psychological symptoms
- Almost always coexist with a severe personality disorder
- History of psychoactive substance abuse

Facts about factitious disorders

Factitious disorders are conditions in which a patient deliberately produces or exaggerates symptoms of a physical or mental illness to assume the role of a sick person. These disorders aren't a form of malingering (pretending illness for a clear benefit such as financial gain). Instead, the patient has a deep-seated need to be seen as ill or injured.

Patients create their symptoms using various methods — injecting themselves with bacteria to produce infections, contaminating urine samples with blood, taking hallucinogens, or other behaviors.

Except for factitious disorders that occur by proxy, these disorders are more common in men than in women. The *Diagnostic and Statistical Manual of Mental Disorders,* Fourth Edition, Text Revision (*DSM-IV-TR*) recognizes four types of factitious disorders, categorized according to the predominant type of symptoms:
- predominantly psychological symptoms
- predominantly physical symptoms
- combined psychological and physical symptoms
- factitious disorder not otherwise specified.

FACTITIOUS DISORDERS WITH PHYSICAL SYMPTOMS

In factitious disorders with physical symptoms (also called *Munchausen syndrome*), the patient convincingly presents with intentionally feigned physical symptoms. These symptoms may be:
- fabricated (as in acute abdominal pain without underlying disease)
- self-inflicted (as by deliberately infecting an open wound)
- an exacerbation or exaggeration of a preexisting disorder (as from taking penicillin despite a known allergy to it)
- a combination of these symptoms.

Some patients with this type of factitious disorder go so far as to have major surgery repeatedly.

History lessons
The typical patient with Munchausen syndrome is an unmarried male who's estranged from his family. His history may include:
- multiple admissions to various hospitals, typically across a wide geographic area
- extensive knowledge of medical terminology

- If patient has a dependent personality, may encourage her to take on the role of a chronic invalid
- In the general population, conversion disorder is rare; however, in general hospitals, roughly 5% to 15% of psychiatric consultations are for conversion disorders
  - Affects two to five times more females than males
  - More prevalent in rural populations and in persons with less education and lower socioeconomic status
  - With males, more prevalent in occupational settings or military service
  - Usually begins in adolescence or early adulthood, although onset can occur at any age
- Conversion disorder is the most common somatoform disorder in children and adolescents
  - May reflect stress in family or in school rather than long-term psychiatric problem

- pathologic lying
- shifting complaints, signs, and symptoms
- poor interpersonal relationships
- refusal of psychiatric examination
- psychoactive substance or analgesic use
- eagerness to undergo hazardous, painful procedures
- evidence of previous treatments such as surgery
- discharge against medical advice to avoid detection.

FACTITIOUS DISORDERS WITH PSYCHOLOGICAL SYMPTOMS

In factitious disorders with psychological symptoms, the patient's symptoms suggest a mental disorder such as schizophrenia. For instance, he may report hallucinations, or he may seem confused or make absurd statements. However, the feigned symptoms represent how he views the mental disorder and seldom conform to those described in the *DSM-IV-TR*.

This disorder almost always coexists with a severe personality disorder. Most patients have a history of psychoactive substance use — and may use such substances to try to elicit the desired symptoms.

FACTITIOUS DISORDERS WITH COMBINED PSYCHOLOGICAL AND PHYSICAL SYMPTOMS

In the combined form of factitious disorder, both psychological and physical symptoms are present, but neither predominates.

FACTITIOUS DISORDERS NOT OTHERWISE SPECIFIED

A patient whose factitious symptoms don't meet the criteria for a specific factitious disorder is diagnosed with factitious disorder not otherwise specified. An example is Munchausen syndrome by proxy, in which the patient's goal is to assume the sick role indirectly.

In Munchausen syndrome by proxy, the person (typically a parent) intentionally produces or causes a physical illness in another person (most commonly a child) through such actions as:
- falsifying the child's medical history
- tampering with laboratory tests to make the child appear sick
- injecting toxic substances into the child
- tampering with treatments (for instance, I.V. or ventilator settings)
- biting or mutilating the child.

- – Usually associated with an overprotective or overinvolved parent with a subconscious need to see child sick
- – Child's symptoms the center of family attention
- Conversion disorder is rarely chronic
  - – In hospitalized patients, generally improves within 2 weeks
  - – In about 90% of patients, recovery within 1 month
  - – In about 20% to 25% of patients, recurrence of symptoms within 1 year
- About one-third of patients with conversion reaction also have somatization disorder (see "Somatization disorder," page 196)

● Causes
- May have both biological and psychological components
- More symptoms on left side of body, suggesting that brain's left hemisphere (where verbal capacities are centralized) somehow blocks impulses carrying painful emotional content from right hemisphere

Common causes of conversion disorder

- Biological and psychological components
- Psychodynamic theory: defense mechanism neutralizes anxiety
- Sudden onset of conversion symptoms

Key signs and symptoms of conversion disorder

- Possible sudden onset of single, debilitating sign or symptom that prevents normal function of affected body part
- Weakness
- Paralysis
- Sensation loss in a specific body part
- Pseudoseizures
- Loss of a special sense, such as vision, hearing, or touch
- Aphonia
- Dysphagia
- Impaired balance or coordination
- Sensation of a lump in the throat
- Symptoms that rarely conform fully to known anatomic and physiologic mechanisms underlying true physical disorder

Diagnosing conversion disorder

- Neurologic evaluation
- Laboratory tests
- Computed tomography
- Magnetic resonance imaging
- Chest X-ray
- Lumbar puncture
- EEG

- Psychodynamic theory: defense mechanism that absorbs and neutralizes the anxiety evoked by unacceptable impulse or wish
  - Involves repression of unconscious intrapsychic conflicts
  - Leads to conversion of anxiety into physical symptom
- In many cases, sudden onset of conversion symptoms—soon after patient experiences traumatic conflict she feels she can't cope with
  - Two theories
    - Achievement of primary gain as the symptom, keeping psychological distress out of conscious awareness
    - Achievement of secondary gain by avoiding a traumatic activity

● **Risk factors**
- History of histrionic personality disorder (marked by excessive emotionality and attention seeking)
  - Children more likely to have conversion disorder if their family members have history of the disorder or are seriously ill or in chronic pain
  - In some children and adolescents, conversion disorder linked to physical or sexual abuse within the family

● **Signs and symptoms**
- In history, possible sudden onset of single, debilitating sign or symptom that prevents normal function of the affected body part
  - Weakness
  - Paralysis
  - Sensation loss in a specific body part
- Pseudoseizures (seizurelike attacks that are thought to be psychogenically produced)
- Loss of a special sense, such as vision (blindness or double vision), hearing (deafness), or touch
- Aphonia (inability to use the voice)
- Dysphagia (difficulty swallowing)
- Impaired balance or coordination
- Sensation of a lump in the throat
- Urine retention
- Possible symptom onset after traumatic event (patient report)
- In many, tendency to not show concern about symptoms or functional limitations (called *la belle indifference*—French for "beautiful indifference"), a hallmark of the disorder
- Symptoms that rarely conform fully to known anatomic and physiologic mechanisms underlying true physical disorder

● **Diagnosis**
- With many, diagnosis considered only after extensive physical examination and laboratory tests fail to reveal physical disorder that fully accounts for symptoms (physical findings inconsistent with complaints); tests depend on symptoms
  - Neurologic evaluation to rule out physical illnesses that affect sensory function (for instance, blindness or anesthesia) or voluntary motor function (such as paralysis or the inability to walk or stand)
  - Laboratory tests to eliminate such conditions as hypoglycemia or hyperglycemia; electrolyte disturbances; renal failure; systemic infection; presence of toxins; and effects of prescribed, over-the-counter, or illicit drugs

– Tests to rule out diseases with vague onset (such as multiple sclerosis or systemic lupus erythematosus)
- In some patients, other diagnostic procedures
  – Computed tomography or magnetic resonance imaging scans (to exclude a space-occupying lesion in the brain or spinal cord)
  – Chest X-ray (to rule out neoplasms)
  – Lumbar puncture for spinal fluid analysis (to rule out infection and other causes of neurologic symptoms)
  – EEG (to help distinguish pseudoseizures from true seizures)
- Diagnosis confirmed if *DSM-IV-TR* criteria met

● Treatment

- A trusting clinician-patient relationship essential; in many cases, simply reassuring the patient that the symptom doesn't indicate a serious underlying disorder makes her feel better and leads to symptom disappearance
- Psychotherapy, family therapy, relaxation training, behavior modification, biofeedback training, or hypnosis, alone or in combination; however, none uniformly effective
  – **Family therapy is treatment of choice for child or adolescent**
  – In hypnosis, hypnotist identifies and explores psychological issues with hypnotized patient; discussion continued after hypnosis session, when patient fully alert
- Narcoanalysis, a type of psychotherapy that uses barbiturates to induce release of suppressed or repressed thoughts
- Benzodiazepines, such as lorazepam and alprazolam

● Nursing interventions

- Establish a supportive relationship that communicates acceptance of the patient but keeps the focus away from her symptoms (helps patient learn to recognize and express anxiety)
  – Conveying a caring attitude that encourages her to share feelings (remember, never force the patient to talk)
  – Encouraging her to seek psychiatric care if she isn't already receiving it
  – Helping the patient identify emotional conflicts that preceded symptom onset (to help clarify the link between the conflict and the symptom without implying that the symptoms are all in her head)
- **Help the patient find appropriate ways to increase her coping ability, reduce anxiety, and enhance self-esteem**
  – Through social interaction (also helps decrease the patient's self-involvement)
  – With constructive coping mechanisms (encourages the patient to relinquish the "sick" role)
- Provide for the patient's physical needs while maintaining the integrity of the affected body system or part
  – Includes allowing the patient to avoid use of affected body part or body system (insisting that she use it would only anger her and impede a therapeutic relationship)
  – Involves ensuring adequate nutrition, even if the patient complains of GI distress
- Include the patient's family in her care, even if they may be contributing to her stress (they're also essential in providing support and helping her regain normal function)

Key treatment options for conversion disorder

- Psychotherapy
- Family therapy
- Relaxation training
- Behavior modification
- Biofeedback training
- Hypnosis

Key nursing interventions for a patient with conversion disorder

- Establish a supportive relationship.
- Help patient find appropriate ways to increase her coping ability, reduce anxiety, and enhance self-esteem.
- Provide for patient's physical needs.
- Include patient's family in her care.

Characteristics of somatization disorder

- Multiple and often vague physical complaints that suggest a physical disorder but have no physical basis
- Complaints may involve any body system and commonly persist or recur for years
- Patients may have impairments in occupational, social, and other functioning; may become extremely dependent in their relationships
- Affects about 0.2% to 2% of general population
- Usually, symptoms begin before age 30

SOMATIZATION DISORDER

● **Defining characteristics**
- Somatization disorder is characterized by multiple and often vague physical complaints that suggest a physical disorder but have no physical basis
- Complaints may involve any body system and commonly persist or recur for years
  - May begin or worsen after job loss, death of close relative or friend, or some other loss
  - May intensify with stress
- Patients with somatization disorder may have impairments in occupational, social, and other functioning and may become extremely dependent in their relationships
  - In many cases, have lifelong history of sickliness and relate to others only through their symptoms (presence of symptoms helps them avoid responsibilities)
  - May increasingly demand help and emotional support, becoming enraged if they feel needs are going unmet
  - May try to manipulate others (even going so far as to threaten or attempt suicide); often desire to be cared for in every aspect of life
- Many patients with somatization disorder attempt to prevent themselves from experiencing pleasure, possibly serving as punishment for underlying feelings of unworthiness and guilt
- Commonly, patients undergo repeated medical evaluations, which (unlike the symptoms themselves) can be potentially damaging and debilitating
  - If dissatisfied with provider or medical care received, seeks out another physician and presses for more tests, treatments, possibly unnecessary surgery
  - Even with a satisfactory relationship with one physician, usually continues to request specialist consultations and referrals
  - Unlike patient with hypochondriasis, isn't preoccupied with belief that she has a specific disease
- The disorder affects an estimated 0.2% to 2% of the general population; it's about 10 times more common in females (possibly reflecting cultural pressures on women or greater social "permission" for women to be physically weak or sickly)
- Usually, symptoms begin before age 30 (commonly in adolescence or early adulthood); few patients are asymptomatic or go more than 1 or 2 years without seeking medical attention
- Somatization disorder is a chronic condition, with a fluctuating course and a poor prognosis
  - Rarely associated with complete, spontaneous remission
  - Most patients disabled for much of their lives
- Somatization disorder often coexists with other psychiatric conditions, including major depression and anxiety
  - In many cases, concomitant antisocial personality disorder, alcohol or substance abuse, and suicidal behavior (although patients rarely complete suicide)

— Increases risk of substance abuse and drug toxicity because of polypharmacy and drug interactions (from prescriptions written by multiple providers)

Causes

- No specific cause; genetic, biological, environmental, and psychological factors may contribute
- May perceive and process pain differently from others; may also have lower pain threshold, which increases sensitivity to physical sensations
- Possible genetic component (tends to run in families)
  - Occurs in 10% to 20% of primary female relatives of patients with the disorder
  - Among primary male relatives, increased incidence of alcoholism, drug abuse, and antisocial personality disorder
- Probably involves underlying feelings of depression, anxiety, or other distress, which the patient doesn't recognize
- Linked with child abuse (particularly sexual) in recent studies

Signs and symptoms

- Involving any body system, but most commonly GI, neurologic, cardiopulmonary, or reproductive
- Many complaining of multiple symptoms at same time (see *Common assessment findings in somatization disorder,* page 198)
- Having history of multiple medical evaluations by different physicians at different health care facilities (sometimes simultaneously), without significant findings
- Reporting complaints and previous medical evaluations in dramatic, vague or, conversely, highly detailed fashion
  - Has complicated medical history (many physical diagnoses considered)
  - May seem quite knowledgeable about tests, procedures, medical jargon
  - May complain that people think she's imagining symptoms
  - Has tendency to disparage previous health care professionals and previous diagnoses and treatments

Diagnosis

- Can't be verified by specific tests
- Physical examination and limited diagnostic tests to rule out physical conditions that may produce vague, confusing symptoms (such as multiple sclerosis, hypothyroidism, hyperparathyroidism, systemic lupus erythematosus, and porphyria)
- Psychological evaluation to rule out related psychiatric disorders (such as depression, schizophrenia with somatic delusions, hypochondriasis, malingering)
- Diagnosis confirmed if *DSM-IV-TR* criteria met

Treatment

- No definitive therapy
- The patient unlikely to acknowledge psychological aspect of her symptoms or to consider psychiatric treatment
- Patient interactions to help her learn to control and cope with her symptoms rather than eliminate them completely
  - Not helpful to tell the patient symptoms are imaginary

Common causes of somatization disorder

- None specific
- May have genetic, biological, environmental, and psychological influence
- May perceive and process pain differently
- May involve underlying feelings of depression, anxiety, distress
- Linked with child abuse

Key signs and symptoms of somatization disorder

- Involves any body system, but most commonly GI, neurologic, cardiopulmonary, or reproductive
- Many sufferers complain of multiple symptoms at same time
- History of multiple medical evaluations by different physicians at different health care facilities, without significant findings
- Complicated medical history
- Patient may seem quite knowledgeable about tests, procedures, medical jargon
- Patient may complain that people think she's imagining symptoms
- Patient has tendency to disparage previous health care professionals and previous diagnoses and treatments

Diagnosing somatization disorder

- Psychological evaluation to rule out related psychiatric disorders

Body systems commonly affected by somatization disorder

- Cardiopulmonary
- Reproductive
- GI
- Central nervous system

Common assessment findings in somatization disorder

Signs and symptoms of somatization disorder may mimic actual disorders and are just as real to the patient as the physical disorders that can cause them. They most commonly involve a few key body systems.

CARDIOPULMONARY SYMPTOMS

- Chest pain
- Dizziness
- Palpitations
- Shortness of breath (without exertion)

FEMALE REPRODUCTIVE SIGNS AND SYMPTOMS

- Excessive menstrual bleeding
- Irregular menses
- Vomiting throughout pregnancy

GI SIGNS AND SYMPTOMS

- Abdominal pain (excluding menstruation)
- Diarrhea
- Flatulence
- Intolerance to foods
- Nausea and vomiting (excluding motion sickness)

PAIN

- In extremities
- In the back
- During urination

PSEUDONEUROLOGIC SIGNS AND SYMPTOMS

- Amnesia
- Blindness
- Difficulty walking, paralysis, or weakness
- Double or blurred vision
- Dysphagia
- Dysuria or urinary retention
- Fainting or loss of consciousness
- Loss of voice or hearing
- Seizures

SEXUAL SIGNS AND SYMPTOMS

- Burning sensation in sexual organs or rectum (except during intercourse)
- Dyspareunia or lack of pleasure during sex
- Impotence
- Sexual indifference

Key treatment options for somatization disorder

- No definitive therapy
- Management focus: preventing unnecessary medical and surgical interventions; turning patient's attention away from symptoms

  – Commonly helpful to tell the patient that, although she doesn't have a serious illness, she'll continue to receive care to ease symptoms
- Management focus: preventing unnecessary medical and surgical interventions and turning the patient's attention away from symptoms
  – Ideally, should have a continuing, supportive relationship with one empathic health care provider rather than multiple providers
  – More providers involved creates greater opportunity for manipulation and unnecessary medical intervention
- Provider supporting healthy and adaptive behaviors, and encouraging patient to move beyond somatization and manage life effectively
- For the patient with a coexisting depressive or anxiety disorder, a possible benefit from antidepressant drugs, such as SSRIs or monoamine oxidase inhibitors, to ease preoccupation with symptoms

● **Nursing interventions**
  • Always remember that your goal is to help the patient manage her symptoms, not eliminate them
  • Acknowledge the patient's symptoms, and support her efforts to function and cope despite distress
    – By avoiding any mention that symptoms are imaginary
    – By informing her of diagnostic test results and their implications
    – By gently pointing out link between stressful events and onset of troublesome symptoms
    – By emphasizing patient's strengths
  • Keep in mind that interpersonal relationships are commonly linked to symptoms and that remedying the symptoms may impair the patient's interactions with others (including family members and health care providers)
  • Negotiate a care plan with input from the patient and, if possible, her family; encourage and help them to understand her need for troublesome symptoms
  • Check your own feelings and attitudes periodically
    – Acknowledging your feelings honestly
    – If appropriate, consulting a psychiatric clinical nurse specialist to help you develop an effective way to deal with your feelings

NCLEX CHECKS

It's never too soon to begin your NCLEX preparation. Now that you've reviewed this chapter, carefully read each of the following questions and choose the best answer. Then compare your responses to the correct answers.

1. The nurse correctly interprets manifestations of physical symptoms caused by psychological distress as indicative of which disorder?
  ☐ **1.** Pain disorder
  ☐ **2.** Somatization
  ☐ **3.** Conversion disorder
  ☐ **4.** Munchausen syndrome

2. A patient states, "Look at this scar. It's so huge and so horrible. How can I ever go out in public again? Everyone will think I'm such a freak." Further assessment reveals a hairline scar about 2" (5 cm) long located just under the patient's chin line on the left side. The patient is observed continually looking at herself in the mirror and touching the area. Based on these findings, the nurse would suspect:
  ☐ **1.** BDD.
  ☐ **2.** conversion disorder.
  ☐ **3.** hypochondriasis.
  ☐ **4.** somatization.

3. A patient with BDD is receiving behavioral therapy that involves the application of a painful stimuli to modify her obsession with a perceived defect. The nurse knows that this technique is a form of:
  ☐ **1.** thought stopping.
  ☐ **2.** aversion therapy.
  ☐ **3.** implosion therapy.
  ☐ **4.** response prevention.

TOP 10

Items to study for your next test on somatoform disorders

1. Six disorders classified as somatoform disorders
2. Major causes and contributing factors associated with somatoform disorders
3. Four psychobiological mechanisms involved with somatoform disorders
4. Four stress-related disorders in children
5. Defining characteristics of BDD
6. Treatment goals for a patient with BDD
7. Common physical, sensory, and motor complaints associated with hypochondriasis
8. Key assessment findings in pain disorder
9. Key treatment options for conversion disorder
10. Common assessment findings in somatization disorder

4. A patient comes to the clinic reporting a sudden onset of paralysis in the legs. A thorough history and physical examination along with numerous diagnostic tests fail to reveal a physical disorder. The history does reveal that the patient had recently been treated for stress after witnessing a multivehicle accident in which several people died. The nurse interprets these findings as suggesting which condition?

☐ **1.** Hypochondriasis
☐ **2.** Somatization disorder
☐ **3.** Conversion disorder
☐ **4.** Pain disorder

5. Misinterpretation of bodily sensations or symptoms is a chief feature of:

☐ **1.** BDD.
☐ **2.** somatization disorder.
☐ **3.** conversion disorder.
☐ **4.** hypochondriasis.

6. Review of the medical record of a 3-year-old child reveals episodes of sleep terrors. The nurse understands that these episodes characteristically involve:

☐ **1.** abnormal repetitions and hesitations with words and speech rhythms.
☐ **2.** involuntary voiding of urine at night.
☐ **3.** arising from bed in an altered state of consciousness and walking with no recollection of dream content.
☐ **4.** sudden awakening in a clouded state of consciousness with the inability to recognize parents and surroundings.

7. When assessing a patient with BDD, the nurse would be alert for manifestations of which additional psychiatric disorders? Select all that apply:

☐ **1.** Depression
☐ **2.** OCD
☐ **3.** Anorexia nervosa
☐ **4.** Bipolar disorder
☐ **5.** Schizophrenia

8. Which intervention would the nurse include in the care plan for a patient with hypochondriasis?

☐ **1.** Engage the patient in conversations that focus on the physical symptoms.
☐ **2.** Challenge the patient's beliefs about the pain and distress caused by the symptoms.
☐ **3.** Respond to the patient's complaints in a matter-of-fact manner.
☐ **4.** Administer antipsychotic agents to control the patient's delusions about her symptoms.

9. After teaching a class about factitious disorders, which statement would lead the instructor to determine that additional teaching is necessary?

☐ **1.** "Factitious disorders, a form of malingering, involve feigning an illness."
☐ **2.** "Patients with factitious disorders have a need to be seen as sick."
☐ **3.** "Contaminating urine samples is one method used to create symptoms."
☐ **4.** "Factitious disorders, except for those by proxy, are more common in men than in women."

10. Which drug would the nurse least expect to administer to a patient with BDD?
- ☐ **1.** Fluvoxamine (Luvox)
- ☐ **2.** Lithium (Eskalith)
- ☐ **3.** Clomipramine (Anafranil)
- ☐ **4.** Paroxetine (Paxil)

ANSWERS AND RATIONALES

1. CORRECT ANSWER: 2

Somatization occurs when a psychological state causes or contributes to the development of physical symptoms. Pain disorder involves complaints of persistent pain resulting predominantly from psychological factors. Conversion disorder is marked by the loss or change in voluntary motor or sensory function, suggesting a physical illness but without any demonstrable physiologic cause. Munchausen syndrome is a factitious disorder in which the patient intentionally feigns physical symptoms, thereby filling a deep-seated need to be seen as ill.

2. CORRECT ANSWER: 1

In BDD, the patient is preoccupied with an imagined or actual slight defect in physical appearance, which is the focus of attention. In conversion disorder, the patient experiences a sudden onset of a single debilitating sign or symptom (such as blindness, muscle weakness, or difficulty swallowing) that prevents normal functioning. With hypochondriasis, the patient has multiple complaints that involve a single body system but that rarely follow a recognizable pattern and aren't associated with abnormal physical findings. Somatization refers to the conversion of emotional or mental states into bodily symptoms.

3. CORRECT ANSWER: 2

In aversion therapy, a painful stimulus is applied to create an aversion to an obsessive thought that leads to an undesirable behavior. Thought stopping involves the use of an intense distracting stimulus to help the patient stop the offending thought and then focus on achieving calmness and muscle relaxation. Implosion therapy (flooding) exposes the patient to images of the perceived flaw for prolonged periods until they no longer cause distress. Response prevention uses distraction, persuasion, or redirection to prevent compulsive behavior.

4. CORRECT ANSWER: 3

In conversion disorder, symptoms suggest a physical disorder, but physical examination and diagnostic tests find no physiologic cause. The symptoms typically arise suddenly—soon after the patient experiences a traumatic conflict with which she's unable to cope. With hypochondriasis, the patient has multiple complaints that involve a single body system but that rarely follow a recognizable pattern and aren't associated with abnormal physical findings. Somatization disorder is characterized by multiple, typically vague physical complaints that suggest a physical disorder but have no physical basis; the symptoms are recurrent. With pain disorder, the patient complains of persistent pain, which becomes the patient's primary focus of attention and causes significant distress.

5. CORRECT ANSWER: 4

A patient with hypochondriasis misinterprets the severity and significance of bodily sensations or symptoms as indications of illness. A patient with BDD is preoccupied with an imagined or slight defect in physical appearance, which becomes the focus of attention and causes much distress. Somatization disorder involves multiple, recurring physical complaints suggesting a physical disorder, but with no real physical basis. In conversion disorder, the patient suddenly develops a single sign or symptom (blindness, muscle weakness, paralysis) that prevents normal functioning. With hypochondriasis, the patient has multiple complaints involving a single body system (GI, reproductive) that typically don't follow a recognizable pattern and aren't supported by physical findings.

6. CORRECT ANSWER: 4

Sleep terrors are considered a normal developmental occurrence in children ages 2 and 3. Typically, the child awakens terrified, in a state of clouded consciousness, typically unable to recognize parents and familiar surroundings. Stuttering refers to abnormal speech rhythms, with repetitions and hesitations at the beginning of words. Functional enuresis describes the involuntary voiding of urine at night. Sleepwalking involves rising calmly from the bed in an altered state of consciousness and walking about with no recollection of dream content.

7. CORRECT ANSWER: 1, 2, 3

The patient with BDD may have additional psychiatric disorders, including depression, OCD, eating disorders (anorexia nervosa, bulimia nervosa), anxiety disorders, agoraphobia, and trichotillomania. BDD isn't typically associated with bipolar disorder or schizophrenia.

8. CORRECT ANSWER: 3

When dealing with hypochondriasis, the nurse should respond to the patient's complaints in a matter-of-fact manner to reduce the secondary gain received from talking about them. The nurse also should engage the patient in conversations that focus on something other than the physical symptoms and should avoid challenging and denying the patient's symptoms because the pain and distress experienced by the patient are real. Benzodiazepines, SSRIs, and TCAs—not antipsychotic agents—may be used to treat the patient with hypochondriasis.

9. CORRECT ANSWER: 1

Factitious disorders are conditions in which the patient deliberately produces or exaggerates symptoms of a physical or mental illness to assume the role of the sick person. These disorders are not a form of malingering. Patients with factitious disorders have a deep-seated need to be seen as ill or injured. Patients create their symptoms using various methods, such as injecting themselves with bacteria to produce infection, contaminating urine samples, and taking hallucinogens. Factitious disorders are more common in men than in women, except for those that occur by proxy.

10. CORRECT ANSWER: 2

Lithium, neuroleptics, trazodone, and benzodiazepines are usually ineffective in treating BDD and may even exacerbate the symptoms. Luvox and Paxil are both SSRIs, which have been used successfully in treating BDD. Anafranil, a TCA, also has proved effective in treating patients with BDD.

8

Dissociative disorders

LEARNING OBJECTIVES

After studying this chapter, you should be able to:

- Describe the general characteristics of dissociation.
- Identify the diagnostic tools clinicians use to evaluate dissociative disorders.
- State the proposed causes of dissociative disorders.
- List common signs and symptoms of dissociative disorders.
- Identify and characterize the different types of dissociative disorders.
- Discuss how to assess, treat, and intervene for patients with various dissociative disorders.

CHAPTER OVERVIEW

Dissociative disorders are marked by disruption of the fundamental aspects of waking consciousness — memory, identity, consciousness, and the general experience and perception of oneself and one's surroundings. The patient uses dissociation as an unconscious defense mechanism to separate anxiety-provoking feelings and thoughts from the conscious mind.

Dissociation is a common occurrence that ranges from normal to pathologic. Normal types of dissociation include daydreams, "highway hypnosis" (a trancelike feeling that can occur when driving), and getting "lost" in a book, movie, or television program to the point that the person doesn't notice the time or his surroundings. Pathologic dissociation occurs in dissociative disorders.

Characteristics of dissociative disorders

- Rare
- Disturbances in the normal waking state
- Affect fundamental aspects of consciousness, memory, identity, self-perception, and perception of the environment
- Result from overwhelming stress caused by a traumatic event that the person witnessed or experienced, or by some intolerable internal conflict

Types of dissociative disorders

- Depersonalization disorder
- Dissociative amnesia
- Dissociative fugue
- Dissociative identity disorder

Theories for dissociative disorders

- Psychological theories
- Biological theories
- Learning theory

UNDERSTANDING DISSOCIATIVE DISORDERS

- **General information**
  - Dissociative disorders are a group of rare disorders characterized by disturbances in the normal waking state
  - Dissociative disorders affect fundamental aspects of consciousness, memory, identity, self-perception, and perception of the environment (patient's surroundings)
  - These disorders result from overwhelming stress caused by a traumatic event that the person witnessed or experienced, or by some intolerable internal conflict
  - The state of dissociation is a poorly understood phenomenon; some experts believe it's a common defense mechanism used by children who have been traumatized, especially by abuse
  - *Diagnostic and Statistical Manual of Mental Disorders,* Fourth Edition, Text Revision (*DSM-IV-TR*) classifies dissociative disorders as four types
    - Depersonalization disorder
    - Dissociative amnesia
    - Dissociative fugue
    - Dissociative identity disorder (DID)
  - Dissociative disorders (especially dissociative amnesia) gained significant attention in recent years, largely as a result of lawsuits involving allegations based on "forgotten" childhood traumas and repressed memories
  - Dissociative disorders tend to affect more females than males; symptoms can arise suddenly or gradually
    - In many cases, involve transient episodes of dissociation
    - May cause functional impairment if episodes persist

CAUSES

- **Psychological theories**
  - Dissociative disorders are believed to be a response to severe trauma or abuse
  - To cope with the trauma or abuse, the patient tries to repress the unpleasant experience from awareness
  - If repression fails, dissociation occurs as a defense mechanism — the patient separates the experience from the conscious mind because it's too traumatic to integrate it

- **Biological theories**
  - Biological theories are most closely linked with depersonalization disorder
  - Depersonalization disorder shares a key symptom — a sense of loss of one's own reality — with certain neurologic disorders (such as epilepsy and tumors), several psychiatric disorders, and the effects of certain drugs (most notably, barbiturates, benzodiazepines, and hallucinogens)

- **Learning theory**
  - According to this theory, dissociative disorders represent a learned response of avoiding stress and anxiety
  - With opportunity and practice, a person can become highly skilled at dissociating

- This learned behavior of forcing the memory from awareness is common in people with a history of abuse

EVALUATION AND DIAGNOSIS

● Physical and psychological evaluation

- Because dissociative disorders can mimic various physical illnesses or other psychiatric disorders, the patient should undergo a complete physical examination
- A mental health evaluation should include a careful personal history from the patient and family members
- The interview should include questions about childhood and adult trauma and past experiences
  - Blackouts or "lost" time
  - Fugues—travel away from home with no memory of what happened on these trips
  - Unexplained possessions
  - Relationship changes
  - Fluctuations in skills and knowledge
  - Unclear or spotty recollection of the life history
  - Spontaneous trances
  - Spontaneous age regression
  - Out-of-body experiences
  - Awareness of other personalities within oneself

● Diagnostic tools

- Several tools are used to aid in diagnosing dissociative disorders (see *Diagnostic tools*)

Diagnostic tools

The Dissociative Experiences Scale is a brief, self-report scale that measures the frequency of dissociative experiences. It involves quantifying experiences for each item. A high score requires further evaluation using the Dissociative Disorders Interview Schedule or the Structured Clinical Interview for Dissociative Disorders (SCID-D).

DISSOCIATIVE DISORDERS INTERVIEW SCHEDULE

- A highly structured interview used to diagnose trauma-related disorders
- Involves having the patient answer questions that the examiner must ask in a precisely designated order
- Usually takes 30 to 45 minutes

SCID-D

- A semi-structured interview that assesses the nature and severity of five dissociative symptoms

- Assesses amnesia, depersonalization, derealization, identity confusion, and identity alteration
- Allows the clinician to diagnose a dissociative disorder based on *DSM-IV-TR* criteria

DIAGNOSTIC DRAWING SERIES

- Used by art therapists to aid the diagnosis of dissociative disorders

---

Characteristics of depersonalization disorder

- Persistent or recurrent feeling of being detached from the person's own mental processes or body
- Patient's self-awareness is altered or temporarily lost
- Patient may perceive change in consciousness as barrier between herself and outside world
- Patient may feel as if she's passively watching mental or physical activity
- Patient may feel that external world is unreal or distorted
- Sudden onset, usually occurring in adolescence or early adulthood
- Symptom of depersonalization is brief and has no lasting effects
- Typically progresses; in many patients becomes chronic, with exacerbations and remissions
- Resolution usually occurs gradually

Common causes of depersonalization disorder

- Exact cause unknown
- Severe stress
- History of physical, mental, or substance abuse
- History of obsessive-compulsive disorder
- Sensory deprivation
- Neurophysiologic factors

DEPERSONALIZATION DISORDER

● Defining characteristics

- Depersonalization disorder is marked by a persistent or recurrent feeling of being detached from the person's own mental processes or body
    - Seldom involves losing complete touch with reality
    - May cause severe distress and sometimes impairs functioning
- During episodes of depersonalization, the patient's self-awareness (or a portion of it) is altered or temporarily lost
    - May be restricted to a single body part (such as a limb) or may encompass the whole self
    - May include feeling as if a body part or the entire body has shrunk or grown
- The patient may perceive the change in consciousness as a barrier between herself and the outside world, feeling as if she's passively watching mental or physical activity or as if the external world is unreal or distorted
- The *experience* of depersonalization occurs in many "normal" people for brief periods (not to be confused with a psychiatric disorder)
    - Sometimes described as feeling "spaced out," as if in a dream, or as looking at the self from the outside
    - Occurs with intoxication, in which person feels out of control of his actions
- In clinical settings, depersonalization is the third leading psychiatric symptom reported
    - Follows life-threatening danger (such as accidents, assaults, and serious illnesses and injuries) in many patients
    - Can occur as a symptom of many psychiatric disorders, and seizure disorders
- Depersonalization symptoms also can arise from meditation or from certain religious or cultural practices
    - Meditative and trancelike states (may mimic symptoms seen in depersonalization disorder)
    - Possession trance, in which a person's customary identity is replaced with a new identity attributed to the influence of a deity, spirit, or power (may display involuntary movements that appear to be beyond the person's experience and control)
- Onset of depersonalization disorder is sudden, usually occurring in adolescence or early adulthood
- The symptom of depersonalization is brief and has no lasting effects; however, the disorder typically progresses and in many patients becomes chronic, with exacerbations and remissions; resolution usually occurs gradually

● Causes

- Exact cause unknown; not studied widely as separate disorder
- Typically occurs in people who have experienced severe stress, such as combat, violent crime, accidents, or natural disasters
- Other factors linked to development
    - Sensory deprivation
    - Neurophysiologic factors, such as epilepsy or a concussion
    - History of physical or mental abuse

– History of substance abuse

– History of obsessive-compulsive disorder

Signs and symptoms

- Feeling detached from her entire being and body, as if watching herself from a distance or living in a dream
- May report sensory anesthesia, loss of self-control, difficulty speaking, and feelings of losing touch with reality
- Obsessive rumination
- Depression
- Anxiety
- Fear of going insane
- Disturbed sense of time
- Slow recall
- Physical complaints, such as dizziness
- Impaired social and occupational functioning

Diagnosis

- Steps to rule out physical disorders, substance abuse, and other dissociative disorders
- Psychological tests and special interviews to aid diagnosis
- Standard tests, including the Dissociative Experiences Scale and the Dissociative Disorders Interview Schedule, to demonstrate presence of dissociation
- Diagnosis confirmed if *DSM-IV-TR* criteria met

Treatment

- Many recover completely, even without treatment
- Warranted when the condition is persistent, recurrent, or distressing
  - Psychotherapy
  - Cognitive-behavior therapy
  - Hypnosis
  - Pharmacologic agents
- Identifying and addressing all stressors linked to onset
- If linked to a traumatic event, psychotherapy to help the patient recognize the event and the anxiety it has evoked; the therapist teaches the patient to use reality-based coping strategies instead of detaching herself from the situation
- Selective serotonin reuptake inhibitors (SSRIs) and the tricyclic antidepressant (TCA) clomipramine (Anafranil); tranquilizers may also be prescribed

Nursing interventions

- Establish a therapeutic, nonjudgmental relationship with the patient
- If she experienced a traumatic event, encourage her to recognize that depersonalization is a defense mechanism she's using to deal with anxiety caused by the trauma
- Help the patient recognize and deal with anxiety-producing experiences by implementing behavioral techniques to cope with stressful situations, if appropriate
- Assist the patient in establishing supportive relationships

Key signs and symptoms of depersonalization disorder

- Feeling detached from entire being and body or loss of touch with reality
- Sensory anesthesia
- Loss of self-control
- Difficulty speaking
- Obsessive rumination
- Disturbed sense of time

Diagnosing depersonalization disorder

- Rule out physical disorders
- Psychological tests and special interviews
- Confirmed if *DSM-IV-TR* criteria met

Key treatment options for depersonalization disorder

- Many recover without treatment
- Treated when condition persistent, recurrent, or distressing
- Psychotherapy
- Cognitive-behavior therapy
- Hypnosis
- Drugs (SSRIs, TCAs)
- Identifying and addressing all stressors linked to onset

Key nursing interventions for a patient with depersonalization disorder

- Establish therapeutic, nonjudgmental relationship with patient.
- Encourage patient to recognize that depersonalization is a defense mechanism.
- Recognize and deal with anxiety-producing experiences.
- Assist patient in establishing supportive relationships.

Characteristics of dissociative amnesia

- Key feature: Inability to recall important personal information that can't be explained by ordinary forgetfulness
- Forgetting basic autobiographical information
- Acute memory loss triggered by severe psychological stress
- Most patients aware that they have "lost" some time

Types of dissociative amnesia

- Localized
- Selective
- Generalized
- Continuous
- Systematized

DISSOCIATIVE AMNESIA

● Defining characteristics

- The key feature of dissociative amnesia is an inability to recall important personal information (usually of a stressful nature) that can't be explained by ordinary forgetfulness
- Commonly, the patient forgets basic autobiographical information, such as her name; people she spoke to recently; and what she said, thought, experienced, or felt recently
- In most cases, the acute memory loss is triggered by severe psychological stress
- Recovery is usually complete and recurrence rare, although the patient may never be able to recall certain life events
- Dissociative amnesia occurs as five main types
  - Localized amnesia: patient can't remember events that took place during a specific period of time—usually, the first few hours after an extremely stressful or traumatic event
  - Selective amnesia: patient can recall some, but not all, of the events during a circumscribed time period (for instance, a soldier may be able to recall only some parts of a violent combat experience)
  - Generalized amnesia: patient suffers prolonged loss of memory—possibly encompassing an entire lifetime
  - Continuous amnesia: patient forgets all events from a given time forward to the present
  - Systematized amnesia: patient's memory loss is limited to a specific type of information (for instance, related to a specific person)
- Most patients with dissociative amnesia are aware that they have "lost" some time
  - Few reports involving "amnesia for amnesia" (in which patient realizes she has lost time only after seeing evidence of things she did but can't recall doing)
  - May or may not be distressing to the patient
- Unlike other types of amnesia, dissociative amnesia doesn't result from an organic disorder (such as a stroke or dementia) or physical trauma (such as a closed head injury)
- The condition occurs most commonly among adolescents and young women; it also may occur in young men after combat
  - May resolve quickly, but in some patients becomes chronic
  - Usually results in complete recovery; however, some never break through the barriers to reconstruct their missing past
  - Prognosis mainly dependent on life circumstances, particular stresses and conflicts associated with the amnesia, and patient's overall psychological adjustment
- During an amnesia episode, patient safety may be an issue because of impaired memory and reduced awareness of surroundings
  - May affect ability to perform self-care
  - May affect family's usual coping ability (may feel helpless to respond to patient's changed behavior), possibly leading to changed routines and strained relationships

– May also place patient at risk for being taken advantage of (such as by con artists and criminals) due to confused state

Causes

- Probably results from severe stress associated with traumatic experience, major life event, or severe internal conflict
- Possible predisposition in some people such as those easily hypnotized
- Possible contributing factors
  - Altered identity
  - Low self-esteem
  - History of a traumatic event
  - History of physical, emotional, or sexual abuse

Signs and symptoms

- During episode, patient may seem perplexed and disoriented, wandering aimlessly
  - Typically can't remember the event that precipitated the episode
  - Usually doesn't recognize her inability to recall information
  - May have mild to severe social impairment
- When episode ends, patient characteristically unaware of memory disturbance

Diagnosis

- Thorough physical examination to rule out organic cause for symptoms (can mimic many physical disorders such as head injury, brain tumor, seizure disorder, or substance use)
  - May include blood and urine tests to rule out drug use
  - May include EEG to rule out seizure disorder
- Psychiatric examination, including appropriate psychological tests
  - Diagnostic Drawing Series
  - Dissociative Experiences Scale
  - Dissociative Disorders Interview Schedule
- Diagnosis confirmed if *DSM-IV-TR* criteria met

Treatment

- Aims to help the patient recognize the traumatic event that triggered the amnesia and the anxiety it has produced
  - Involves establishing a supportive, trusting therapeutic relationship
  - Requires an accepting environment, which may in itself enable the patient to gradually recover missing memories
- Teaching of reality-based coping strategies by the psychotherapist
  - Includes filling in memory gaps to restore continuity of the patient's identity and sense of self
  - Once gaps have been filled in, helps the patient to clarify the trauma or conflicts, and to resolve problems associated with the amnesia episode
- When the need to recover memories is urgent, questioning the patient under hypnosis or in a drug-induced, semi-hypnotic state
  - Must be used cautiously, as the circumstances that triggered the memory loss are likely to be highly distressing to the patient
  - Considered controversial; external corroboration is required to validate the accuracy of "recovered" memories
- Drugs, including benzodiazepines, such as alprazolam (Xanax) and lorazepam (Ativan), and SSRIs

---

Common causes of dissociative amnesia

- Stress caused by traumatic experience
- Predisposition
- History of physical, emotional, or sexual abuse

Key signs and symptoms of dissociative amnesia

- Patient may seem perplexed and disoriented or wander aimlessly
- Can't remember event that precipitated episode
- Doesn't recognize inability to recall information
- When episode ends, unaware of memory disturbance

Diagnosing dissociative amnesia

- Physical examination to rule out organic cause of symptoms
- Psychiatric examination, including psychological tests
- Confirmed if *DSM-IV-TR* criteria met

Key treatment options for dissociative amnesia

- Helping patient recognize traumatic event trigger
- Teaching of reality-based coping strategies by psychotherapist
- When recovery is urgent, questioning patient under hypnosis or in a drug-induced, semi-hypnotic state
- Drugs (benzodiazepines and SSRIs)

Key nursing interventions for a patient with dissociative amnesia

- Establish therapeutic, nonjudgmental relationship.
- Encourage patient to verbalize feelings of distress.
- Help patient recognize that memory loss is a defense mechanism.
- Help patient deal with anxiety-producing experiences.
- Teach and assist patient in using reality-based coping strategies.
- Teach family members techniques for dealing with patient's memory loss.

Characteristics of dissociative fugue

- Sudden, unexpected travel away from home or workplace
- Inability to recall past
- Confusion about personal identity
- Occasional formation of new identity during episode
- Degree of impairment varies with duration of fugue and nature of personality state evoked
- Upon return to pre-fugue state, patient may have no memory of events that occurred during fugue
- Usually resolves rapidly

Common causes of dissociative fugue

- Precise cause unknown
- Follows extremely stressful event
- Heavy alcohol use (possible predisposing factor)

● Nursing interventions

- Establish a therapeutic, nonjudgmental relationship
- Encourage the patient to verbalize feelings of distress
  - Should avoid trying to elicit forgotten memories
  - Must keep in mind that only a mental health professional with competence in addressing unconscious memories should attempt technique
- Help the patient to recognize that memory loss is a defense mechanism used to deal with anxiety and trauma
- Help the patient deal with anxiety-producing experiences
- Teach and assist the patient in using reality-based coping strategies to deal with stress, rather than strategies that distort reality
- Teach the family about the disorder, encourage them to talk about their frustrations, and give them techniques for dealing with their family member's memory loss

DISSOCIATIVE FUGUE

● Defining characteristics

- Dissociative fugue is marked by a patient's sudden, unexpected travel away from her home or workplace, along with an inability to recall her past; the patient is typically confused about her personal identity
- Occasionally, the patient forms a new identity during a dissociative fugue
  - Assumes a new name, takes up a new residence, and engages in social activities with no hint that she has a mental disorder
  - New identity is typically more outgoing and less inhibited than the former one was
- The degree of impairment varies with the duration of the fugue and the nature of the personality state it invokes
- Travel may range from brief trips lasting hours or days to complex wandering for weeks or months; in some cases, the patient travels thousands of miles
- During the fugue, the patient may appear normal and attract no attention; however, she may show signs of distress if awareness of the memory loss develops
  - May begin to feel confused about her identity, or her original identity may return
  - May be brought to the attention of the police or taken to a hospital
- Upon return to the pre-fugue state, the patient may have no memory of the events that took place during the fugue
- Dissociative fugue is rare; it occurs in about 0.2% of the population
  - Most common among those who have experienced war, accidents, violent crimes, and natural disasters
  - May also occur in those with DID
- Dissociative fugue usually resolves rapidly
  - Good prognosis for complete recovery
  - Can recur; patients with frequent episodes may more appropriately be diagnosed with DID

● Causes

- Precise cause unknown; typically follows extremely stressful event (heavy alcohol use may be predisposing factor)

- With many fugues, seem to represent disguised wish fulfillment; some appear to protect patient from suicidal or homicidal impulses
- Also may be mechanism patient uses to unconsciously absolve herself from accountability for her actions, or to reduce her exposure to a hazard; viewed by some as form of malingering

● **Signs and symptoms**
- Often asymptomatic during fugue; others may suspect only if certain behaviors displayed
  - Seems confused about her identity or puzzled about her past
  - Grows confrontational when new identity (or absence of identity) is challenged
- Possible symptoms after fugue
  - Depression
  - Discomfort
  - Grief
  - Shame
  - Intense internal conflict
  - Suicidal or aggressive impulses
  - Confusion, distress, or even terror due to failure to remember events during fugue

● **Diagnosis**
- During a suspected fugue, psychiatric examination to aid in diagnosis (sometimes doesn't help)
  - May reveal that patient has assumed new, more uninhibited identity
  - May not be evident if patient has traveled to distant location, set up new residence, and developed well-integrated network of social relationships (if new personality is still evolving, patient may even avoid social contact)
- Psychosocial history to check for episodes of violent behavior
- May not be able to diagnose until fugue ends (patient resumes pre-fugue identity and may then show signs of distress at finding herself in unfamiliar circumstances)
- Thorough physical examination to rule out medical disorders (such as seizure disorder), or medication or substance use as the cause of symptoms
- Diagnosis confirmed if *DSM-IV-TR* criteria met

● **Treatment**
- Psychotherapy to help the patient recognize the traumatic event that triggered the fugue state, and to develop reality-based strategies for coping with anxiety; a trusting relationship is crucial for successful therapy
- Hypnosis to prompt the patient to recall events and feelings and, ultimately, to assist her in recovering her memory
- Cognitive therapy to help the patient to examine maladaptive thought patterns and to link them to irrational behaviors such as fleeing
- Group therapy to provide ongoing support and to help the patient gain self-esteem and increase socialization
- Family therapy to explore the patient's traumatic experiences while teaching family members about the disorder
- Creative therapies, such as music or art therapy, to permit the patient to explore emotions in a safe environment

---

Key signs and symptoms of dissociative fugue

- Often asymptomatic during fugue
- Confusion about identity or puzzled about past
- Confrontational when new identity (or absence of identity) is challenged
- Depression
- Discomfort
- Grief
- Shame
- Intense internal conflict
- Suicidal or aggressive impulses
- Confusion, distress, even terror due to failure to remember events during fugue

Diagnosing dissociative fugue

- Psychiatric examination (during suspected fugue)
- Psychosocial history to check for episodes of violent behavior
- May not be able to diagnose until fugue ends
- Physical examination to rule out medical disorders
- Confirmed if *DSM-IV-TR* criteria met

Key treatment options for dissociative fugue

- Psychotherapy
- Establishing trusting relationship
- Hypnosis
- Cognitive therapy
- Group therapy
- Family therapy
- Creative therapies, such as music or art therapy

Key nursing interventions for a patient with dissociative fugue

- Encourage patient to identify emotions that occur under stress.
- Monitor patient for signs of overt aggression toward self or others.
- Teach patient effective coping skills.
- Encourage patient to use available social support systems.

Characteristics of DID

- Marked by two or more distinct identities or subpersonalities
- Identities or subpersonalities recurrently take control of patient's consciousness and behavior
- Each identity may exhibit unique behavior patterns, memories, and social relationships
- In many cases, primary personality is religious, with strong moral sense, while subpersonalities are radically different
- Primary personality may be unaware of subpersonalities
- Subpersonalities are more likely aware of existence of other personalities
- Transition from one personality to another triggered by stress or meaningful social or environmental cue in many patients

Common causes of DID

- Strong connection between DID and history of severe childhood abuse

● **Nursing interventions**
- Encourage the patient to identify emotions that occur under stress
- If the patient is resolving a dissociative fugue state, monitor her for signs of overt aggression toward herself or others
- Teach the patient effective coping skills
- Encourage her to use available social support systems
- Teach the patient's family about the disorder

DISSOCIATIVE IDENTITY DISORDER

● **Defining characteristics**
- DID is marked by two or more distinct identities or subpersonalities (or alters) that recurrently take control of the patient's consciousness and behavior; each identity may exhibit unique behavior patterns, memories, and social relationships
  - Formerly called *multiple personality disorder*
  - Considered the most severe type of dissociative disorder
- In many cases, the primary personality is religious, with a strong moral sense, while the subpersonalities are radically different
  - May behave aggressively and lack sexual inhibitions
  - May have a different gender, sexual orientation, religion, or race than that of the primary personality
  - May even differ in hand dominance, vocal qualities, intelligence level, and EEG readings
- The primary personality may be unaware of the subpersonalities and may wonder about lost time and unexplained events; however, subpersonalities are more likely to be aware of the existence of the other personalities, and may even interact with one another
- The transition from one personality to another is triggered by stress or a meaningful social or environmental cue in many patients
  - Usually occurs suddenly (within seconds to minutes)
  - Can take hours or days
- The exact incidence of DID is unknown (estimates range from 1 in 500 to 1 in 5,000 persons, or between 250,000 and 2.5 million people in the United States); it's four times more common in women than it is in men
- DID tends to be chronic
  - May lead to severe social and occupational impairment, depending on the nature of the subpersonalities and their interrelationships
  - Associated with overlapping mental disorders (generalized anxiety disorder, borderline personality disorder, mood disorder) in one or more of the subpersonalities in many patients
  - May provoke suicide attempts, self-mutilation, externally directed violence, and psychoactive drug dependence

● **Causes**
- No single known cause; may result primarily from trauma or extreme stress — especially when experienced before age 15
- Strong connection between DID and history of severe childhood abuse (identified in research), suggesting victims of severe trauma and abuse develop DID as survival mechanism

– Begins when child is exposed to overwhelming trauma or abuse
– Leads to evolution of multiple personalities that allow child to dissociate herself from the traumatic situation
– Results in linking the dissociative contents with one of many possible influences that shape personality organization
- Additional factors that may contribute to DID
  – Genetic predisposition
  – Lack of nurturing experiences to assist in recovering from abuse
  – Low self-esteem

Signs and symptoms

- Lack of recall beyond ordinary forgetfulness (may be reported by family or friends)
- Pronounced changes in facial presentation, voice, and behavior
- Hallucinations, particularly auditory and visual
- Posttraumatic symptoms (flashbacks, nightmares, exaggerated startle response)
- Recurrent depression
- Sexual dysfunction and difficulty forming intimate relationships
- Sleep disorders
- Eating disorders
- Somatic pain disorders
- Substance abuse
- Guilt and shame
- Suicidal tendencies or other self-harming behaviors
  – Excessive risk-taking
  – Unprotected sex with multiple partners
  – Self-neglect
  – Excessive drinking, smoking, or eating

Diagnosis

- For many patients, correct diagnosis only after months or even years in the mental health system; common misdiagnoses: schizophrenia and bipolar disorder with psychotic episodes
- Medical history revealing unsuccessful psychiatric treatment, periods of amnesia, and disturbances in time perception
- Standard tests that demonstrate presence of dissociation: Diagnostic Drawing Series, Dissociative Experiences Scale, Dissociative Disorders Interview Schedule, SCID-D
- Diagnosis confirmed if *DSM-IV-TR* criteria met

Treatment

- Long-term process, taking 5 years or longer
- Goal to integrate all of the patient's personalities and to prevent the personality from splitting again
- After stabilizing the patient, decreasing the degree of dissociation, enhancing cooperation and co-consciousness among the subpersonalities, and ultimately merging them into one personality (done by the therapist)
  – May address the different personalities separately
  – Attempts to build a strong relationship with each subpersonality
  – Ultimately strives for an increased connectedness (the measure of success)

Key signs and symptoms of DID

- Lack of recall beyond ordinary forgetfulness
- Pronounced changes in facial presentation, voice behavior
- Hallucinations, particularly auditory and visual
- Suicidal tendencies or other self-harming behaviors

Diagnosing DID

- Correct diagnosis only after months or even years in mental health system
- Medical history revealing unsuccessful psychiatric treatment, periods of amnesia, and disturbances in time perception
- Standard tests that demonstrate presence of dissociation
- Confirmed if *DSM-IV-TR* criteria met

Key treatment options for DID

- Long-term process
- Goal: To integrate all of patient's personalities and prevent personality from splitting again
- After stabilization, decreasing degree of dissociation, enhancing cooperation and co-consciousness among subpersonalities, and ultimately merging them into one personality
- Family and couples therapy
- Hypnosis
- Drugs (benzodiazepines, SSRIs, and TCAs)

The don'ts of DID therapy

- *Don't* encourage patient to create new personalities.
- *Don't* suggest that patient adopt names for subpersonalities.
- *Don't* encourage subpersonalities to function more autonomously.
- *Don't* encourage patient to ignore certain subpersonalities.
- *Don't* exclude unlikable subpersonalities from therapy.

Promoting recovery from DID

Integrating the subpersonalities is the goal of therapy for a patient with dissociative identity disorder (DID). Certain actions by the therapist and caregivers can promote connectedness among the subpersonalities, but the actions listed here are counterproductive. Refer to this list of "Don'ts" when caring for a patient with DID:

- *Don't* encourage the patient to create additional subpersonalities.
- *Don't* suggest that she adopt names for unnamed subpersonalities.
- *Don't* encourage subpersonalities to function more autonomously.
- *Don't* encourage the patient to ignore certain subpersonalities.
- *Don't* exclude unlikable subpersonalities from therapy.

- Treating all of the patient's personalities with equal respect and empathetic concern, whether disagreeable or congenial (see *Promoting recovery from DID*)
- Clearly delineating boundaries
- Family and couples therapy
- Hypnosis
  - Helps the patient revisit the traumatic experience
  - Manages crises (for instance, reducing spontaneous flashbacks and reorienting the patient to reality)
  - Strengthens the patient's ego
  - Stabilizes the patient between therapy sessions
  - Ongoing hypnosis treatment controversial
    - Overconfidence of patients and therapists may skew accuracy of information derived during hypnotic trance
    - Therapists must minimize use of leading questions to reduce risk that patient will alter details of what she recalls during hypnosis
    - Informed consent required before use; patient must receive explanation of benefits, risks, and limitations (including information that anything the patient recalls while in a trance isn't likely to be admissible evidence in legal actions)
- Drugs, including benzodiazepines, SSRIs, and TCAs

Key nursing interventions for a patient with DID

- Establish trusting relationship with each subpersonality.
- Help patient identify each subpersonality.
- Encourage patient to identify emotions that occur under stress.
- Teach patient effective defense mechanisms and coping skills.
- Stress importance of continuing with psychotherapy, and patient for what to expect.
- Monitor patient for violence directed at others.
- Monitor patient for suicidal ideation and behavior; implement precautions as needed.

● **Nursing interventions**

- Establish a trusting relationship with each subpersonality; keep in mind that the patient with a history of abuse may have difficulty trusting others
- Promote interventions that help the patient identify each subpersonality, keeping in mind the ultimate goal of integration
- Encourage the patient to identify emotions that occur under stress
- Recognize and acknowledge even small gains made by the patient
- Teach the patient effective defense mechanisms and coping skills, including use of available social support systems
- Stress the importance of continuing with psychotherapy, and prepare her for what to expect
  - The need for prolonged therapy, with alternating successes and failures
  - The possibility that one or more of the subpersonalities may resist treatment
- Monitor the patient for violence directed at others
- Monitor the patient for suicidal ideation and behavior, and implement precautions as needed

NCLEX CHECKS

It's never too soon to begin your NCLEX preparation. Now that you've reviewed this chapter, carefully read each of the following questions and choose the best answer. Then compare your responses to the correct answers.

1. When caring for a patient with a dissociative disorder, the nurse should understand that the defense mechanism typically used to block traumatic experiences is:
- ☐ **1.** projection.
- ☐ **2.** reaction-formation.
- ☐ **3.** denial.
- ☐ **4.** repression.

2. The nurse would expect a patient to report feelings of a dreamlike state or being a detached observer when assessing for which disorder?
- ☐ **1.** Dissociative fugue
- ☐ **2.** Dissociative amnesia
- ☐ **3.** Depersonalization disorder
- ☐ **4.** DID.

3. After teaching a group of students about dissociative disorders, the instructor determines that teaching has been successful when the students correctly identify multiple personality disorder as:
- ☐ **1.** dissociative fugue.
- ☐ **2.** depersonalization disorder.
- ☐ **3.** dissociative amnesia.
- ☐ **4.** DID.

4. When assessing a patient with DID, which factor would the nurse identify as least likely to contribute to its development?
- ☐ **1.** History of seizures
- ☐ **2.** Emotional, physical, or sexual abuse
- ☐ **3.** Genetic predisposition
- ☐ **4.** Extreme stress and trauma

5. When would the nurse expect the signs and symptoms of dissociative fugue to be most pronounced?
- ☐ **1.** Weeks before the fugue episode
- ☐ **2.** Hours before the fugue episode
- ☐ **3.** During the fugue episode
- ☐ **4.** After the fugue episode

6. The nurse is assessing a patient with a suspected dissociative disorder. Which areas should the nurse cover when interviewing the patient and family? Select all that apply:
- ☐ **1.** Changes in relationships
- ☐ **2.** Spotty recollections about life history
- ☐ **3.** Blackouts
- ☐ **4.** Out-of-body experiences
- ☐ **5.** Daydreaming
- ☐ **6.** Spontaneous age regression

TOP 10

Items to study for your next test on dissociative disorders

1. Common features of the four major types of dissociative disorders
2. Signs and symptoms that differentiate dissociative disorders
3. Theories explaining the development of dissociative disorders
4. Characteristics of normal dissociation
5. Factors that contribute to development of dissociation
6. Ways to recognize and assess dissociative disorders
7. Diagnostic tests used to identify dissociative disorders
8. Treatment options for various dissociative disorders
9. Pharmacologic and supportive measures to treat dissociative disorders
10. Helpful nursing interventions for patients with dissociative disorders

7. A patient is using a self-report scale in which she assigns a number to the frequency of her dissociative experiences. The nurse correctly identifies this as which type of diagnostic tool?

- ☐ **1.** Dissociative Disorders Interview Schedule
- ☐ **2.** Dissociative Experiences Scale
- ☐ **3.** SCID-D
- ☐ **4.** Diagnostic Drawing Series

8. Which medication would the nurse expect the physician to prescribe for a patient with depersonalization disorder?

- ☐ **1.** Clomipramine (Anafranil)
- ☐ **2.** Lithium (Eskalith)
- ☐ **3.** Chlorpromazine (Thorazine)
- ☐ **4.** Fluphenazine (Prolixin)

9. Assessment reveals that a patient with dissociative amnesia has had amnesia from a specific time through the present. The nurse documents that the patient is experiencing:

- ☐ **1.** selective amnesia.
- ☐ **2.** generalized amnesia.
- ☐ **3.** systematized amnesia.
- ☐ **4.** continuous amnesia.

10. The following nursing interventions are planned for a patient with dissociative amnesia. Order the interventions in ascending chronological order, based on priority. Use all the options.

1. Assist the patient in verbalizing feelings of distress.
2. Establish a therapeutic, non-judgmental relationship.
3. Help the patient to recognize memory loss as a defense mechanism for anxiety.
4. Teach the patient how to use reality-based coping strategies.
5. Assist the patient in coping with anxiety-producing experiences.

ANSWERS AND RATIONALES

1. CORRECT ANSWER: 4
Repression is the defense mechanism typically used to block traumatic experiences. Projection, reaction-formation, and denial are irrelevant to these disorders.

2. CORRECT ANSWER: 3
Depersonalization disorder is characterized by a sense of being in a dreamlike state or being a detached observer. Dissociative fugue is marked by sudden unexpected travel away from one's home or workplace, along with an inability to recall one's past and confusion about one's personal identity. Dissociative amnesia involves an inability to recall important personal information that can't be explained by ordinary forgetfulness. DID involves two or more distinct identities or subpersonalities that recurrently take control of the patient's consciousness and behavior.

3. CORRECT ANSWER: 4
DID, formerly known as *multiple personality disorder*, is characterized by the emergence of two or more distinct identities or subpersonalities that assume control of the patient's consciousness and behavior on a recurring basis. In dissociative fugue, the patient suddenly and unexpectedly travels away from home or her workplace in a confused state, is unable to recall her past and personal identity, and sometimes assumes a new identity. In depersonalization disorder, the patient experiences a dreamlike state or a feeling of being a detached observer. With dissociative amnesia, the patient typically suffers from an inability to recall important personal information that can't be explained by ordinary forgetfulness.

4. CORRECT ANSWER: 1
A history of seizures hasn't been linked to the development of DID. Contributing factors may include severe trauma; emotional, physical, or sexual abuse; genetic predisposition; lack of nurturing experiences to recover from abuse; and low self-esteem.

5. CORRECT ANSWER: 4
After a fugue, the patient may experience depression, grief, shame, intense conflict, confusion, terror, or suicidal or aggressive impulses. In contrast, a fugue in progress is rarely recognized. There are no warning signs of an impending fugue episode.

6. CORRECT ANSWER: 1, 2, 3, 4, 6
During the assessment interview of a patient with a dissociative disorder, the nurse should focus on questioning the patient and family about changes in relationships, spotty recollections about life history, blackouts or lost time, out-of-body experiences, and spontaneous age regression. Daydreaming is a normal type of dissociation that isn't considered pathologic.

7. CORRECT ANSWER: 2
The Dissociative Experiences Scale is a brief, self-report scale that measures the frequency of dissociative experiences. The patient quantifies her experience by assigning a number for each item in the scale. The Dissociative Disorders Interview Schedule is a highly structured interview tool used to diagnose trauma-related disorders. SCID-D is a semi-structured interview tool that assesses the nature and severity of five dissociative symptoms. The Diagnostic Drawing Series tests the patient by asking her to draw a tree and a picture of how she's feeling.

8. CORRECT ANSWER: 1

Clomipramine, a TCA, has been moderately successful in treating patients with depersonalization disorders. SSRIs also may be used for this disorder. Lithium is commonly used to treat mood disorders, specifically bipolar disorders. Chlorpromazine and fluphenazine are conventional antipsychotics used to treat schizophrenia.

9. CORRECT ANSWER: 4

In continuous amnesia, the patient forgets all events from a given time forward to the present. With selective amnesia, the patient can recall some, but not all, of the events during a circumscribed time period. With generalized amnesia, the patient suffers prolonged loss of memory, possibly encompassing a lifetime. With systematized amnesia, the patient's memory loss is limited to a specific time block of information.

10. CORRECT ANSWER:

2. Establish a therapeutic, non-judgmental relationship.
1. Assist the patient in verbalizing feelings of distress.
3. Help the patient to recognize memory loss as a defense mechanism for anxiety.
5. Assist the patient in coping with anxiety-producing experiences.
4. Teach the patient how to use reality-based coping strategies.

The first priority is to establish a nonjudgmental, therapeutic relationship. Without this, the other interventions would be ineffective. Once a therapeutic relationship is established, then the nurse would assist the patient to verbalize feelings of distress. However, the nurse wouldn't try to elicit forgotten memories. Next, the nurse would help the patient recognize the use of memory loss as a defense mechanism for anxiety, and assist her in coping with anxiety-producing experiences. Lastly, the nurse would teach the patient how to use reality-based coping strategies (rather than memory loss) to deal with anxiety.

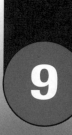

9

Personality disorders

LEARNING OBJECTIVES

After studying this chapter, you should be able to:

- Name the three clusters of personality disorders.
- Identify the major features of personality disorders.
- Discuss the proposed causes of personality disorders.
- Differentiate among the various types of personality disorders.
- Identify assessment findings and nursing interventions for patients with personality disorders.
- Discuss the recommended treatments for patients with personality disorders.

CHAPTER OVERVIEW

A personality disorder exists when personality traits—behavior patterns that reflect how a person perceives and relates to others and himself—become rigid, maladaptive, and fixed. The disorder affects the person's cognition, behavior, and style of interacting with others.

When mild, a personality disorder may have little effect on a person's social, family, or work life. However, if symptoms get worse—as they commonly do during times of increased stress—the disorder can seriously interfere with emotional, psychological, social, and occupational functioning. Severe personality disorders can result in hospitalization, poor work performance, lost productivity, domestic violence, child abuse, and imprisonment. Their emotional toll—unhappiness, disturbed or unhealthy relationships, and even suicide—is equally staggering.

Characteristics of personality disorders

- Pervasive pattern of behavior and thinking that differs markedly from norms of patient's cultural or ethnic background
- Disturbances in self-image
- Inappropriate range of emotions
- Poor impulse control
- Maladaptive ways of perceiving self, others, and world
- Long-standing problems in personal relationships
- Reduced occupational functioning

Personality disorder clusters

- Cluster A: paranoid, schizoid, and schizotypal disorders
- Cluster B: antisocial, borderline, histrionic, and narcissistic disorders
- Cluster C: avoidant, dependent, and obsessive-compulsive disorders

UNDERSTANDING PERSONALITY DISORDERS

- **General information**
  - Personality disorders are a group of disorders characterized by a pervasive pattern of behavior and thinking that differs markedly from the norms of the patient's cultural or ethnic background
  - Most people with personality disorders share several features
    - Disturbances in self-image
    - Inappropriate range of emotions
    - Poor impulse control
    - Maladaptive ways of perceiving self, others, and the world
    - Long-standing problems in personal relationships, ranging from dependency to withdrawal and isolation
    - Reduced occupational functioning, ranging from compulsive perfectionism to intentional self-sabotage
  - Because people with personality disorders don't have the same personal and societal expectations as do others, they typically have difficulty getting along with others, who are forced to adjust to their behaviors and expectations
    - May be irritable, demanding, hostile, fearful, or manipulative
    - Typically have inadequate coping mechanisms, trouble dealing with everyday stresses, and strained relationships
  - If others don't or can't adjust, people with the disorder may become angry, frustrated, depressed, or withdrawn
    - May prompt a vicious cycle of persistent maladaptive behavior until needs are met
    - May further anger those around them

- **Personality disorder clusters**
  - The *Diagnostic and Statistical Manual of Mental Disorders*, Fourth Edition, Text Revision (*DSM-IV-TR*) groups personality disorders into three clusters
    - Cluster A — paranoid, schizoid, and schizotypal personality disorders (characterized by odd or eccentric behavior)
    - Cluster B — antisocial, borderline, histrionic, and narcissistic personality disorders (characterized by dramatic, emotional, or erratic behavior)
    - Cluster C — avoidant, dependent, and obsessive-compulsive personality disorders (marked by anxious or fearful behavior)
  - Each disorder produces characteristic signs and symptoms, which may vary among patients and even within the same patient at different times

- **Incidence and disease course**
  - Personality disorders are relatively common, affecting an estimated 10% to 15% of the U.S. population
  - Gender plays a role in their prevalence
    - Antisocial and obsessive-compulsive personality disorders more common in men
    - Borderline, dependent, and histrionic personality disorders more prevalent in women
  - Personality disorders are lifelong conditions, with onset in adolescence or early adulthood

- – Cluster A and B disorders tending to grow less intense in middle-age and later life
- – Cluster C disorders tending to become exaggerated in middle and later life; patients more susceptible to substance abuse, impulse control, and suicidal behavior, which may shorten lifespan
- Personality disorders commonly overlap with other psychiatric disorders, such as substance abuse, and mood and anxiety disorders

CAUSES

General information
- The exact cause of personality disorders is unknown
- Most likely, they represent a combination of genetic, biological, social, psychological, developmental, and environmental factors

Genetic factors
- Genetic factors influence the biological basis of brain function as well as basic personality structure
- In turn, personality structure affects how a person responds to and interacts with life experiences and the social environment
- Over time, each person develops distinctive ways of perceiving the world and of feeling, thinking, and behaving

Biological factors
- Some researchers suspect that poor regulation of the brain circuits that control emotion increases the risk for a personality disorder—when combined with such factors as abuse, neglect, or separation
- For a biologically predisposed person, the major developmental challenges of adolescence and early adulthood (such as separation from the parents, identity, and independence) may trigger a personality disorder

Psychodynamic theories
- Psychodynamic theories propose that personality disorders stem from deficiencies in ego and superego development
- These deficiencies may relate to mother-child relationships marked by unresponsiveness, overprotectiveness, or early separation

Social theories
- Personality disorders reflect responses learned through the processes of reinforcement, modeling, and aversive stimuli
- With even low levels of stress, chronic trauma or long-term stressors may create new neurochemical pathways
- As a result the person "acts out" old patterns

EVALUATION

Physical examination
- A patient with a suspected personality disorder should undergo a physical examination to rule out an underlying physical or organic cause for his symptoms
- Personality change may be the first sign of a serious neurologic, endocrine, or other physiologic illness that may be reversible if detected early

---

Common causes of personality disorders

- Exact cause unknown
- Most likely, disorders represent combination of genetic, biological, social, psychological, developmental, and environmental factors

Evaluating personality disorders

- Physical examination: to rule out underlying physical or organic cause
- Psychological examination
- – MMPI-2
- – MCMI-III
- – Structured Clinical Interview for *DSM-IV-TR* for Axis II Disorders
- – Confirmed only if *DSM-IV-TR* criteria are met
- Substance screening

Key treatment options for personality disorders

- Focus: enhancing patient's coping skills, solving short-term problems, and building relationship skills
- Psychotherapy
- Adjunctive medication

Drug therapy according to cluster

- Cluster A: may benefit from antidepressants and low-dose antipsychotic agents
- Cluster B: for marked mood reactivity, impulsivity, or rejection hypersensitivity, anticonvulsant mood-stabilizing agents and MAO inhibitors
- Cluster C: may benefit from antianxiety agents

Characteristics of antisocial personality disorder

- Chronic antisocial behavior that violates others' rights or generally accepted social norms
- Predisposes affected person to criminal behavior
- Impulsivity and recklessness
- Egocentricity
- Disregard for the truth
- Lack of remorse or empathy
- Irritability and aggression
- Inability to tolerate boredom and frustration
- Inability to maintain consistent, responsible functioning at work or school or as a parent

● **Psychological examination**
- A psychological evaluation can exclude other psychiatric disorders—or it may suggest additional ones
- Psychological tests, such as the Minnesota Multiphasic Personality Inventory-2 (MMPI-2) and the Millon Clinical Multiaxial Inventory-III (MCMI-III), may support or guide the diagnosis; the Structured Clinical Interview for *DSM-IV-TR* for Axis II Disorders also aids diagnosis
- Official diagnosis of a personality disorder is confirmed only if the criteria established in *DSM-IV-TR* are met
- Some patients meet the criteria for more than one personality disorder, making diagnosis a particular challenge

● **Substance screening**
- Toxicology screening may be warranted
- Intoxication with certain substances can mimic the features of a personality disorder

TREATMENT

● **General information**
- Personality disorders are among the most challenging psychiatric disorders to treat because the personality is an integral part of what defines the individual and his self-perceptions
- Rather than cure, treatment typically focuses on enhancing the patient's coping skills, solving short-term problems, and building relationship skills through psychotherapy and education

● **Psychotherapy**
- Traditionally, long-term psychotherapy has been the treatment of choice
- Effective psychotherapy always requires a trusting relationship with the therapist

● **Adjunctive medication**
- Many patients also receive drugs to relieve associated symptoms, such as acute anxiety or depression
- Drugs are used only as an adjunct to psychotherapy—not as a cure for the personality disorder
  - Cluster A disorders: may benefit from antidepressants and low-dose antipsychotic agents
  - Cluster B disorders: patients who suffer marked mood reactivity, impulsivity, or rejection hypersensitivity may respond well to anticonvulsant mood-stabilizing agents and monoamine oxidase (MAO) inhibitors
  - Cluster C disorders: may benefit from antianxiety agents

ANTISOCIAL PERSONALITY DISORDER

● **Defining characteristics**
- Antisocial personality disorder is characterized by chronic antisocial behavior that violates others' rights or generally accepted social norms, which predisposes the affected person to criminal behavior

- Additional features are common in people with this disorder
    - Impulsivity and recklessness
    - Egocentricity
    - Disregard for the truth
    - Lack of remorse or empathy
    - Irritability and aggression
    - Inability to tolerate boredom and frustration
- A person with antisocial personality disorder is typically unable to maintain consistent, responsible functioning at work, at school, or as a parent
- In the general population, the prevalence of antisocial personality disorder is about 2% to 3%, affecting up to four times as many males as it does females
    - In prison populations, may be as high as 50%
    - History of arrest in roughly half of those with the disorder
- During adolescence, common coexisting disorders include conduct disorder and oppositional defiant disorder

Causes
- Possible biological factors (may underlie low arousal, poor fear conditioning, and decision-making deficits)
    - Poor serotonin regulation in certain brain regions, which may decrease behavioral inhibition
    - Reduced autonomic activity and developmental or acquired abnormalities in the prefrontal brain systems
- Possible genetic influence: more common in first-degree biological relatives than in general population
- Other possible causes or risk factors: attention-deficit-hyperactivity disorder, large families

Risk factors (related to childhood exposure)
- Substance abuse
- Criminal behavior
- Physical or sexual abuse
- Neglectful or unstable parenting
- Social isolation
- Transient friendships
- Low socioeconomic status

Signs and symptoms
- Long-standing pattern of disregarding others' rights and society's values
- Repeatedly performing unlawful acts
- Reckless disregard for own or others' safety
- Deceitfulness
- Lack of remorse or empathy
- Consistent irresponsibility
- Power-seeking behavior
- Destructive tendencies
- Impulsivity and failure to plan ahead
- Superficial charm
- Manipulative behavior for self-gratification
- Inflated, arrogant self-appraisal
- Irritability and aggressiveness
- Inability to maintain close personal or sexual relationships

Common causes of antisocial personality disorder
- Biological factors
- Poor serotonin regulation
- Reduced autonomic activity and acquired abnormalities in frontal lobe
- Possibly genetic

Key childhood risk factors for antisocial personality disorder
- Substance abuse
- Criminal behavior
- Physical or sexual abuse
- Neglectful or unstable parenting
- Social isolation
- Transient friendships
- Low socioeconomic status

Key signs and symptoms of antisocial personality disorder
- Long-standing pattern of disregarding others' rights and society's values
- Repeatedly performing unlawful acts
- Reckless disregard for own or others' safety
- Deceitfulness
- Lack of remorse or empathy
- Consistent irresponsibility
- Power-seeking behavior
- Destructive tendencies
- Impulsivity and failure to plan ahead
- Superficial charm
- Inflated, arrogant self-appraisal

Personality and projective tests

- BDI
- Draw-a-Person Test
- MMPI-2
- Sentence-Completion Test
- Thematic Apperception Test

Personality and projective tests

Personality and projective tests elicit patient responses that provide insight into mood, personality, or psychopathology. These tests include the Beck Depression Inventory (BDI), Draw-a-Person Test, Minnesota Multiphasic Personality Inventory-2 (MMPI-2), Sentence-Completion Test, and Thematic Apperception Test.

BDI
A self-administered, self-scored test, the BDI asks patients to rate how often they experience symptoms of depression, such as poor concentration, suicidal thoughts, feelings of guilt, and crying. Questions focus on cognitive symptoms such as impaired decision-making and physical symptoms such as appetite loss.

You may help patients complete the BDI by reading the questions, but be careful not to influence their answers. Instruct patients to choose the answer that describes them most accurately.

Scoring
The sum of 21 items gives the total, with a maximum possible score of 63.
- A score of 11 to 16 indicates mild depression.
- A score of 17 or above indicates moderate depression.

If you suspect depression, a BDI score of 17 or above may provide objective evidence of the need for treatment. To monitor the patient's depression, repeat the BDI during the course of treatment.

DRAW-A-PERSON TEST
In the Draw-a-Person Test, the patient draws two human figures (one of each gender). The psychologist interprets the drawings systematically and correlates the interpretation with diagnosis. This test also provides an estimate of a child's developmental level.

MMPI-2
The MMPI-2 is a structured, paper-and-pencil test that provides a practical way to assess personality traits and ego function in adolescents and adults. Most patients who read English need little assistance in completing it. The

Diagnosing antisocial personality disorder

- Differentiated from simple criminal activity, adult antisocial behavior, or other behaviors that don't support diagnosis
- Formal psychological testing
- Confirmed if *DSM-IV-TR* criteria met

- Disconnection between feelings and behaviors
- Possible evidence of substance abuse

● **Diagnosis**
- Disorder differentiated from simple criminal activity, adult antisocial behavior, or other behaviors that don't support diagnosis (not all criminals have antisocial personality disorder)
- Formal psychological testing, as with the MMPI-2 (see *Personality and projective tests*)
- Diagnosis confirmed if *DSM-IV-TR* criteria met

● **Treatment**
- Intensive psychoanalytic approaches aren't indicated; they may be unfamiliar with feelings associated with emotional states
- Therapy focusing on helping the patient make connections between his feelings and behaviors, by gaining better access to and experiencing such feelings
    – Reinforcing appropriate behaviors
    – Helping the patient develop victim empathy

MMPI—the original version of this test— was developed at the University of Minnesota and was introduced in 1942. The MMPI-2 was released in 1989 and was subsequently revised in early 2001.

The MMPI-2 has 567 questions and takes 60 to 90 minutes to complete. (A short form consists of the first 370 questions of the long-form version.) Questions are designed to evaluate the thoughts, emotions, attitudes, and behavioral traits that comprise personality.

Interpreting the results

A psychologist translates the patient's answers into a psychological profile, and then combines the profile with data gathered from the interview. Test results shed light on the patient's coping strategies, defenses, personality strengths and weaknesses, sexual identification, and self-esteem. The MMPI-2 may also identify certain personality disturbances or mental deficits caused by neurologic problems.

A patient's test pattern may strongly suggest a diagnostic category. If the results reveal a risk for suicide or violence, monitor the patient's behavior. If

he has frequent somatic complaints (indicating possible hypochondria), evaluate his physical status. If the complaints lack medical confirmation, help the patient explore how these symptoms might signal emotional distress.

SENTENCE-COMPLETION TEST

In the Sentence-Completion Test, the patient completes a series of partial sentences. A sentence might begin, "When I get angry, I…" The response may reveal the patient's fantasies, fears, aspirations, or anxieties.

THEMATIC APPERCEPTION TEST

In the Thematic Apperception Test, the patient views a series of pictures depicting ambiguous situations, and then tells a story describing each picture. The psychologist evaluates these stories systematically to help analyze the patient's personality, particularly regarding interpersonal relationships and conflicts.

– Experiencing intense affect usually a sign of progress
• Psychotherapy: usual treatment of choice; options include individual psychotherapy, group therapy, family therapy, and self-help support groups (drug or alcohol rehabilitation may also be needed)
  – Solid therapist-patient rapport essential for establishing therapeutic relationship
  – Fears about confidentiality pose obstacle to patient's trust
  – Honesty needed about disclosure of information to courts
• Individual psychotherapy in a forensic or prison setting
  – Rarely seek evaluation or treatment on their own; more likely court-mandated or result of family pressure
  – Threats (reporting lack of motivation to courts, prison warden) especially ineffective in antisocial patients mandated to have therapy (not effective motivators in any setting)
  – In confined settings, alternative life issues should be focus of therapy
    • Goals the patient can pursue after his release from custody
    • Improving social or family relationships

Key treatment options for antisocial personality disorder

• Focus: helping patient make connections between his feelings and behaviors by gaining better access to and experiencing such feelings
• Psychotherapy (treatment of choice)
• Group therapy
• Family therapy
• Self-help support groups
• Inpatient hospitalization (rare)
• Specialized treatment programs
• Drugs (such as lithium, beta-adrenergic blockers, anticonvulsants)

• Learning new coping skills
• Outpatient psychotherapy focusing on discussing the patient's antisocial behavior and lack of feelings
  – Threats remain ineffective as motivator
  – Therapist should help patient find good reasons to want to work on problems
• Group therapy after the patient overcomes his initial fears about joining a group
  – Should consist exclusively of people with antisocial personality disorder (gives patient better reason to contribute and share)
  – Group leader must ensure that group doesn't become "how-to" course in criminal behavior or forum for bragging about criminal exploits
• Family therapy to help the family understand the patient's antisocial behavior
  – Should encourage open discussion, especially regarding confusion, guilt, temptation to make restitution for patient's criminal acts, and frustrations of being with someone who's ill but resists treatment
• Inpatient hospital care rarely required; however, hospitalization may be necessary for treatment of a crisis or major depression
  – May be intensive and expensive
  – Rarely sought out by patients themselves
  – Community follow-up needed after discharge to maintain treatment gains (support from hospital staff, other professionals, self-help support group)
• Specialized treatment programs
• Drugs to treat disorganized thinking, to stabilize mood swings, or to ease the acute symptoms of concurrent psychiatric disorders
  – Possible use of lithium (Eskalith), beta-adrenergic blocker, such as propranolol (Inderal), or anticonvulsant, such as carbamazepine (Tegretol), to control aggressive outbursts

● **Nursing interventions**
• Set limits on the patient's behavior
  – Using a straightforward, matter-of-fact approach
  – Clearly conveying your expectations of the patient, as well as the consequences if he fails to meet them
  – Establishing a behavioral "contract" to communicate to the patient that other behavior options are available
  – Holding the patient responsible for his behavior to promote the development of a collaborative relationship
  – Encouraging and reinforcing positive behavior (see *Setting limits effectively*)
• Anticipate manipulative efforts (keep in mind that the patient may seem charming and convincing); help the patient identify such behaviors so he can learn that other people aren't extensions of himself
• Expect the patient to refuse to cooperate in an effort to gain control
• Avoid power struggles and confrontations to maintain the opportunity for therapeutic communication
• Avoid defensiveness and arguing
• Observe for physical and verbal signs of agitation
• Help the patient manage his anger

Setting limits effectively

Follow these guidelines to set limits effectively.

CHOOSE YOUR BATTLES WISELY

- Choose your battles wisely by setting limits only as needed.
- Set limits when you first sense that the patient is violating others' rights; don't tolerate his behavior for several days and then launch an angry tirade.
- Avoid using limits as punishment or retaliation; don't set limits only when you're angry or under stress as this reaction will thwart your efforts to build a therapeutic relationship.
- Let the patient express his feelings about what the limits mean to him; he may perceive them as a message that you no longer like him, or may feel increased anxiety because he isn't used to external controls.

FOCUS ON BEHAVIOR

- Establish limits strictly for the patient's *behavior*, not his feelings; if you focus on such feelings as anger, the patient may sense that his emotions are unacceptable.

- If the patient oversteps the limits, explain that although you don't accept his behavior, you do accept him as a person.
- Make sure the patient knows exactly what behavior you expect.
- Apply the rules consistently and, when possible, offer alternatives to unacceptable behavior.

ENSURE CONSISTENCY

- Inform other staff members of the limits you've set; otherwise, a manipulative patient may try to split the staff into factions he can pit against one another.
- Apply the same principles when working with the patient's family; many patients come from families that have had little success in establishing discipline, and family members need to learn that rules can be enforced in a way that communicates love, caring, and acceptance.

> ### Guidelines for setting limits
> - Choose your battles wisely.
> - Focus on behavior.
> - Ensure consistency.

- Teach the patient social skills, and reinforce appropriate behavior
- Encourage the patient to express his feelings, analyze his own behavior, and be accountable for his actions

AVOIDANT PERSONALITY DISORDER

● Defining characteristics

- Avoidant personality disorder is marked by feelings of inadequacy, extreme social anxiety, social withdrawal, and hypersensitivity to others' opinions
- People with this disorder have low self-esteem and poor self-confidence; they dwell on the negative and have difficulty viewing situations and interactions objectively
  - To rationalize their avoidance of new situations, exaggerate potential difficulties involved
  - May create fantasy worlds to substitute for the real one
- The avoidant person yearns for social relationships but fears being rejected or embarrassed in front of others

> ### Characteristics of avoidant personality disorder
> - Feelings of inadequacy
> - Extreme social anxiety
> - Social withdrawal
> - Hypersensitivity to others' opinions
> - Low self-esteem
> - Poor self-confidence
> - Patient dwells on negative and has difficulty viewing situations and interactions objectively

Psychiatric disorders associated with avoidant personality disorder

- Social phobia
- Schizoid or dependent personality disorder
- Agoraphobia
- Obsessive-compulsive disorder
- Generalized anxiety disorder
- Dysthymia
- Major depressive disorder
- Somatoform disorders
- Dissociative disorder
- Schizophrenia

Common causes of avoidant personality disorder

- Combined genetic, biological, environmental, and other factors
- Evidence for genetic and biological causes is limited
- Genetic and biological theories linked to temperament
- Overly critical parenting style
- Significant environmental influences during childhood

Key signs and symptoms of avoidant personality disorder

- Shyness, timidity, and social withdrawal behavior meant to drive others away
- Reluctance to speak or, conversely, overly talkative
- Constant mistrust or wariness of others
- Difficulty starting and maintaining relationships
- Perfectionism
- Rejection of those not living up to own high standards
- Limited emotional expression
- Low self-esteem
- Self-consciousness
- Reluctance to take personal risks or engage in new activities

- – Isn't willing to enter into social relationships without assurance of uncritical acceptance
  - – Seeks out jobs that require little contact with others
- Many people with avoidant personality disorder also have other psychiatric disorders
  - – Social phobia
  - – Schizoid or dependent personality disorder
  - – Agoraphobia
  - – Obsessive-compulsive disorder
  - – Generalized anxiety disorder
  - – Dysthymia
  - – Major depressive disorder
  - – Somatoform disorders
  - – Dissociative disorder
  - – Schizophrenia
- Avoidant personality disorder is found in an estimated 0.5% to 1.0% of the general adult population; it affects males and females equally, and develops by early adulthood

Causes

- Most likely results from combination of genetic, biological, environmental, and other factors; however, evidence for genetic and biological causes is limited
- Psychodynamic view attributes disorder to overly critical parenting style
- Genetic and biological theories
  - – Disorder closely linked to temperament
  - – In studies of children younger than age 2, some have apparently inborn tendency to withdraw from new situations or people
  - – Roughly 10% of toddlers habitually fearful and withdrawn when exposed to new people and situations
  - – Some evidence that timid temperament in infancy may predispose to later avoidant personality disorder
  - – Overstimulation or excess of incoming information may be cause of inherited tendency to be shy
    - • Can't cope with excess information and withdraws in defense
    - • May stem from low autonomic arousal threshold (certain structures in brain's limbic system may have lower threshold of arousal and more pronounced response when activated)
- Environmental factors
  - – Full development of disorder possibly resulting from significant environmental influences during childhood (such as rejection by the parents or peers)
  - – Rejection appears intense or frequent; thought to wear down self-esteem

Signs and symptoms

- Shyness, timidity, and social withdrawal behavior or appearance that's meant to drive others away (gives patient sense of control)
- Reluctance to speak or, conversely, overly talkative
- Constant mistrust or wariness of others
- Testing of others' sincerity
- Difficulty starting and maintaining relationships
- Perfectionism

- Rejection of people who don't live up to his impossibly high standards
- Limited emotional expression
- Tenseness and anxiety
- Low self-esteem
- Feelings of being unworthy of successful relationships
- Self-consciousness
- Loneliness
- Reluctance to take personal risks or engage in new activities
- May also report frequent escapes into fantasy, such as by excessive reading, watching television, or daydreaming

Diagnosis
- No specific diagnostic tests; patient should undergo psychological evaluation and personality and projective tests
- Diagnosis confirmed if *DSM-IV-TR* criteria met

Treatment
- People rarely seeking treatment unless something goes wrong in their lives to indicate they aren't coping adequately
- Psychotherapy only for high-functioning patients, while others benefit from a combination of medication and psychotherapy
- Goal: to improve social interaction and increase confidence in interpersonal relationships using various techniques
  - Enhancing self-esteem
  - Improving social interaction and increasing confidence in interpersonal relationships
  - Desensitizing reaction to criticism
  - Decreasing resistance to change
  - Improving coping
  - Achieving cognitive restructuring
  - Developing appropriate affect and expression of emotions
- Individual psychotherapy (the preferred treatment): most effective when it's short-term and focused on solving specific life problems
  - May consider group therapy as patient progresses through individual therapy
  - May be difficult to establish solid therapist-patient relationship; patient may terminate therapy early
  - Successful ending to relationship is important (reinforces possibility of new relationships)
- Self-help support groups; however, such groups may be difficult to find, and patients are likely to avoid them because of their social anxiety
- Medications as an adjunct to psychotherapy if a patient has moderate to severe functional impairments
  - Commonly positive response to MAO inhibitors (especially phenelzine [Nardil]) to improve confidence and assertiveness in social settings)
  - May also use medications for such symptoms as anxiety and depression
  - Medications may interfere with effective psychotherapeutic management if patient feels disconnected from emotions

Nursing interventions
- Offer persistent, consistent, and flexible care; take a direct, involved approach to gain the patient's trust

Diagnosing avoidant personality disorder
- Psychological evaluation
- Personality and projective tests
- Confirmed if *DSM-IV-TR* criteria met

Key treatment options for avoidant personality disorder
- Goal: to improve social interaction and increase confidence in interpersonal relationships
- Psychotherapy (only for high-functioning patients)
- Individual psychotherapy (preferred treatment)
- Self-help support groups
- Adjunctive medications

Key nursing interventions for a patient with avoidant personality disorder

- Offer persistent, consistent, and flexible care.
- Take direct, involved approach to gain patient's trust.
- Monitor for signs of dependency.
- Assess patient for signs of depression.
- Prepare patient for upcoming procedures well in advance.
- Inform patient when you will and won't be available if he needs assistance.
- Initially give patient explicit directives rather than asking him to make decisions.
- Teach patient relaxation and stress-management techniques.

Characteristics of borderline personality disorder

- Poor regulation of emotions
- Pattern of instability in interpersonal relationships, mood, behavior, and self-image
- Difficulty distinguishing reality from misconceptions of world
- Alternating extremes of anger, anxiety, depression, and emptiness
- Possible cognitive problems, conflicts with others, or brief, psychotic-like experiences
- Feeling bad or unworthy, misunderstood, mistreated, bored, or empty
- Impulsivity
- Intense and stormy relationships (alternates between black/white view of others)
- Extreme sensitivity to rejection
- Patient may resort to self-destructive behaviors
- Commonly triggered by fear of abandonment

- Be aware that the patient may become dependent on the few staff members he feels he can trust; monitor for signs of dependency, avoid actions that foster dependency, and encourage self-care
- Assess the patient for signs of depression because social impairment increases the risk for mood disorders
- Prepare the patient for upcoming procedures well in advance (giving him plenty of time to adjust) as patients with avoidant personality disorder don't handle surprises well
- Inform the patient when you will and won't be available if he needs assistance
- Initially, give the patient explicit directives rather than asking him to make decisions; gradually encourage him to make easy decisions, and continue to provide support and reassurance as his decision-making ability improves
- Encourage the patient's expression of feelings, analysis of behavior, and accountability for his actions
- Teach the patient relaxation and stress-management techniques to help him manage his anxiety level and cope in times of stress

BORDERLINE PERSONALITY DISORDER

Defining characteristics

- A disorder of poor regulation of emotions, borderline personality disorder is marked by a pattern of instability in interpersonal relationships, mood, behavior, and self-image
- People with this disorder can experience it in various ways
  - In most cases, have difficulty distinguishing reality from their own misperceptions of the world (for instance, have difficulty viewing events and relationships from perspectives of others)
  - Commonly have alternating extremes of anger, anxiety, depression, and emptiness (intense bouts of emotion typically last only hours or, at most, a day)
  - May have cognitive problems due to overwhelming emotions
  - May cause conflicts with others
  - May have brief, psychotic-like experiences
- Distortions in cognition and sense of self can lead to frequent changes in long-term goals, jobs and career plans, friendships, values, and even sex identity
- A person with this disorder may see herself as fundamentally bad or unworthy, feeling misunderstood, mistreated, bored, and empty, with little idea of who she really is
- People with borderline personality disorder tend to act impulsively, without considering the consequences
  - May include promiscuity, substance abuse, and eating or spending binges
  - May prompt outbursts of intense anger that leads to violence (easily triggered when others criticize or thwart their impulsive acts)
- A person with borderline personality disorder tends to have intense and stormy relationships, alternating between a "black" and "white" view of others
- Perceptions of family members and friends may shift suddenly, from great admiration and love to intense anger and dislike (called *splitting*)

- Considered a defense mechanism meant to protect patient from perception of dangerous anxiety and intense affects
- Instead of offering real protection, leads to destructive behavior and turmoil
- A person with this disorder is extremely sensitive to rejection, possibly reacting with anger and distress to even mild separations from loved ones (such as with vacations, business trips, or a sudden change in plans)
  - May resort to self-destructive behaviors, such as self-mutilation (cutting or burning), substance abuse, eating disorders, and suicide attempts to escape inner turmoil
  - Commonly triggered by fear of abandonment
- Borderline personality disorder affects 2% to 3% of the general population, about 11% of psychiatric outpatients, and nearly 20% of psychiatric inpatients; it's three times more common in females than it is in males
- The disorder usually begins in early childhood and peaks in adolescence and early adulthood
  - In late teens and early 20s, high use of health care resources
  - By 30s and 40s, some stability achieved in work and personal life (although significant areas of dysfunction remain) in up to 60% of patients
- Borderline personality disorder commonly overlaps with other personality disorders as well as bipolar disorder, depression, anxiety disorders, and substance abuse

Causes

- Precise cause unknown; several theories being investigated
- Possible genetic component (five times more common in first-degree relatives of people with the disorder)
- Possible biological factors
  - Dysfunction in brain's limbic system or frontal lobe
  - Decreased serotonin activity
  - Increased activity in alpha-2-noradrenergic receptors
- Factors may appear more common in patients than in general population
  - Prolonged separation from parents
  - Other major losses early in life
  - Physical, sexual, or emotional abuse or neglect

Signs and symptoms

- Four main categories of major signs and symptoms
  - Unstable relationships
  - Unstable self-image
  - Unstable emotions
  - Impulsivity
- Most acute when patient feels isolated and without social support, causing him to make frantic efforts to avoid being alone
- Possible assessment findings
  - Pattern of unstable and intense interpersonal relationships
  - Intense fear of abandonment, as displayed in clinging and distancing maneuvers
  - Rapidly shifting attitudes about friends and loved ones
  - Desperate attempts to maintain relationships

Common causes of borderline personality disorder

- Precise cause unknown
- Possible genetic component
- Dysfunction in brain's limbic system or frontal lobe
- Decreased serotonin activity
- Increased activity in alpha-2-noradrenergic receptors

Key signs and symptoms of borderline personality disorder

- Unstable relationships
- Unstable self-image
- Unstable emotions
- Impulsivity
- Most acute when patient feels isolated and without emotional support
- Intense fear of abandonment
- Rapidly shifting attitudes
- Manipulation
- Dissociation
- Uncertainty about major issues
- Rapid, dramatic mood swings
- Acting out
- Chronic feelings of emptiness
- Unpredictable, self-damaging behavior

- Unstable perceptions of relationships, with estrangement over ordinary disagreements
- Manipulation, as in pitting people against one another
- Limited coping skills
- Dissociation (separating objects from their emotional significance)
- Transient, stress-related paranoid ideation or severe dissociative symptoms
- Inability to develop a healthy sense of oneself
- Uncertainty about major issues (such as self-image, identity, life goals, sexual orientation, values, career choices, or types of friends)
- Imitative behavior
- Rapid, dramatic mood swings—from euphoria to intense anxiety to rage—within hours or days
- Acting out of feelings instead of expressing them appropriately or verbally
- Inappropriate, intense anger or difficulty controlling anger
- Chronic feelings of emptiness
- Unpredictable, self-damaging behavior (such as driving dangerously, gambling, sexual promiscuity, overeating, overspending, and abusing substances)
- Self-destructive behavior

● Diagnosis
- Standard psychological tests, possibly revealing high degree of dissociation
- Diagnosis confirmed if *DSM-IV-TR* criteria met

● Treatment
- May be multifaceted
- Psychotherapy: treatment of choice; while the disorder can be hard to treat, individual and group therapies are at least partially effective for many patients
  - Patient's unstable relationships and intense anger causing difficulty in establishing therapeutic relationship with health care professionals
  - Patient failing to respond to therapeutic efforts, and making considerable demands on caregiver's emotional resources, especially when suicidal and other self-harming behaviors prominent
  - Requires carefully assessing and monitoring of suicide potential throughout entire treatment course; may require medication and hospitalization if at high risk
  - Initially, may require implementing a no-harm contract to help assess risk of suicide and self-harm and to establish caring therapeutic relationship (contract is no assurance that patient won't harm herself; therapeutic value is in assessing patient's risk of self-harm, and demonstrating concern for patient's well being)
- Structured therapeutic setting
  - Requires establishing boundaries for the relationship when therapy begins (patient may initially try to test therapist's limits)
  - Requires cooperation of everyone involved in patient's care to maintain consistent boundaries
- Psychosocial treatment called *dialectical behavior therapy* (see *Dialectical behavior therapy*)

Diagnosing borderline personality disorder
- Standard psychological tests
- Confirmed if *DSM-IV-TR* criteria met

Key treatment options for borderline personality disorder
- Psychotherapy (treatment of choice)
- Structured therapeutic setting
- Psychosocial treatment (dialectical behavior therapy)
- Social learning theory and conflict resolution therapies
- Inpatient hospitalization (rare)
- Partial hospitalization and day treatment programs
- Milieu therapy
- Self-help support groups
- Drugs

Dialectical behavior therapy

During the past 15 years, a psychosocial treatment called *dialectical behavior therapy* (DBT) – developed specifically to treat borderline personality disorder – has proven effective in helping patients cope with the disorder.

In this comprehensive approach, the patient is taught to better control her life and emotions through self-knowledge, emotion regulation, and cognitive restructuring.

TREATMENT MODES

DBT involves four primary modes of treatment:
- Individual therapy
- Group skills training
- Telephone contact with the therapist
- Therapist consultation

INDIVIDUAL THERAPY SESSIONS

The main work of therapy occurs in individual therapy sessions. (The therapist may add group therapy and other treatment modes as appropriate.) Between sessions, the patient is offered telephone contact with the therapist, providing help and support in applying the skills she's learning to real-life situations (and to help prevent self-injury).

THERAPEUTIC HIERARCHY

In individual therapy sessions, goals are dealt with according to the following hierarchy:
- Decreasing suicidal behaviors
- Decreasing behaviors that interfere with therapy
- Decreasing behaviors that interfere with the quality of life
- Improving behavioral skills
- Decreasing behaviors related to posttraumatic stress
- Improving self-esteem
- Working on individual goals negotiated with the patient

SKILLS TRAINING

Skills training usually is carried out in a group. In the group, patients learn:
- Core mindfulness skills (meditation-like techniques)
- Interpersonal effectiveness skills (focusing on effective ways to achieve one's objectives with others)
- Emotion-modulation skills (ways of changing distressing emotional states)
- Distress-tolerance skills (techniques for coping with the emotional states that can't be changed for the time being)

- Social learning theory and conflict resolution therapies to treat borderline personality disorder; however, these solution-focused therapies may neglect the patient's core problems (such as difficulty expressing appropriate emotions and problems forming emotional attachments to others because of faulty cognitions)
- Hospitalization rarely indicated; long-term care in a hospital setting rarely appropriate
  - During episode of acute depression or another crisis, patient may be seen in an emergency department, inpatient unit, or local community health center
  - Due to costs of hospitalization, patient encouraged to instead find additional social support within the community; resources include telephone or personal contact with therapist or physician, self-help support groups (including those available though the Internet), and crisis hotlines

Guidelines for milieu therapy

- Explain purpose of therapy to patient.
- Tell patient what you expect of her.
- Explain how she can participate in therapeutic community.
- Regularly evaluate patients' symptoms and therapeutic needs.
- Encourage patient to keep a schedule typical of life outside hospital.
- Encourage patient to interact with others.
- Encourage patient to keep follow-up appointments with therapist.

Pharmacologic options for treating borderline personality disorder

- Antidepressants: SSRIs or MAO inhibitors
- Antianxiety agent: buspirone
- Antipsychotic drugs: risperidone and olanzapine
- Antimanic medications: valproate or lithium
- Naltrexone

Milieu therapy

Whether it takes place in the hospital or in a community setting, milieu therapy uses the patient's setting or environment to help her overcome psychiatric disorders. If your patient is undergoing this type of therapy, follow these guidelines.

PATIENT PREPARATION
Explain the purpose of milieu therapy to the patient. Tell her what you expect of her, and explain how she can participate in the therapeutic community. Orient her to the community's routines such as the schedule for various activities. Introduce her to other patients and staff.

MONITORING AND AFTERCARE
Regularly evaluate the patient's symptoms and therapeutic needs. Oversee her activities, encouraging her to keep a schedule typical of life outside the hospital. Encourage her to interact with others so she doesn't become withdrawn or feel secluded. Point out the importance of respecting others and her environment.

HOME CARE INSTRUCTIONS
When the patient returns to the outside community, encourage her to keep follow-up appointments with her therapist.

- Partial hospitalization and day treatment programs to provide a safe environment, offering support, feedback, and structure for a short time or during the day (the patient usually returns home in the evening)
    - May be more appropriate than inpatient hospitalization during times of increased stress or difficulty coping
    - Encourages patient to be less dependent on others to solve problems
- Milieu therapy (see *Milieu therapy*)
- Self-help support groups to help patients to cope better on their own, thereby avoiding situational crises
    - Allow patients to try out new coping skills
    - Teach patients to regulate emotions
    - Help patients develop new and healthier social relationships
    - Teach effective techniques to reduce stress and anxiety
- Drugs to relieve specific symptoms, especially during a crisis
    - Antidepressants, such as selective serotonin-reuptake inhibitors (SSRIs) (for example, fluoxetine [Prozac]) or MAO inhibitors, to treat depression
    - Antianxiety drugs such as buspirone (BuSpar), to ease anxiety
    - Antipsychotic drugs, such as risperidone or olanzapine, to ease dissociative symptoms or self-destructive impulses
    - Antimanic medications, such as valproate (Depakote) or lithium, to treat mood swings
    - Naltrexone (ReVia) to reduce self-mutilating behaviors
    - Dosages should be kept low and prescriptions monitored closely — accompanied by psychosocial intervention

● Nursing interventions

- Encourage the patient to take responsibility for herself; don't try to rescue her from the consequences of her actions (except suicidal and self-mutilating behaviors)

- Convey empathy and support, but don't try to solve problems she can solve herself
- Maintain a consistent approach in all interactions with the patient, and ensure that other team members use the same approach
- Avoid sympathetic, nurturing responses
- Recognize and avoid unconsciously reinforcing behaviors used to manipulate people
- Set appropriate expectations for social interactions, and praise the patient when she meets these expectations
- To promote trust, respect the patient's personal space
- Be aware that the patient may idealize some staff members and devalue others
- Don't take sides in the patient's disputes with staff members
- Avoid defensiveness and arguing
- Try to limit the patient's interactions to assigned staff to decrease splitting behaviors; remember that using only a few consistent staff members helps to maintain continuity of care
- If the patient is taking medications, monitor her for "cheeking" (holding medications in the cheek) or hoarding medications for overdose at a later time
- Monitor prescriptions closely; the patient may overdose impulsively if she has an adequate drug supply
- Encourage the patient to express her feelings, analyze her behavior, and be accountable for her actions
- Help the patient develop problem-solving skills
- Teach and encourage relaxation techniques
- Suggest that the patient start an exercise regimen (exercise promotes stability by decreasing mood swings and aiding the release of anger)

DEPENDENT PERSONALITY DISORDER

- **Description**
  - Dependent personality disorder is characterized by an extreme need to be taken care of, which leads to submissive, clinging behavior and fear of separation or rejection
  - People with this disorder let others make important decisions for them and have a strong need for constant reassurance and support
    - Elicit caregiving by engaging in dependent behavior
    - Feel helpless and incompetent, complying passively and transferring responsibility to others
    - Seek others to dominate and protect them
  - Some stay in abusive relationships and are willing to tolerate mistreatment
    - May become suicidal when the breakup of a romantic relationship is imminent
    - Urgently seeks another relationship as a source of care and support after a close relationship ends
  - Behaviors typically arise from the perception that the patient can't function adequately without others
    - Craves attention and validation

Common causes of dependent personality disorder

- Exact cause unknown
- Possible link with authoritarian or overprotective parenting
- Childhood trauma
- Closed family system that discourages outside relationships
- Childhood physical or sexual abuse
- Social isolation

Key signs and symptoms of dependent personality disorder

- Submissiveness
- Self-effacing, apologetic manner
- Low self-esteem
- Lack of self-confidence
- Lack of initiative
- Incompetence and need for constant assistance
- Intense, unremitting need to be loved in stable, long-term relationship that goes through minimal change
- Feelings of pessimism, inferiority, and unworthiness
- Hypersensitivity to criticism
- Clinging, demanding behavior
- Dependence on a number of people
- Avoidance of change and new situations

- May repeatedly request attention to her complaints over such issues as her lifestyle, social relationships, lack of meaning in life, or medical problems
- Overly sensitive to disapproval, the patient often feels helpless and depressed
    - Belittles her own abilities and is racked with self-doubt
    - Views criticism and disapproval as proof that she's worthless
- A dependent person is likely to avoid positions of responsibility; if her job requires independent initiative she may suffer occupational impairments
    - In females, associated with pattern of submissiveness
    - In males, associated with pattern of autocratic behavior
- Dependent personality disorder occurs in about 1.5% of the general population; it affects slightly more females than it does males
    - In mental health clinics, among the most commonly reported personality disorders
    - Concurrent personality disorder (commonly borderline or avoidant) found in an estimated 80% of patients
    - Coexisting mood disorders, including depression (most common), anxiety disorders, somatoform disorders, and dissociative disorders, found in many

● Causes

- Exact cause unknown; tends to run in families (may have genetic component)
- Possible link with authoritarian or overprotective parenting, leading to high levels of dependency
    - May cause child to believe she can't function without others' guidance and protection
    - May lead to child maintaining relationships by giving into others' demands
- Contributing factors
    - Childhood trauma
    - Closed family system that discourages outside relationships
    - Childhood physical or sexual abuse
    - Social isolation

● Signs and symptoms

- Submissiveness
- Self-effacing, apologetic manner
- Low self-esteem
- Lack of self-confidence
- Lack of initiative
- Incompetence and a need for constant assistance
- Intense, unremitting need to be loved in a stable, long-term relationship that goes through minimal change
- Anxiety and insecurity, especially when deprived of a significant relationship
- Feelings of pessimism, inferiority, and unworthiness
- Hypersensitivity to criticism
- In females, little need to overtly control or compete with others
- Clinging, demanding behavior
- Use of cajolery, bribery, promises to change, and even threats, all to maintain key relationships

- Fear and anxiety over losing a relationship or being alone
- Dependence on a number of people, any one of whom could substitute for the other
- Difficulty making everyday decisions without advice and reassurance
- Avoidance of change and new situations
- Exaggerated fear of losing support and approval
- Possible complaints of fatigue, lethargy, and depression

● Diagnosis

- Psychological evaluation and psychological and projective tests, as indicated
- Medical evaluation and diagnostic tests to rule out underlying medical conditions (somatic complaints)
- Diagnosis confirmed if *DSM-IV-TR* criteria met

● Treatment

- Outpatient mental health clinics
  - Rarely seek treatment for dependency or help in making decisions
  - Typically complain of anxiety, tension, or depression
- Individual psychotherapy, behavioral therapy, and support groups, and medication to manage associated symptoms
- Psychotherapy (the treatment of choice) to promote autonomy and self-efficacy
  - Short-term most effective (focus is helping patient solve specific life problems)
  - Long-term therapy contraindicated (reinforces dependent relationship with therapist)
- Individual and group therapy (the patient may use a group setting to find new dependent relationships)
- Therapy: patient may be needy and seek tremendous reassurance and attention — especially between therapy sessions
  - At the start of therapy, requires setting boundaries as to how the treatment will be conducted — includes setting appropriate times to contact the therapist between sessions and establishing clearly defined goals that, once attained, mark the end of therapy
- Assertiveness training (behavior modification using assertiveness techniques)
- Self-help support groups to allow patients to share their experiences and feelings, and put to use their newly learned skills; such groups shouldn't be used as the sole treatment because they may encourage dependent relationships
- Medications to treat associated symptoms, such as low energy, fatigue, and depression
  - In some patients, good response to antidepressants, including SSRIs, tricyclic drugs, and MAO inhibitors
  - In a crisis, possible use of benzodiazepine antianxiety drugs (such as alprazolam [Xanax], lorazepam [Ativan], and clonazepam [Klonopin]); however, benzodiazepine abuse potential requires limited use and monitoring

---

Diagnosing dependent personality disorder

- Psychological evaluation
- Psychological and projective tests
- Medical evaluation and diagnostic tests
- Confirmed if *DSM-IV-TR* criteria met

Key treatment options for dependent personality disorder

- Outpatient mental health clinics
- Psychotherapy (treatment of choice)
- Individual and group therapy
- Assertiveness training
- Self-help support groups
- Medications for associated symptoms
- In crisis, possible use of benzodiazepines

Key nursing interventions for a patient with dependent personality disorder

- Offer persistent, consistent, and flexible care.
- Take direct, involved approach to gain patient's trust.
- Give patient as much opportunity as possible to control her treatment.
- Verify patient's approval before initiating specific treatments.
- Encourage activities that require decision-making.
- Help patient establish and work toward goals to promote sense of autonomy.
- If patient has physical complaints, don't minimize, dismiss or, conversely, encourage them.

Characteristics of histrionic personality disorder

- Pervasive pattern of excessive emotionality and attention-seeking behavior
- Patient drawn to momentary excitements and fleeting adventures
- Charming, dramatic, and expressive
- Style of speech excessively impressionistic; gestures exaggerated
- Must be center of attention at all times
- Patient may have no sense of who he is
- Patient commonly changes attitudes and values based on views held by significant others
- Difficulty in developing and sustaining satisfactory relationships
- Fidelity and loyalty often lacking

● **Nursing interventions**
- Offer persistent, consistent, and flexible care; take a direct, involved approach to gain the patient's trust
- Give the patient as much opportunity as possible to control her treatment; offer options and allow her to choose, even if she chooses all of them
- Verify the patient's approval before initiating specific treatments
- Try to limit caregivers to a few consistent staff members to increase the patient's sense of security
- Encourage activities that require decision-making (such as balancing a checkbook, planning meals, and paying bills), and help the patient establish and work toward goals to promote a sense of autonomy
- If the patient has physical complaints, don't minimize, dismiss or, conversely, encourage them; instead, use a simple, matter-of-fact approach
- Help the patient express her ideas and feelings assertively
- Be aware that, outwardly, the patient may seem compliant — perhaps overly compliant — with suggestions for treatment; however, despite her passivity, she may fail to make real gains in therapy because her compliance is usually superficial
- Monitor the patient's medication regimen
  - Teaching her about prescribed medications, including exactly what each medication is prescribed for
  - Emphasizing that there are no magical drug effects
  - If the patient is receiving benzodiazepines, checking for signs and symptoms of physiologic and psychological dependence

HISTRIONIC PERSONALITY DISORDER

● **Defining characteristics**
- Patients with histrionic personality disorder characteristically have a pervasive pattern of excessive emotionality and attention-seeking behavior, and are drawn to momentary excitements and fleeting adventures
- Charming, dramatic, and expressive, such patients can be easily hurt, vain, demanding, capricious, excitable, self-indulgent, and inconsiderate
  - Typically come across as manipulative and phony (words and expressed feelings seem shallow and simulated, not real or deep)
  - Can shift instantly from rage to friendliness
- Their style of speech is excessively impressionistic, if not theatrical, and their gestures are exaggerated
  - Use grandiose language to describe everyday events
  - Value words more for their emotional content than for their factual accuracy
- People with histrionic personality disorder need to be the center of attention at all times
  - Exaggerate illnesses to gain attention
  - Interrupt others so they can dominate conversation
  - Seek constant praise

– Place great emphasis on physical appearance, commonly dressing provocatively and behaving seductively

– Consumed with superficialities, devoting little time or attention to their internal lives

• With limited self-knowledge, these patients may have no sense of who they are, aside from their identification with others; they commonly change their attitudes and values based on the views of significant others

– Rarely gain an understanding of others

– Devote intense observation skills to determining which behaviors, attitudes, or feelings are most likely to win others' admiration and approval

– View relationships as closer or more significant than really are

• Because they don't view others realistically, people with histrionic personality disorder have difficulty developing and sustaining satisfactory relationships (relationships that start out seeming ideal may end up as disasters)

– Tendency to idealize the significant other early in relationship, sometimes seeing connection as more intimate than it really is

– If significant other starts pulling back from patient's incessant demands, patient may become dramatic and demonstrative in attempt to bind other person to the relationship

– To avoid rejection, may resort to crying, coercion, temper tantrums, assault, and suicidal gestures

• Despite their attempts to bind others to them, many patients with histrionic personality disorder often lack fidelity and loyalty

• Histrionic personality disorder affects an estimated 2% to 3% of the general population; it's more commonly diagnosed in women, but may be just as common in men

• Without treatment, the disorder can lead to social, occupational, and functional impairments

– Many able to function at a high level and succeed at work (although frequent disruption of intimate relationships is common)

– Commonly coexists with somatoform and mood disorders

Causes

• Cause unknown

• Possible genetic component (hysterical traits more common in relatives of those with disorder)

• Little research on biological origins

• Childhood events may play role

• Psychoanalytic theories: focus is on seductive and authoritarian attitudes by fathers of patients

Signs and symptoms

• Constant craving for attention, stimulation, and excitement

• Intense affect

• Shallow, rapidly shifting expression of emotions

• Flirtatious, seductive behavior

• Vanity, over-investment in appearance, exhibitionism

• Exaggerated, vague speech

• Self-dramatization

• Impulsivity

Common causes of histrionic personality disorder

• Exact cause unknown
• Possibly genetic component
• Childhood event may play a role
• Seductive or authoritative attitude of father

Key signs and symptoms of histrionic personality disorder

• Constant craving for attention, stimulation, and excitement
• Intense affect
• Shallow, rapidly shifting expression of emotions
• Flirtatious, seductive behavior
• Vanity, over-investment in appearance, exhibitionism
• Exaggerated, vague speech
• Self-dramatization
• Impulsivity
• Suggestibility and impressionability
• Egocentricity, self-indulgence, and lack of consideration for others
• Somatic preoccupation and symptoms
• Use of alcohol or drugs to quickly alter negative feelings
• Depression
• Suicidal gestures and threats

- Suggestibility and impressionability
- Egocentricity, self-indulgence, and lack of consideration for others
- Intolerance of frustration, disappointment, and delayed gratification; impatience
- Intolerance of being alone
- Dread of growing old
- Suppression or denial of internal distress, weakness, depression, or hostility
- May be manipulative or angry with others
  - Divisive, demanding behavior
  - Angry outbursts and tantrums
  - Sudden enraged, despairing, or fearful states
- Somatic (physical) preoccupation and symptoms
- Use of alcohol or drugs to quickly alter negative feelings
- Depression
- Suicidal gestures and threats

Diagnosis

- No specific diagnostic tests; personality and projective tests can be helpful
- Must rule out physiologic disorders in patients with somatic complaints
- Diagnosis confirmed if *DSM-IV-TR* criteria met

Treatment

- Rarely seeks treatment unless a crisis occurs or a situational factor causes functional impairments and ineffective coping
- Goal to relieve the worst elements of the patient's behavior, rather than to cure her
- Psychotherapy (treatment of choice)
  - Focuses on solving problems in patient's life rather than producing long-term personality changes
  - Individual therapy preferred over group or family therapy, and self-help groups (group environment may trigger dramatic, attention-seeking behavior)
  - While establishing rapport and trust, therapist must avoid dependent situation with needy patient who sees therapist as her rescuer
  - Insight-oriented and cognitive approaches not especially effective (patients have little capacity or inclination to examine unconscious motives and thoughts)
  - Therapist must try to help patient view her interactions objectively, and explore and clarify emotions
    - Must be aware of patient's use of suppression, disavowal, denial, and avoidance to block information that could cause emotional distress
    - Should focus on issues that patient usually avoids (to help her live with reality on its terms)
    - Requires regular assessment for suicidal potential (all suicidal thoughts and plans should be taken seriously)
    - Should establish a "no self-harm" contract that specifies under what conditions patient may contact therapist when she feels like hurting herself (contract doesn't guarantee that self-destructive behavior will be prevented)

Diagnosing histrionic personality disorder

- Personality and projective tests
- Physiologic disorders must be ruled out
- Confirmed if *DSM-IV-TR* criteria met

Key treatment options for histrionic personality disorder

- Goal: to relieve worst elements of behavior, rather than cure patient
- Psychotherapy (treatment of choice)
- Focus: solving problems in patient's life rather than producing long-term personality changes
- Individual therapy
- Medications for relief of associated symptoms

• Medications to relieve associated symptoms, such as anxiety or depression; careful monitoring is required during therapy
  – In a crisis, may seek drugs for self-destructive or harmful purposes
  – May respond to side effects of medications with intense, dramatic overreactions

● **Nursing interventions**
  • Give the patient choices in care options, and incorporate her wishes into the treatment plan as much as possible; increasing her sense of self-control may help lower anxiety
  • Anticipate the patient's tendency to try to "win over" caregivers (may be responsive and cooperative, at least initially)
  • Teach the patient appropriate social skills, and reinforce appropriate behavior
  • Help the patient learn to think more clearly
  • Promote the patient's expression of feelings, analysis of her behavior, and accountability for her actions
  • Encourage warmth, genuineness, and empathy
  • Teach the patient stress-reducing techniques, such as deep breathing and an exercise regimen
  • Help her to manage crises and the feelings that trigger them
  • Monitor the patient for suicidal thoughts and behavior

NARCISSISTIC PERSONALITY DISORDER

● **Defining characteristics**
  • A person with narcissistic personality disorder is self-centered, self-absorbed, and lacking in empathy for others; he typically takes advantage of people to achieve his own ends, and uses them without regard to their feelings
    – Has inflated sense of himself and intense need for admiration
    – Tries to maintain image of perfection and invincibility to prevent others from discovering weaknesses and imperfections (beneath the image, basically insecure with low self-esteem)
  • The narcissist expects to be recognized as superior
    – Preoccupied with fantasies of brilliance and unlimited success or power
    – Believes he's special and entitled to favored treatment
    – Expects others to comply with wishes automatically, and believes he should associate only with other special or high-status people
  • Many narcissists are driven and achievement-oriented
  • The narcissist's delusion of greatness may be shattered by a threat to his ego, making him feel as though his life is unraveling, and possibly triggering a panic attack
    – Physical illness
    – Loss of a job or relationship
    – Feelings of emptiness and depression despite material wealth and success
  • Narcissistic personality disorder is found in less than 1% of the general population and affects about three times as many males as it does females
    – Develops by early adulthood but may not be identified until midlife, when person experiences sense of loss of opportunity or faces personal limitations

---

Common causes of narcissistic personality disorder

- Exact cause unknown
- Psychodynamic theory: child's basic needs go unmet
- Ambivalent self-perception

Key signs and symptoms of narcissistic personality disorder

- Arrogance or haughtiness
- Self-centeredness
- Unreasonable expectations of favorable treatment
- Grandiose sense of self-importance
- Exaggeration of achievements and talents
- Constant desire for attention and admiration
- Lack of empathy and concern toward those he offends
- Taking advantage of others to achieve goals

Diagnosing narcissistic personality disorder

- Psychological evaluation
- Personality and projective testing
- Confirmed if *DSM-IV-TR* criteria met

Key treatment options for narcissistic personality disorder

- Long-term psychotherapy (treatment of choice)
- Group therapy not effective because patient typically dominates group
- Possible hospitalization for severe symptoms
- Longer-term therapy for those who lack motivation for outpatient treatment

---

- In many cases, occurs in those with histrionic or borderline personality disorder

● **Causes**
  - Exact cause unknown
  - Psychodynamic theory proposes disorder arises when child's basic needs go unmet
  - Also theorized that patients have ambivalent self-perception
    - Develops from idealized (or overidealized) view of the self coexisting with deep feelings of inferiority and low self-esteem (grandiose image is effort to cover feelings of inferiority)
    - Begins during childhood, when patient received little encouragement and support from parents, and internalized process by looking for these feelings within himself

● **Signs and symptoms**
  - Arrogance or haughtiness
  - Self-centeredness
  - Unreasonable expectations of favorable treatment
  - Grandiose sense of self-importance
  - Exaggeration of achievements and talents
  - Preoccupation with fantasies of success, power, beauty, brilliance, or ideal love
  - Constant desire for attention and admiration
  - Lack of empathy or concern toward those he offends
  - Taking advantage of others to achieve own goals
  - May also exhibit rage, shame, or humiliation in response to criticism
  - In severe cases, may have self-destructive tendencies and poor reality testing

● **Diagnosis**
  - No specific diagnostic tests; patient should undergo psychological evaluation and personality and projective testing
  - Diagnosis confirmed if *DSM-IV-TR* criteria met

● **Treatment**
  - Most seeking treatment only in a crisis and terminate it as soon as their symptoms ease
  - Those not terminating treatment may be seeking help for depression or interpersonal difficulties
  - Long-term psychotherapy (treatment of choice) to help establish a strong alliance between the patient and therapist
    - Should focus on making small, not large, changes in personality traits
    - Includes placing the patient's exaggerated self-importance in perspective, helping him develop empathy, and teaching him how to handle slights and rejections without feeling extremely threatened
  - Group therapy not effective because the patient typically dominates the group
    - May be tiring to others, who have to hear about his accomplishments and talents
    - May drop out of group if criticized by others
  - Hospitalization may be necessary for severe symptoms, such as self-destructive behavior and poor reality testing; when needed, it should be brief, and treatment should be symptom-specific

- Longer-term therapy for those who lack motivation for outpatient treatment or for those with destructive, acting-out, and chaotic lifestyles
  - May involve intensive milieu therapy, individual psychotherapy, family involvement, or specialized residential environment
  - May be appropriate for patients with severe ego weakness, helping them to improve self-concept

● **Nursing interventions**
- Convey respect and acknowledge the patient's sense of self-importance so he can reestablish a coherent sense of self
- Avoid reinforcing either pathologic grandiosity or weakness
- Focus on the patient's positive traits or on his feelings of pain, loss, or rejection
- If the patient makes unreasonable demands or has unreasonable expectations, tell him so in a matter-of-fact way
- Remain nonjudgmental (a critical attitude may make him even more demanding and difficult)
- Don't avoid the patient (this could increase his maladaptive attention-seeking behavior)
- Avoid defensiveness and arguing
- Offer persistent, consistent, and flexible care; this includes taking a direct, involved approach to gain the patient's trust
- Teach the patient social skills, and reinforce appropriate behavior

OBSESSIVE-COMPULSIVE PERSONALITY DISORDER

● **Defining characteristics**
- Obsessive-compulsive personality disorder is marked by a pervasive desire for perfection and order at the expense of openness, flexibility, and efficiency
  - Characteristically involves viewing the world as black and white
  - Associated with relentless anxiety about not getting things perfect
  - Interferes with interpersonal relationships and daily routines
- The patient with obsessive-compulsive personality disorder places a great deal of pressure on himself and others not to make mistakes
  - May have a constant sense of righteous indignation and feel anger and contempt for anyone who disagrees with him
  - Believes his way of doing something is the only right way
  - May force himself and others to follow rigid moral principles and to conform to extremely high standards of performance
  - May insist on literal compliance with authority and rules
- A person with obsessive-compulsive personality disorder has an overwhelming need to control the environment but agonizes over the process
  - May suffer severe procrastination and indecisiveness because he can't determine with certainty which choice is correct
  - May have difficulty starting a task because of his need to sort out the priorities correctly

Key nursing interventions for a patient with narcissistic personality disorder
- Avoid reinforcing either pathologic grandiosity or weakness.
- Focus on patient's positive traits or on his feelings of pain, loss, or rejection.
- If patient makes unreasonable demands or has unreasonable expectations, tell him so in a matter-of-fact way.
- Remain nonjudgmental.
- Don't avoid patient.
- Avoid defensiveness and arguing.

Characteristics of obsessive-compulsive personality disorder
- Pervasive desire for perfection and order at expense of openness, flexibility, and efficiency
- Involves viewing the world as black and white
- Patient places great deal of pressure on himself and others not to make mistakes
- Patient has overwhelming need to control environment but agonizes over the process
- Lifelong pattern of rigid thinking may lead to poor social skills
- Many patients have one or both of the other cluster C personality disorders

Common causes of obsessive-compulsive personality disorder

- Possible genetic or familial cause
- Patient viewed as needing control as a defense against feelings of powerlessness

Key signs and symptoms of obsessive-compulsive personality disorder

- Behavioral, emotional, and cognitive rigidity
- Perfectionism
- Severe self-criticism
- Indecisiveness
- Controlling manner
- Cool, distant, formal manner
- Emotional constriction
- Bouts of intense anger when things stray from patient's idea of how things "should be"
- Difficulty incorporating new information into life
- Chronic sense of time pressure and inability to relax
- Preoccupation with orderliness, neatness, and cleanliness

Diagnosing obsessive-compulsive personality disorder

- Psychological evaluation
- Personality and projective tests
- Confirmed if *DSM-IV-TR* criteria met

- A lifelong pattern of rigid thinking may lead to poor social skills; symptoms may cause extreme distress and may interfere with the patient's occupational and social functioning
- Many patients with obsessive-compulsive personality disorder have one or both of the other cluster C personality disorders (avoidant and dependent personality disorders); some also have paranoid personality disorder as well as various types of anxiety, somatoform, and depressive disorders
- Obsessive-compulsive personality disorder affects about 1.5% of the general population—about twice as many males as females
  - In psychiatric settings, occurs in about 5% to 10% of patients
  - Higher incidence among oldest children in a family, and in those whose occupations require attention to detail and methodical perseverance

● Causes
- Possible roles of genetic and developmental factors; tendency to run in families suggested by twin and adoption studies
- Psychodynamic theories: patients viewed as needing control as a defense against feelings of powerlessness or shame

● Signs and symptoms
- Behavioral, emotional, and cognitive rigidity
- Perfectionism
- Severe self-criticism
- Indecisiveness
- Controlling manner
- Difficulty expressing tender feelings
- Poor sense of humor
- Cool, distant, formal manner
- Solemn, tense demeanor
- Emotional constriction
- Excessive discipline
- Aggression, competitiveness, and impatience
- Bouts of intense anger when things stray from the patient's idea of how things "should be"
- Indirect expression of anger despite apparent undercurrent of hostility
- Difficulty incorporating new information into life
- Chronic sense of time pressure and inability to relax
- Preoccupation with orderliness, neatness, and cleanliness
- Scrupulousness about morality, ethics, or values
- Miserliness and hoarding of money and other possessions
- Findings reported by patients
  - Signs and symptoms of depression
  - Sexual dysfunction
  - Physical complaints (commonly stemming from overwork)
  - Psychosomatic complaints

● Diagnosis
- Psychological evaluation, including personality and projective tests
- Diagnosis confirmed if *DSM-IV-TR* criteria met

Treatment

- Typically, seeks treatment only if depressed, unproductive, or under extreme stress (circumstances that tax his limited coping skills)
- Individual psychotherapy, possibly in conjunction with medication
- Discussion of the nature of the disease process and explanation of typical treatments by the therapist in a businesslike, factual manner, rather than giving vague impressions
- Patient likely to adhere to treatment rigorously and strive to be a good patient because he views himself as conscientious, honest, motivated, and hard-working
- Long-term work on changing the personality commonly unrealistic because the inherent nature of obsessive-compulsive personality disorder makes it especially resistant to change
- Effective psychotherapy centering on short-term symptom relief and support for existing coping mechanisms
  - Replacing maladaptive coping skills with effective ones as therapy progresses
  - Examining social relationships
  - Identifying the patient's feelings (likely to be out of touch with his emotions)
- Creative techniques to help the patient truly experience his feelings
  - Encouraging the patient to express how various situations, events, and daily occurrences make him feel (versus simply describing his feelings)
  - Having the patient keep a daily journal of feelings to help him remember how he felt at any given time
- Cognitive approaches rarely work (patients are likely to use this type of therapy as a means of verbally attacking the therapist or otherwise taking the focus off themselves)
- Group therapy usually intolerable for the patient because of the social contact necessary for healthy group dynamics; group members may ostracize the patient if he points out their deficits and perceived incorrect ways of doing things
- Generally, poor response to medication; if a patient suffers from depression, however, SSRIs or other antidepressants may be helpful

Nursing interventions

- Offer persistent, consistent, and flexible care; involves taking a direct, involved approach to gain the patient's trust
- Let the patient control his own treatment plan by giving him choices whenever possible
- Maintain a professional attitude; avoid informality as the patient demands strict attention to detail
- Recognize and respect the patient's need for physical and emotional distance
- Be prepared for long monologues centering on the patient's goals and ambitions, and reasons that family members, friends, and work subordinates need to be rigidly controlled; try to remain attentive
- Use tolerance and ordinary kindness when dealing with the patient (remember that he's used to causing exasperation in others but doesn't fully understand why)

Key treatment options for obsessive-compulsive personality disorder

- Individual psychotherapy
- Possible adjuvant medications
- Cognitive approaches rarely work
- Group therapy intolerable
- Generally, poor response to medication

Key nursing interventions for a patient with obsessive-compulsive personality disorder

- Let patient control his own treatment plan by giving him choices whenever possible.
- Avoid informality as patient demands strict attention to detail.
- Recognize and respect patient's need for physical and emotional distance.
- Be prepared for long monologues; try to remain attentive.
- Use tolerance and ordinary kindness when dealing with patient.
- Avoid defensiveness and arguing.
- Don't brush aside issues that patient thinks are important in an effort to get on with affective issues.
- Don't pressure patient to focus on emotions before he's ready; it will alienate him.
- Remember that patient's defensive structure is a cover for his vulnerability to shame, humiliation, and dread.

Characteristics of paranoid personality disorder

- Distrust of other people
- Constant, unwarranted suspicion that others have sinister motives
- Patient places excessive trust in own knowledge and abilities
- Patient searches for hidden meanings and hostile intentions in everything others say and do
- Patient quick to challenge loyalties of friends and loved ones

Common causes of paranoid personality disorder

- Exact cause unknown
- Possibly genetic influence
- May be a result of inadequate or poorly established parent-child attachment

Key signs and symptoms of paranoid personality disorder

- Suspicion and distrust of others' motives (hallmark sign)
- Refusal to confide in others
- Inability to collaborate with others
- Hypersensitivity
- Inability to relax
- Detachment and social isolation

- Avoid defensiveness and arguing
- Don't brush aside issues that the patient thinks are important in an effort to get on with affective issues; pressuring him to focus on emotions before he's ready will alienate him
- If appropriate, encourage the patient to record his feelings in a journal
- Remember that the patient's defensive structure (which makes him seem arrogant and argumentative) is a cover for his vulnerability to shame, humiliation, and dread
- Teach the patient social skills and reinforce appropriate behavior
- Teach him about prescribed medications
- Encourage him to continue therapy for optimal results

PARANOID PERSONALITY DISORDER

● **Defining characteristics**
  - Paranoid personality disorder is marked by a distrust of other people and a constant, unwarranted suspicion that others have sinister motives
  - Persons with paranoid personality disorder place excessive trust in their own knowledge and abilities
  - They search for hidden meanings and hostile intentions in everything others say and do
  - Patients are quick to challenge the loyalties of friends and loved ones
    - May seem cold and distant
    - Commonly shift blame to others and carry long grudges
    - Have a tendency to drive people away
    - Have few friends (only bolsters suspicions of conspiracy against them)
  - The prevalence of paranoid personality disorder is estimated at 0.5% to 2.5% of the general population
  - In clinical samples and, possibly, in the general population, paranoid personality disorder is more common in males

● **Causes**
  - Specific cause unknown
  - Possible genetic influence suggested by higher incidence in families with a member with schizophrenia
  - May result (at least partly) from inconsistent attachment or poorly established or maintained parent-child attachments, which can produce profound insecurity in the child

● **Signs and symptoms**
  - Suspicion and distrust of others' motives (hallmark sign)
  - Refusal to confide in others
  - Inability to collaborate with others
  - Hypersensitivity
  - Inability to relax (hypervigilance)
  - Need to be in control
  - Self-righteousness
  - Detachment and social isolation

- Poor self-image
- Sullenness, hostility, coldness, and detachment
- Humorlessness
- Anger, jealousy, and envy
- Bad temper, hyperactivity, and irritability
- Lack of social support systems

Diagnosis

- MMPI-2 and other psychological tests for diagnosis
- Diagnosis confirmed if *DSM-IV-TR* criteria met

Treatment

- Few seek treatment on their own; however, when they do, health care providers may have difficulty establishing rapport because of these patients' suspicious, distrustful nature
- Challenge of engaging the patient in a collaborative working relationship based on trust
- Individual psychotherapy preferred over group therapy (patient has a suspicious nature)
- Psychotherapy involving a simple, honest, businesslike approach rather than an insight-oriented approach
  - Initially focuses on the current problem that brought the patient to therapy
  - As therapy progresses and patient begins developing trust, may focus on disclosing paranoid ideations
- Pharmacologic therapy
  - Should be limited to briefest course possible
  - Antipsychotic drugs (such as olanzapine [Zyprexa] or risperidone [Risperdal]) to treat severe agitation or delusional thinking (given in one-tenth to one-fourth the usual dosage used in psychotic patients)
  - SSRIs, such as fluoxetine, to treat irritability, anger, and obsessional thinking
  - Antianxiety drugs to treat severe anxiety that interferes with normal functioning
- Because of patient's distrust of medications and resentment of the suggestion that antipsychotic agent is needed, some therapists delay considering medication until the patient asks about it
- Thorough teaching about possible adverse effects so he doesn't grow more suspicious if these occur

Nursing interventions

- Use a straightforward, honest, professional approach rather than a casual or friendly approach
- Offer persistent, consistent, and flexible care
- Provide a supportive, nonjudgmental environment in which the patient can safely explore his feelings; avoid defensiveness and arguing
- Establish a therapeutic relationship by actively listening and responding
- Avoid inquiring too deeply into his life or history unless it's relevant to clinical treatment

Guidelines for effectively interviewing a patient with paranoid personality disorder

- Start interview with a broad, empathic statement.
- Explore normal behaviors before discussing abnormal ones.
- Phrase questions sensitively to ease patient's anxiety.
- Ask patient to clarify vague statements.
- If patient rambles, help him focus on most pressing problem.
- Interrupt a nonstop talker as tactfully as possible.
- Express empathy toward a tearful, silent, or confused patient who has trouble describing a problem.

Guidelines for an effective interview

Establishing a rapport with a patient with a personality disorder can be difficult. These guidelines and examples may offer some help:

- Start the interview with a broad, empathic statement: "You look distressed. Tell me what's bothering you today."
- Explore normal behaviors before discussing abnormal ones: "What do you think has allowed you to cope with the pressures of your job?"
- Phrase questions sensitively to ease the patient's anxiety: "Things were going well at home and then you became depressed. Tell me about that."
- Ask the patient to clarify vague statements: "Explain to me what you mean when you say, 'They're all after me.'"
- If the patient rambles, help him focus on his most pressing problem: "You've talked about several problems. Which one bothers you the most?"
- Interrupt a nonstop talker as tactfully as possible: "Thank you for your comments. Now let's move on."
- Express empathy toward a tearful, silent, or confused patient who has trouble describing a problem: "I realize it's difficult for you to talk about this."

- Don't challenge the patient's paranoid beliefs; such beliefs are delusional and aren't reality-based, so it's useless to argue them from a rational point of view
- Avoid situations that threaten the patient's autonomy
- Be aware that the patient may not respond well to interviewing (see *Guidelines for an effective interview*)
- Use humor cautiously (a paranoid patient may misinterpret a remark that was meant to be humorous)
- Encourage the patient to interact socially to expose him to others' perceptions and realities and to promote development of social skills
- Help the patient identify negative behaviors that interfere with his relationships so he can see how his behavior affects others
- Encourage the patient's expression of feelings, analysis of his behavior, and accountability for his actions
- Respect the patient's need for physical and emotional distance
- Assess the patient's coping skills, and encourage him to use any existing (effective) coping skills; teach him effective strategies to alleviate stress and reduce anxiety
- Teach the patient about his prescribed medications
- Encourage him to continue drug therapy for optimal results

SCHIZOID PERSONALITY DISORDER

● **Defining characteristics**
- Schizoid personality disorder is characterized by detachment and social withdrawal

Characteristics of schizoid personality disorder

- Detachment and social withdrawal
- Patient is loner, with solitary interests and occupations
- No close friends
- Maintains social distance
- Seems unconcerned about others' praise or criticism
- Functions adequately in everyday life but doesn't develop many meaningful relationships

- People with this disorder are commonly described as loners, with solitary interests and occupations and no close friends; typically, they maintain a social distance even from family members, and seem unconcerned about others' praise or criticism
- Most people with this disorder function adequately in everyday life but don't develop many meaningful relationships
  - Fare poorly in groups
  - May excel in positions requiring only minimal contact with others
- Some people have additional personality disorders — most commonly schizotypal, paranoid, or avoidant personality disorder
- The disorder occurs in only about 0.7% of the general population; although it affects more men than women, more impairment is seen in women

Causes

- Exact cause unknown; may be inherited
- Sustained history of isolation during infancy and childhood
- Circumstances that interfere with warm, effective early parenting
- Parental modeling of interpersonal withdrawal, indifference, and detachment

Signs and symptoms

- Emotional detachment
- Social withdrawal
- Lack of strong emotions and little observable change in mood
- Indifference to others' feelings, praise, or criticism
- Strong preference for solitary activities
- Avoidance of activities that involve significant interpersonal contact
- Little desire for or enjoyment of close relationships
- Lack of close friends or confidants other than immediate family members
- No desire to be part of a family
- Little or no interest in sexual experiences with another person
- Inability to experience pleasure
- Shyness, distrust, and discomfort with intimacy
- Loneliness
- Feelings of utter unworthiness coexisting with feelings of superiority
- Self-consciousness and feeling ill at ease with people
- Oversensitivity to slights

Diagnosis

- No specific diagnostic tests; requires full psychological evaluation along with personality and projective tests (such as the MMPI-2 and MCMI-III)
- Must be distinguished from schizotypal and avoidant personality disorders, which also involve social isolation and withdrawal
- Diagnosis confirmed if *DSM-IV-TR* criteria met

Treatment

- Typically won't seek treatment unless under great stress
- Initially can't — or has no desire to — form relationship with therapist or other health care professional
- Based on individual and group therapy, and focuses on several goals
  - Helping the patient find the most comfortable solitary niche and cultivate satisfying hobbies that allow him to be on his own

---

Common causes of schizoid personality disorder

- Exact cause unknown
- Sustained history of isolation in infancy and childhood
- Circumstances that interfere with warm, effective early parenting
- Parental modeling of interpersonal withdraw, indifference, and detachment

Key signs and symptoms of schizoid personality disorder

- Emotional detachment
- Social withdrawal
- Lack of strong emotions
- Little observable change in mood
- Indifference to others' feelings, praise, or criticism
- Lack of close friends or confidants
- Inability to experience pleasure
- Feelings of utter worthlessness coexisting with feelings of superiority
- Oversensitivity to slights

Diagnosing schizoid personality disorder

- Psychological evaluation
- Personality and projective tests
- Must be distinguished from schizotypal and avoidant personality disorders
- Confirmed if *DSM-IV-TR* criteria met

- – Decreasing his resistance to change
  - – Reducing social isolation and improving social interaction
  - – Enhancing self-esteem
- Short-term individual psychotherapy, focusing on solving the patient's immediate concerns or problems (long-term psychotherapy for the patient with schizoid personality has a poor outcome and isn't recommended)
  - – Developing rapport and trusting therapeutic relationship with patient is usually slow, gradual process
  - – Therapist must make every effort to help him feel secure, acknowledge boundaries to avoid confrontations
  - – When patient opens up, may reveal fantasies, imaginary friends, and fears of unbearable dependency; may also fear growing dependent on the therapist, preferring to remain in fantasy and isolation (therapist should bring such feelings into proper focus)
  - – Therapist must strive to provide stability and support without smothering patient; some acting-out behaviors expected and should be tolerated
- Cognitive restructuring (cognitive therapy) to deal with illogical thoughts that impede the patient's coping ability and functioning; the goal is help the patient learn to identify his pattern of thoughts, emotions, and behavior, then change his thinking to benefit his mental health
- Incorporating group therapy into the treatment plan after the patient has developed adequate social skills and a tolerance for interacting within a group setting; initially, the patient is typically quiet, seeing little or no reason for social interaction
  - – Anticipate patient's behavior and avoid pressuring to participate more fully until ready
  - – Protect patient from criticism by other group members
  - – Encourage group to tolerate patient's initial silence
  - – When appropriate, encourage more supportive members to help patient overcome fear of closeness and feeling of isolation
- Self-help support groups to promote healthier social relationships, enhance functioning, cope better with unexpected stressors, and reduce fears of closeness and feelings of isolation; the setting allows the patient to try out new coping skills and learn that social attachments don't have to be rife with rejection or fear
- Medications for overlapping psychiatric disorders, such as major depression, or if the patient needs relief from other acute symptoms
  - – For patients with psychotic ideations, possible benefit from low-dose treatment with atypical antipsychotic, such as olanzapine or risperidone
  - – Long-term drug treatment generally avoided

● Nursing interventions
- Respect the patient's need for privacy, and slowly build a trusting therapeutic relationship so he finds more pleasure than fear in relating to you
- Offer persistent, consistent, flexible care; take a direct, involved approach to gain the patient's trust
- Recognize the patient's need for physical and emotional distance; remember that he needs close human contact but is easily overwhelmed
- Teach the patient social skills and reinforce appropriate behavior

- Encourage the patient to express his feelings, analyze his own behavior, and take accountability for his action; give him plenty of time to express his feelings as pushing him to do so before he's ready may cause him to retreat
- Avoid defensiveness and arguing

SCHIZOTYPAL PERSONALITY DISORDER

● **Defining characteristics**
- Schizotypal personality disorder is marked by odd thinking and behavior, a pervasive pattern of social and interpersonal deficits, and acute discomfort with others
- Schizotypal patients commonly exhibit eccentric behavior and have difficulty concentrating for long periods
  - May have peculiar mannerisms and dress
  - May have unusual speech that's overly elaborate, vague, metaphorical, and hard to follow
  - May have magical thinking, strange fantasies, odd beliefs (such as thinking they have extrasensory abilities), unusual perceptions and bodily illusions, social isolation, and paranoid ideas
- Some experts think schizotypal personality disorder represents mild schizophrenia; however, schizotypal patients aren't psychotic (for example, they don't generally experience hallucinations, delusions, or grossly disorganized thought and speech)
- During times of extreme stress, some patients do experience cognitive or perceptual disturbances
  - Not as fully developed as in schizophrenia
  - Generally short-lived, resolving with use of an appropriate antipsychotic drug
- Typically, schizotypal patients have severe social anxiety, usually because they're paranoid about others' motivations
  - May relate to others in a stiff or inappropriate way
  - May fail to respond to normal interpersonal cues
- Some people with this disorder marry; most have no more than one person they relate to closely
- The disorder takes a chronic course and in some patients progresses to schizophrenia
  - Major depression found in about 30% to 50% of patients
  - Another personality disorder (especially paranoid or avoidant personality disorder) found in many patients
- Schizotypal personality disorder is found in about 3% of the general population; it's slightly more common in men than it is in women

● **Causes**
- Possible genetic basis; family, twin, and adoption studies show increased risk in people with family history of schizophrenia
- Manifestation of schizotypal personality disorder versus schizophrenia possibly determined by environmental factors such as severe stress
- Some evidence of poor regulation of dopamine pathways in the brain in patients with disorder

Characteristics of schizotypal personality disorder

- Odd thinking and behavior
- Pervasive pattern of social and interpersonal deficits
- Acute discomfort with others
- Eccentric behavior and difficulty concentrating for long periods
- Cognitive or perceptual disturbances during times of extreme stress
- Severe social anxiety because of paranoia about others' motivations

Common causes of schizotypal personality disorder

- Possible genetic basis
- Environmental factors such as stress
- Possible poor regulation of dopamine pathways in brain
- Deficits in attention and information processing
- Ego boundary problems
- Parents likely had inadequate parenting skills and poor communication skills

Key signs and symptoms of schizotypal personality disorder

- Disturbed thinking
- Behavioral disturbances

Diagnosing schizotypal personality disorder

- Personality tests such as MMPI-2 and MCMI-III
- Confirmed if *DSM-IV-TR* criteria met

Key treatment options for schizotypal personality disorder

- Psychoanalytic intervention
- Cognitive-behavioral therapy
- Individual therapy (preferred)
- Group therapy
- Antipsychotic agents (low-dose)

- Psychological and cognitive theories (focus on deficits in attention and information processing)
  - Typically perform poorly on tests that assess continuous performance tasks (require ability to maintain attention on one object and look at new stimuli selectively)
  - Tend to do poorly on tasks involving emotionally laden words, suggesting cognitive bias toward neutral words
- Two psychoanalytic theories
  - Patients with disorder have ego boundary problems
  - Patients raised by parents with inadequate parenting skills, poor communication skills

● **Signs and symptoms**
- Disturbed thinking
  - Inaccurate beliefs that others' behavior or environmental phenomena are meant to have an effect on the patient
  - Odd beliefs or magical thinking (such as thinking that one's thoughts or desires can influence the environment or cause events to occur)
  - Unusual perceptual experiences, including bodily illusions
  - Vague, circumstantial, metaphorical, overly elaborate, or stereotypical speech or thinking
  - Unfounded suspicion of being followed, talked about, persecuted, or under surveillance
- Behavioral disturbances
  - Odd or eccentric behavior or appearance
  - Inappropriate or flat affect
  - Lack of close relationships other than those with immediate family members
  - Social isolation
  - Excessive social anxiety that doesn't abate with familiarity
  - Sense of feeling different and not fitting in easily with others

● **Diagnosis**
- No specific tests for identifying and diagnosing
- Personality tests, such as the MMPI-2 and MCMI-III, help to determine disorder type, severity
- Diagnosis confirmed if *DSM-IV-TR* criteria met

● **Treatment**
- Individual psychotherapy, family therapy, group therapy, cognitive-behavioral therapy, self-help measures, and medications
- Social skills training and other behavioral approaches that emphasize the basics of social interactions
- Psychoanalytic intervention focusing on defining ego boundaries
- Cognitive-behavioral therapy attempting to help the patient interpret his odd beliefs, and teach him valuable coping and interpersonal skills
- Individual therapy (preferred)
  - Includes establishing a warm, supportive, patient-centered approach
  - Requires avoiding any direct challenge of patient's delusional or inappropriate thoughts

- Group therapy as the patient progresses; initially, tolerating a group may be difficult due to distrust and suspiciousness
- Low-dose antipsychotic agents, such as clozapine (Clozaril), to treat psychotic symptoms
- SSRIs shown effective for mood or anxiety symptoms

● **Nursing interventions**
- Offer persistent, consistent, flexible care; be sure to take a direct, involved approach to promote the patient's trust
- Keep in mind that the patient is easily overwhelmed by stress
- Give him plenty of time to make difficult decisions, or decisions that seem difficult only to the patient
- Be aware that the patient may relate unusually well to certain staff members but not at all to others; remind staff not to take this personally
- Recognize and respect the patient's need for physical and emotional distance
- Teach the patient social skills and reinforce appropriate behavior
- Encourage the patient's expression of feelings, self-analysis of behavior, and accountability for actions
- Avoid defensiveness and arguing

NCLEX CHECKS

It's never too soon to begin your NCLEX preparation. Now that you've reviewed this chapter, carefully read each of the following questions and choose the best answer. Then compare your responses to the correct answers.

1. The nurse understands that the personality disorder characterized primarily by mistrust is commonly classified as:
- ☐ **1.** paranoid personality disorder.
- ☐ **2.** antisocial personality disorder.
- ☐ **3.** dependent personality disorder.
- ☐ **4.** schizotypal personality disorder.

2. For most patients with personality disorders, the treatment of choice is usually:
- ☐ **1.** group therapy.
- ☐ **2.** individual psychotherapy.
- ☐ **3.** self-help support groups.
- ☐ **4.** inpatient therapy.

3. When assessing a patient with a personality disorder, the nurse notes ideas of reference and magical thinking, leading her to suspect which personality disorder?
- ☐ **1.** Borderline personality disorder
- ☐ **2.** Schizotypal personality disorder
- ☐ **3.** Schizoid personality disorder
- ☐ **4.** Histrionic personality disorder

4. Which finding would the nurse identify as the most prominent characteristic of borderline personality disorder?
- ☐ **1.** Suspiciousness
- ☐ **2.** Reckless disregard for others
- ☐ **3.** Instability in personal relationships
- ☐ **4.** Unlawful behavior

Key nursing interventions for a patient with schizotypal personality disorder

- Remember that patient is easily overwhelmed by stress.
- Give patient ample time to make difficult decisions, or decisions that seem difficult only to patient.
- Recognize and respect patient's need for physical and emotional distance.
- Teach patient social skills and reinforce appropriate behavior.

TOP 10

Items to study for your next test on personality disorders

1. Characteristics of a healthy personality
2. Types of personality disorders
3. Characteristics of cluster A personality disorders
4. Characteristics of cluster B personality disorders
5. Characteristics of cluster C personality disorders
6. Assessment of personality disorders
7. Mental health issues associated with personality disorders
8. Treatment of personality disorders
9. Nursing interventions for personality disorders
10. Appropriate medications to be used with personality disorders

5. A patient with dependent personality disorder reports physical complaints. Which action would be most appropriate?

☐ **1.** Overlooking the symptoms
☐ **2.** Encouraging her to talk about her symptoms
☐ **3.** Disregarding the symptoms until emotional issues are explored
☐ **4.** Exploring symptoms in a matter-of-fact way

6. The physician prescribes risperidone (Risperdal) 0.5 mg daily for a patient with paranoid personality disorder who's experiencing delusional thinking. The pharmacy has only 0.25-mg tablets of Risperdal available. How many tablets should the nurse administer?

_____

7. The nurse instructs a group of students about clusters of personality disorders, and knows her teaching was successful when the group identifies which disorders as belonging to cluster B? Select all that apply:

☐ **1.** Antisocial personality disorder
☐ **2.** Avoidant personality disorder
☐ **3.** Borderline personality disorder
☐ **4.** Dependent personality disorder
☐ **5.** Histrionic personality disorder
☐ **6.** Paranoid personality disorder

8. Which characteristic would the nurse most likely identify as common to all personality disorders?

☐ **1.** Positive self-image
☐ **2.** Adequate impulse control
☐ **3.** Appropriate range of emotions
☐ **4.** Personal relationship problems

9. Which nursing intervention is appropriate to include in the care plan of a patient with schizoid personality disorder?

☐ **1.** Push the patient to express and discuss his feelings.
☐ **2.** Sit as close to the patient as possible.
☐ **3.** Ensure the patient's privacy.
☐ **4.** Encourage the patient to respond quickly.

10. While assessing a patient with borderline personality disorder, the nurse notes that the patient tends to view others and situations as extremes of good and bad. The nurse documents this finding as:

☐ **1.** dissociation.
☐ **2.** splitting.
☐ **3.** dialectical behavior.
☐ **4.** milieu.

ANSWERS AND RATIONALES

1. CORRECT ANSWER: 1

Paranoid personality disorder is characterized by an extreme distrust of others. Patients with this disorder avoid relationships in which they aren't in control or have the potential of losing control. Antisocial personality disorder is marked by behavior that violates the rights of others or violates social norms. A patient with dependent personality disorder characteristically has an extreme need to be taken care of, leading to submissive, clinging behavior, and fear of separation or rejection. In schizotypal personality disorder, the patient typically has a pervasive pattern of social and interpersonal deficits along with discomfort around others.

2. CORRECT ANSWER: 2

Individual psychotherapy is usually the treatment of choice for patients with personality disorders. Other therapies, such as group therapy, self-help support groups, and inpatient therapy, are usually not as effective.

3. CORRECT ANSWER: 2

Schizotypal personality disorder is marked by ideas of reference, odd beliefs, or magical thinking, among other features. Borderline personality disorder is characterized by marked instability involving relationships, self-image, and emotions as well as impulsivity. Schizoid personality disorder includes the hallmark symptoms of detachment, social withdrawal, indifference to others' feelings, and restricted emotional range. Histrionic personality disorder is characterized by a pervasive pattern of emotionality and attention-seeking behavior.

4. CORRECT ANSWER: 3

The prominent characteristic of borderline personality disorder is the patient's instability with personal relationships, mood, behavior, and self-image. Suspiciousness is most commonly associated with paranoid personality disorder. Reckless disregard for others and unlawful behavior are typically associated with antisocial personality disorder.

5. CORRECT ANSWER: 4

The nurse should explore the patient's symptoms in a matter-of-fact way—evaluating them promptly, but avoiding any lengthy discussion about them with the patient. Overlooking symptoms or disregarding them until emotional issues are explored is inappropriate.

6. CORRECT ANSWER: 2

Rationale: Using the formula, D/H × V, set up the problem as follows:

$$\frac{0.5 \text{ mg}}{0.25 \text{ mg}} \times 1 \text{ tablet}$$

Then solve:

$$2 \times 1 \text{ tablet} = 2 \text{ tablets}.$$

7. CORRECT ANSWER: 1, 3, 5

Cluster B personality disorders include antisocial, borderline, histrionic, and narcissistic personality disorders. Avoidant and dependent personality disorders are included in cluster C. Paranoid personality disorder is categorized as cluster A.

8. CORRECT ANSWER: 4

All personality disorders share certain common features, including problems with personal relationships (typically long-standing), disturbances in self-image, poor impulse control, and an inappropriate range of emotions.

9. CORRECT ANSWER: 3

The patient with schizoid personality disorder is typically described as a loner and, therefore, needs privacy. The nurse should respect this need and should proceed slowly to build a trusting, therapeutic relationship; this way, the patient experiences more pleasure than fear in relating to others. This patient also needs time to express his feelings; pushing him before he's ready for discussions or encouraging quick responses may cause him to retreat. The need for distance (physical and emotional) is part of the patient's pathology; therefore, sitting close to him would be inappropriate.

10. CORRECT ANSWER: 2

Splitting is a defense mechanism whereby the patient views others as either extremely good or extremely bad. Dissociation refers to the separation of objects from their emotional significance. Dialectical behavior is a psychosocial approach used in the treatment of borderline personality disorder. Milieu is a type of therapy that uses the patient's setting or environment to help him overcome a psychiatric disorder.

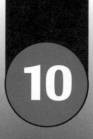

10

Eating disorders

CHAPTER OVERVIEW

Eating disorders are severe disturbances in eating behavior accompanied by distortions in body image and self-perception. The two main eating disorders, anorexia nervosa and bulimia nervosa, share such features as dieting and preoccupation with weight and shape. Additionally, anorexia nervosa and bulimia nervosa can occur simultaneously.

UNDERSTANDING EATING DISORDERS

● **Patient characteristics**
  • Eating disorders can occur in people of all ages and of all economic, ethnic, and educational backgrounds, but they're most prevalent in industrialized societies

Characteristics of eating disorders

- Occur in people of all ages and all economic, ethnic, and educational backgrounds
- Most prevalent in industrialized societies
- Typical sufferer is white, middle-class female in her teens or 20s
- Physically and psychologically debilitating
- Can lead to suicide or death from physical complications
- Sufferers face social obstacles (ostracism and isolation)
- Can establish vicious cycle leading to further isolation

Common causes of eating disorders

- Combination of components
- Tend to run in families
- Neurochemical factors
- Low self-esteem
- Conflicts over identity, role development, and body image
- Fears concerning sexuality
- Chaotic families
- Unrealistic expectations for appearance, equating being thin with being successful, powerful, and popular

- The typical sufferer is a white, middle-class female in her teens or 20s

● Effects of eating disorders
- An eating disorder can be physically and psychologically debilitating
- Extreme cases can lead to suicide or death from physical complications
- The risk of mortality is especially high if the disorder is long-standing or the patient has an overlapping psychiatric problem, such as substance abuse or depression
- People with eating disorders face social obstacles
  - May be ostracized because of peers (others don't know how to approach them; most boys aren't comfortable dating them)
  - Can establish a vicious cycle that leads to further isolation

CAUSES

● General information
- Theories explaining the cause of eating disorders encompass such factors as genetics, biology, psychodynamics, and social and family influences
- A combination of components is involved

● Genetic and biological theories
- Eating disorders tend to run in families, with female relatives most commonly affected
  - Increased risk (10 to 20 times higher) among girls whose female siblings already have the disorder
  - Suggests that genetic factors may predispose some people to eating disorders (or to accepting society's bias toward thinness)
- Neurochemical factors have also been linked to eating disorders; however, it's unclear whether these factors cause, accompany, or follow the development of the eating disorder

● Psychological factors
- Low self-esteem
- Conflicts over identity, role development, and body image
- Fears concerning sexuality
- Chaotic families with few rules or boundaries
- Parental overemphasis on, or excessive worry over, the child's weight
- Overly close mother-daughter relationship (in bulimia nervosa)
- Sexual abuse

● Social influences
- Society sets unrealistic expectations for appearance, equating being thin with being successful, powerful, and popular
- These expectations are conveyed through omnipresent images of thin, beautiful people on television and in films, magazines, and other media

ANOREXIA NERVOSA

● **Defining characteristics**
- Anorexia nervosa is a self-starvation syndrome in which the person relentlessly pursues thinness—sometimes to the point of fatal emaciation—as she becomes preoccupied with food and body image
- Despite extreme thinness, the person with anorexia nervosa thinks she's fat because she has a distorted body image
- Generally, a person is deemed to have anorexia nervosa when her weight drops to less than 85% of ideal body weight
- Anorexia nervosa occurs in two main forms
  - Restricting type: Patient limits food intake
  - Binge-eating or purging type: Patient engages in regular binge-eating or purging behaviors (including self-induced vomiting or misuse of laxatives, diuretics, or enemas) along with limiting her food intake
- Although more than 90% of those with anorexia nervosa are adolescents and women, the condition has also been diagnosed in males, in children as young as age 7, and in women up to age 80
  - Conservatively, found in about 0.5% to 1% of females in late adolescence or early adulthood
  - Across the lifespan, estimated to occur in 0.5% to 3.7% of all females
- About half of all patients with anorexia nervosa have additional psychiatric disorders
- The prognosis varies, but improves if the patient is diagnosed early or seeks help voluntarily
- Mortality is estimated to be about 5%; suicide accounts for about one-third of those deaths

● **Complications**
- Resulting from the malnutrition, dehydration, and electrolyte imbalances caused by prolonged starvation, vomiting, and laxative abuse
- Increased susceptibility to infection
- Hypoalbuminemia and subsequent edema or hypokalemia from malnutrition—possibly leading to ventricular arrhythmias and renal failure
- Coupled with laxative abuse, poor nutrition and dehydration that produce bowel changes similar to those of chronic inflammatory bowel disease
- Consequences of frequent vomiting
  - Esophageal erosion
  - Ulcers, tears, and bleeding
  - Tooth and gum erosion
  - Dental caries
- Amenorrhea (cessation of menstrual periods) when the patient loses about 25% of her normal body weight; prolonged amenorrhea can lead to estrogen deficiency (which raises the risk of calcium deficiency and osteoporosis) and infertility
- Life-threatening cardiovascular complications
  - Heart failure
  - Decreased left ventricular muscle mass and chamber size
  - Reduced cardiac output

Characteristics of anorexia nervosa
- Self-starvation syndrome
- Relentless pursuit of thinness sometimes to point of fatal emaciation
- Preoccupation with food and body image
- Despite extreme thinness, sufferer thinks she's fat because of distorted body image
- Weight drops to less than 85% of ideal body weight

Types of anorexia nervosa
- Restricting type: patient limits food intake
- Binge-eating or purging type: patient engages in regular binge-eating or purging behaviors along with limiting food intake

Key complications of anorexia nervosa
- Increased susceptibility to infection
- Hypoalbuminemia and subsequent edema or hypokalemia
- Poor nutrition and dehydration
- Bowel changes
- Esophageal erosion
- Ulcers, tears, and bleeding
- Tooth and gum erosion
- Dental caries
- Amenorrhea
- Estrogen deficiency
- Infertility
- Heart failure
- Decreased left ventricular muscle mass and chamber size
- Reduced cardiac output
- Hypotension
- Bradycardia
- ECG changes
- Sudden death

– Hypotension
– Bradycardia
– Electrocardiography (ECG) changes, such as nonspecific ST intervals, T wave changes, and prolonged PR intervals
– Sudden death, possibly from ventricular arrhythmias

● Causes

- Exact cause unknown; probable combination of genetic, biological, behavioral, environmental, and psychological factors (family dynamics also play role)
- Genetic factors
  - Identical twins at greater risk than fraternal twins are
  - Female siblings of anorexics more likely to have the disorder than male siblings are
- Biological factors
  - Study findings: Below-normal levels of the neurotransmitters serotonin and norepinephrine, and above-normal levels of cortisol (a "stress" hormone) and vasopressin
  - Findings suggest link to inadequate production of norepinephrine and serotonin
  - Findings also suggest possible role of stress (increases cortisol levels, thereby increasing risk for disorder)
- Behavioral and environmental theories
  - Societal standards of ideal body shape and constant pressure to be thin implicated as contributing to disorder
  - Occurs mainly in Western and industrialized countries, in which media (television, films, magazines) typically equate cultural image of beauty and health with thinness
  - May have great influence on development of self-image (many first learn about eating disorders through friends and media)
  - Suggests that eating behaviors are learned response to strong social pressures, which are bolstered by society's expectation that women stay thin
- Psychological factors
  - Prevailing view that low self-esteem, perfectionism, and sense of powerlessness underlie anorexia nervosa
  - Disorder is both symptom of and defense against feelings of inadequacy, to which patient responds
    - Develops perfectionistic tendencies to compensate for her low self-esteem
    - Becomes extremely self-critical in response to failure or rejection, which further weakens her fragile self-esteem
    - Expresses painful feelings of inadequacy through her eating because she doesn't know how to deal with feelings directly
    - Strives for a sense of power and control through caloric restriction because she feels powerless and unable to control her life or environment
    - Believes that, if she can control her eating, she'll be in control of her world, and that if she achieves the "perfect" body, she'll lead the "perfect" life
  - Refusal to eat is possible subconscious effort to avoid dealing issues surrounding sexuality

---

Common causes of anorexia nervosa

- Identical twins at greater risk
- Female siblings of anorexics more likely to have disorder
- Below-normal levels of serotonin and norepinephrine; above-normal levels of cortisol
- Stress
- Pressure from societal standards of ideal body shape
- Learned response to strong social pressures
- Low self-esteem
- Perfectionism
- Sense of powerlessness
- Feelings of inadequacy
- Possible subconscious effort to avoid dealing with sexuality issues
- Family dynamics

   – Family dynamics
- Tend to be chaotic and place high value on achievement
- Have trouble resolving conflict and expressing anger directly
- Possible abuse (sexual, emotional, physical); one aggressive parent and one passive parent; mother who's superficially powerful in family, but is actually weak; father who's distant and withholds feelings as daughter becomes adolescent

Signs and symptoms

- Key feature: self-imposed starvation despite obvious emaciation
- Usual history findings: 15% or greater weight loss with no organic reason, coupled with morbid dread of being fat and compulsion to be thin
- Physical findings
  - Emaciated appearance
  - Skeletal muscle atrophy
  - Loss of fatty tissue
  - Breast tissue atrophy
  - Blotchy or sallow skin
  - Lanugo (a covering of soft, fine hair) on the trunk
  - Dryness or loss of scalp hair
  - Hypotension
  - Bradycardia
  - Painless salivary gland enlargement
  - Fatigue
  - Sleep difficulties
  - Cold intolerance and hypothermia
  - Peripheral edema
  - Constipation
  - Bowel distention
  - Slow reflexes
  - Loss of libido
  - Amenorrhea
- Psychosocial findings
  - Preoccupation with body size
  - Distorted body image
  - Descriptions of herself as "fat"
  - Dissatisfaction with a particular aspect of appearance
  - Low self-esteem
  - Social isolation
  - Perfectionism
  - Ritualism
  - Inflexible thinking
  - Paradoxical obsession with food, such as preparing elaborate meals for others
  - Social regression, including poor sexual adjustment and fear of failure
  - Feelings of despair, hopelessness, and worthlessness
  - Suicidal thoughts
- Behavioral findings
  - Wearing oversized clothing in an effort to disguise body size
  - Layering clothing or wearing unseasonably warm clothing to compensate for cold intolerance and loss of adipose tissue

---

Key signs and symptoms of anorexia nervosa

- Self-imposed starvation despite obvious emaciation (key feature)
- 15% or greater weight loss with no organic reason
- Morbid dread of being fat and compulsion to be thin
- Emaciated appearance
- Skeletal muscle atrophy
- Loss of fatty tissue
- Blotchy or sallow skin
- Lanugo
- Dryness or loss of scalp hair
- Hypotension
- Painless salivary gland enlargement
- Amenorrhea
- Preoccupation with body size; distorted body image
- Low self-esteem
- Suicidal thoughts
- Wearing oversized clothing
- Layering clothing or wearing unseasonably warm clothing
- Restless activity and vigor
- Avid exercising with no apparent fatigue

– Restless activity and vigor (despite undernourishment)
– Avid exercising with no apparent fatigue
– Outstanding academic or athletic performance

Diagnosis

- Should be suspected in any young woman who isn't overweight with extreme or sudden weight loss (diagnosis missed in many patients because some are secretive about symptoms)
- Complete physical examination, including laboratory tests to help rule out endocrine, metabolic, and central nervous system abnormalities; cancer; malabsorption syndrome; and other disorders that cause physical wasting (such as acquired immunodeficiency syndrome)
- Possible findings in a patient who has lost more than 30% of her normal weight
    – Blood testing: below-normal hemoglobin, platelet count, white blood cell count, and levels of serum luteinizing hormone, follicle-stimulating hormone, serum creatinine, uric acid, cholesterol, total protein, albumin, sodium, potassium, chloride, calcium, and fasting blood glucose (from malnutrition); prolonged bleeding time (from thrombocytopenia); decreased erythrocyte sedimentation rate and triiodothyronine level (from a lower basal metabolic rate); and elevated serum amylase levels (unless pancreatitis is present) and blood urea nitrogen
    – Urinalysis: dilute urine (from the kidney's impaired ability to concentrate urine)
    – ECG readings irregular (possibly revealing nonspecific changes in ST intervals and T waves, prolonged PR intervals, and ventricular arrhythmias)
- Differential diagnosis to rule out other psychiatric disorders
    – Substance abuse (especially with stimulants, such as cocaine and amphetamines)
    – Anxiety disorders (especially obsessive-compulsive disorder and social phobia)
    – Body dysmorphic disorder
    – Mood disorders (such as major depression and bipolar disorder)
    – Schizophrenia
- Diagnosis confirmed if *Diagnostic and Statistical Manual of Mental Disorders, Fourth Edition, Text Revision* (*DSM-IV-TR*) criteria met

Treatment

- Aims to promote weight gain, correct malnutrition, and resolve the underlying psychological dysfunction
- Psychotherapy that addresses the underlying problems of low self-esteem, guilt, anxiety, and depression
- All forms of psychotherapy, from psychoanalysis to hypnotherapy
- Psychotherapy (specifically, cognitive behavioral therapy), most effective when coupled with weight restoration within 10% of normal; this may include the use of several treatment measures
    – Reasonable diet, with or without liquid supplements
    – Vitamin and mineral supplements
    – Activity curtailment, as needed (such as for arrhythmias or other physical reasons)
    – Behavior modification, with privileges based on weight gain

– Group, family, or individual psychotherapy
– Antidepressant medications
- Outpatient treatment; hospitalization in a medical or psychiatric unit is required when a patient exhibits certain signs or symptoms
  – Rapid weight loss (15% or more of normal body mass)
  – Persistent bradycardia (heart rate of 50 beats/min or less)
  – Systolic blood pressure of 90 mm Hg or lower
  – Hypothermia (core body temperature of 97° F [36.1° C] or lower)
  – Electrolyte imbalances, cardiac arrhythmias
  – Suicidal ideation
  – Persistent sabotage or disruption of outpatient treatment
  – Denial of the disorder and the need for treatment

Nursing interventions

- Help the patient to modify her body image misperceptions through cognitive and behavioral strategies
- During hospitalization, regularly monitor the patient's vital signs, nutritional status, and fluid intake and output
- Help her establish a target weight, and support her efforts to achieve this goal
- Negotiate an adequate food intake with the patient; make sure she understands that she must comply with this contract or lose privileges
- Frequently offer small portions of food or drinks
- Monitor the patient for suicide potential
- Maintain one-on-one supervision of the patient during meals and for 1 hour afterward to ensure that she's complying with the dietary treatment program (remember that for a hospitalized patient with anorexia nervosa, food is considered a medication)
  – Allow patient to maintain control over types and amounts of food she eats
  – Teach her to keep food journal (chronicling types of foods she eats, eating frequency, feelings associated with eating and exercise)
- Be aware that during an acute anorexic episode, nutritionally complete liquids are more acceptable because they don't require the patient to select foods (something patients with anorexia nervosa commonly find difficult)
- If tube feedings or other special feeding measures become necessary, explain these measures to the patient; anticipate the need to discuss her fears or reluctance, and limit discussion about the food itself
  – Weigh the patient daily (before breakfast or morning feeding, if possible) on the same scale, at the same time, and while she's wearing the same clothing
  – Before weighing her, observe her to detect added objects in her pockets or elsewhere or the intake of large amounts of fluids meant to falsely increase her weight
  – Keep in mind that her weight should increase from morning to night
  – Anticipate a weight gain of about 1 lb per week
- If edema or bloating progresses with treatment, reassure her that this swelling is temporary (otherwise, she may fear that she's getting fat and may stop complying with the treatment plan)
- Encourage the patient to recognize and assert her feelings freely; if she understands that she can be assertive, she gradually may learn that expressing her true feelings won't result in losing control or love

Key nursing interventions for a patient with anorexia nervosa *(continued)*

- Advise family members to avoid discussing food with patient.
- Remember that patient uses exercise, preoccupation with food, ritualism, manipulation, and lying as mechanisms to preserve control in her life.
- For outpatient who requires hospitalization, maintain contact with treatment team.
- Refer patient and family to Anorexia Nervosa and Related Eating Disorders, Inc.

Characteristics of bulimia nervosa

- Episodes of binge-eating followed by feelings of guilt, humiliation, depression, and self-condemnation
- Frequent binging
- Recurrent use of compensatory measures to prevent weight gain

Key complications of bulimia nervosa

- Not usually incapacitating
- Gastric rupture during periods of binge-eating
- Dental caries, erosion of tooth enamel, parotitis, and gum infections
- Dehydration or electrolyte imbalances
- Chronic, irregular bowel movements and constipation from laxative use
- Increased risk of suicide and psychoactive substance abuse

- Explain to the patient how improved nutrition can reverse the effects of starvation and prevent complications
- Advise family members to avoid discussing food with the patient; explain that nagging her to eat won't help, and might actually impede her progress
- Remember that the patient with anorexia nervosa uses exercise, preoccupation with food, ritualism, manipulation, and lying as mechanisms to preserve the only control she thinks she has in her life
- If an outpatient requires hospitalization, maintain contact with her treatment team to promote a smooth return to the outpatient setting
- Anticipate the need for therapy to uncover and correct dysfunctional patterns
- Refer the patient and her family to Anorexia Nervosa and Related Eating Disorders, Inc. *(www.anred.com)*, a national organization that can help them understand what anorexia nervosa is, convince them that they need help, and help them find a psychotherapist or medical physician who's experienced in treating this disorder

BULIMIA NERVOSA

● Defining characteristics
- Bulimia nervosa is characterized by episodes of binge-eating followed by feelings of guilt, humiliation, depression, and self-condemnation
  - Includes frequent binging (consuming abnormally large portions of food within a specific time period); in severe cases, can have several binge episodes in one day
  - Involves recurrent use of compensatory measures to prevent weight gain (such as self-induced vomiting, diuretic or laxative use, dieting, fasting, or a combination of these measures)
- The typical patient with bulimia nervosa is a young woman who's of normal weight or slightly obese with a history of extended dieting, excessive exercise, and use of diuretics, diet pills, laxatives, and steroids
  - As dieting continues, may experience a growing impulse to eat restricted foods
  - Eventually (usually after an anxiety-producing situation), eats to excess, temporarily relieving the impulse
  - Fears that food will turn to fat; may cause her to panic, inducing vomiting or using diuretics or laxatives (or both) to prevent weight gain
- Bulimia nervosa has been diagnosed in about 3% of the female population; however, up to 15% of females have some symptoms of the disorder (may be a gross underestimation because many sufferers are able to hide their symptoms)
- About 8 or 9 out of every 10 bulimia patients are female
- The condition usually begins in adolescence or early adulthood and may coexist with anorexia nervosa

● Complications
- Not usually incapacitating unless devoting an excessive amount of time to binge-eating and purging
- Gastric rupture during periods of binge-eating

- Dental caries, erosion of tooth enamel, parotitis, and gum infections from repetitive vomiting
  - In rare instances, can lead to esophageal inflammation and rupture
  - If ipecac syrup is used to induce vomiting, may suffer heart failure
- Dehydration or electrolyte imbalances (including metabolic alkalosis, hypochloremia, and hypokalemia), increasing the risk of arrhythmias and sudden death
- Chronic, irregular bowel movements and constipation from laxative use
- Increased risk for suicide and psychoactive substance abuse

Causes

- Exact cause unknown; as with anorexia nervosa, interplay of genetic, biological, behavioral, environmental, family, and psychosocial factors suspected
- Genetic and biological factors
  - Eating disorders shown more common in first-degree, biological relatives of people with bulimia (suggests frequency related to genetics, but possible importance of family influences as well)
  - Specific area of chromosome 10p linked to families with history of bulimia nervosa, providing strong evidence for genetic role in determining susceptibility
  - Role of altered serotonin levels in brain suggested by some studies
- Society's overemphasis on appearance and thinness recognized as integral in development of the disorder
- Other possible contributing factors
  - Family disturbances or conflict
  - Sexual abuse
  - Learned maladaptive behavior
  - Struggle for control or self-identity

Signs and symptoms

- History typically includes eating (in a discrete period of time) amount of food considerably larger than most people would eat
- During binge-eating episodes, sense of lack of control; patient continues to eat until interrupted by abdominal pain, sleep, or another person
- In most cases, patient states preference for foods that are sweet, soft, and high in calories and carbohydrates
- Physical findings
  - Thin, normal, or slightly overweight appearance, with history of frequent weight fluctuations
  - Weight within normal range (through use of diuretics, laxatives, vomiting, and exercise)
  - Persistent sore throat and heartburn (from vomited stomach acids)
  - Calluses or scarring on back of hands and knuckles (from forcing the hand down the throat to induce vomiting)
  - Salivary gland swelling, hoarseness, throat lacerations, and dental erosion (from repetitive vomiting)
  - Tooth staining or discoloration, loss of dental enamel, and increased dental caries (from repeated vomiting)
  - Abdominal and epigastric pain (from acute gastric dilation)
  - Amenorrhea from weight loss, hormonal imbalance

Common causes of bulimia nervosa

- More common in first-degree, biological relatives of people with bulimia
- Specific area of chromosome 10p linked to families with history of bulimia
- Possible role of altered serotonin levels in brain
- Society's emphasis on appearance and thinness
- Family disturbances or conflict
- Sexual abuse
- Learned maladaptive behavior
- Struggle for control or self-identity

Key signs and symptoms of bulimia nervosa

- Persistent sore throat, heartburn
- Callused or scarring on back of hands and knuckles
- Tooth staining or discoloration, loss of dental enamel, and increased dental caries
- History of eating amount of food larger than what most people would eat
- During binge-eating episodes, sense of lack of control
- Thin, normal, or slightly overweight appearance, with history of frequent weight fluctuations
- Abdominal and epigastric pain
- Amenorrhea
- Fluid and electrolyte imbalances
- Perfectionism
- Distorted body image
- Exaggerated sense of guilt
- Feelings of alienation
- Image as "perfect"
- Poor impulse control
- Low tolerance for frustration
- Peculiar eating habits or rituals
- Excessive exercise regimen
- Withdrawal from friends and usual activities
- Frequent weighing

– Fluid and electrolyte imbalances from repeated purging and use of diuretics and laxatives

- Psychosocial findings
  – Perfectionism
  – Distorted body image
  – Exaggerated sense of guilt
  – Feelings of alienation
  – Recurrent anxiety
  – Signs and symptoms of acute or chronic depression
  – Image as the "perfect" student, mother, career woman, or daughter (a child may be distinguished for participating in competitive activities, such as ballet or gymnastics)
  – Poor impulse control
  – Low tolerance for frustration
  – Self-consciousness
  – Difficulty expressing such feelings as anger
  – Impaired social or occupational adjustment
  – History of childhood trauma (especially sexual abuse)
  – History of unsatisfactory sexual relationships
  – Parental obesity
- Behavioral findings (typical)
  – Evidence of binge-eating, such as disappearance of large amounts of food over short periods, or presence of containers and wrappers
  – Evidence of purging, including frequent trips to the bathroom after meals, sounds and smells of vomiting, and presence of diuretics and laxatives
  – Peculiar eating habits or rituals
  – Excessive, rigid exercise regimen despite poor weather, fatigue, illness, or injury
  – Complex schedule (to make time for binge-and-purge sessions)
  – Withdrawal from friends and usual activities
  – Hyperactivity
  – Frequent weighing

Diagnosis

- Medical evaluation to rule out upper GI disorder that can cause repeated vomiting
- Psychological evaluation and Beck Depression Inventory to identify depression and other psychiatric disorders
- History to help determine seriousness of condition (if patient is honest about duration and extent of behavior)
- Laboratory tests to determine presence and severity of complications
  – Serum electrolyte studies revealing above-normal bicarbonate levels and decreased potassium and sodium levels
  – Blood glucose testing possibly detecting hypoglycemia
  – Baseline ECG showing cardiac arrhythmias (if the patient has severe electrolyte disturbances)
- Diagnosis confirmed if *DSM-IV-TR* criteria met

Treatment

- Early treatment is crucial; over time, the patient's behavior pattern becomes more deeply ingrained and more resistant to change; also, patients treated

---

Diagnosing bulimia nervosa

- Medical evaluation to rule out upper GI disorder
- Psychological evaluation and Beck Depression Inventory
- History
- Laboratory tests (serum electrolytes, blood glucose, baseline ECG)
- Confirmed if *DSM-IV-TR* criteria met

early in the disease course are more likely to recover fully than are those who delay treatment for years
- Most effective treatment centers on the issues that cause the behavior, not the behavior itself
- Individual, group, and family therapy; nutrition counseling; and (in many cases) medications
- High degree of structure and a behavioral treatment plan based on the patient's weight and eating behaviors
- Continuing treatment for several years; long-term psychotherapy and medical follow-up are essential
- Psychotherapy to break the binge-purge cycle and help the patient regain control over her eating behavior
  - May be inpatient or outpatient
  - Usually includes cognitive and behavior modification therapy, possibly in highly structured psychoeducational group meetings
  - In individual psychotherapy and family therapy, eating disorder addressed as symptom of unresolved conflict (approach may help patient understand the basis of her behavior, and teach her self-control strategies)
- Tricyclic antidepressant (TCA) such as imipramine (Tofranil), or a selective serotonin reuptake inhibitor (SSRI) such as paroxetine (Paxil) (adjunct to psychotherapy)
- Participating in a self-help group, such as Overeaters Anonymous, or a drug rehabilitation program (if she has a concurrent substance abuse problem)
- Hospitalization (medical or psychiatric) if binge-eating and purging have caused serious physical harm
  - Provides means for control and around-the-clock observation of all eating and elimination (urination, bowel movements, and vomiting)
  - Physical health determines degree of control that must be imposed on eating and total environment
  - As symptoms abate and eating behaviors and weight stabilize, patient gradually resumes control over her eating

Nursing interventions
- Engage the patient in a therapeutic alliance to obtain commitment to treatment
- Promote an accepting, nonjudgmental atmosphere; control your reactions to the patient's behavior and feelings
- Establish a contract with the patient that specifies the amount and types of food she must eat at each meal
- Supervise the patient during mealtimes and for a specified period afterward (usually 1 hour)
  - Includes setting a time limit for each meal
  - Helps to create a pleasant, relaxed eating environment (company during mealtime)
- Identify the patient's elimination patterns
- Teach the patient to keep a journal to monitor high-risk situations that cue maladaptive eating and purging behaviors
- Encourage her to recognize and verbalize her feelings about her eating behavior
- Encourage the patient to talk about stressful issues, such as achievement, independence, socialization, sexuality, family problems, and control

---

Key treatment options for bulimia nervosa
- Centering on issues that cause the behavior, not the behavior itself
- Psychotherapy
- TCAs or SSRIs
- Self-help groups
- Hospitalization

Key nursing interventions for a patient with bulimia nervosa
- Engage patient in therapeutic alliance to obtain commitment to treatment.
- Establish contract with patient that specifies amount and type of food she must eat at each meal.
- Set a time limit for each meal.
- Identify patient's elimination patterns.
- Teach patient to keep journal to monitor high-risk situations that cue binging and purging behaviors.
- Encourage patient to recognize and verbalize her feelings about her eating behavior.
- Explain risks of laxative, emetic, and diuretic abuse.
- Provide assertiveness training.
- Assess and monitor patient's suicide potential.
- Refer patient and family to American Anorexia/Bulimia Association or Anorexia Nervosa and Related Eating Disorders, Inc.

Medication guidelines for a patient with bulimia nervosa

TCAs
- Advise patient to take drug with food.
- Caution patient to avoid alcoholic beverages and sunlight exposure.
- Instruct patient not to stop taking medication.
- Caution patient about risk of overdose.

SSRIs
- Teach patient how to recognize signs of central serotonin syndrome.
- Advise patient to withdraw from the medication gradually.

 TIME-OUT FOR TEACHING

Medication guidelines for patients with bulimia nervosa

The treatment plan for a patient with bulimia nervosa may include the use of a tricyclic antidepressant (TCA) or a selective serotonin reuptake inhibitor (SSRI). Be sure to address this information when you teach your patient about her prescribed medication.

FOR THE PATIENT RECEIVING A TCA
- Advise her to take the drug with food.
- Caution her to avoid alcoholic beverages, sunlight exposure, heat lamps, and tanning beds.
- Instruct her not to stop taking the medication unless her physician approves.
- Caution her about the risk of overdose.
- Advise her to withdraw from the medication gradually.

FOR THE PATIENT TAKING AN SSRI
- Teach her how to recognize signs of central serotonin syndrome (abdominal pain, diarrhea, sweating, fever, myoclonus, irritability and, in severe cases, hyperpyrexia and cardiovascular shock).
- Advise her to withdraw from the medication gradually.

- Explain to the patient the risks of laxative, emetic, and diuretic abuse
- Provide assertiveness training to help the patient gain control over her behavior and achieve a realistic and positive self-image
- Assess and monitor the patient's suicide potential
- Instruct the patient about medication therapy, as appropriate (see *Medication guidelines for patients with bulimia nervosa*)
- Offer support, and encourage the patient stay in treatment
- Refer the patient and family to the American Anorexia/Bulimia Association, or to Anorexia Nervosa and Related Eating Disorders, Inc. *(www.anred.com)* for more information and support

NCLEX CHECKS

It's never too soon to begin your NCLEX preparation. Now that you've reviewed this chapter, carefully read each of the following questions and choose the best answer. Then compare your responses to the correct answers.

1. The nurse is preparing a presentation about the risks and complications of anorexia nervosa for a local community group of parents with adolescents. Which complication of this eating disorder should she identify as the most serious?
- ☐ **1.** High risk of mortality
- ☐ **2.** Coexisting depression
- ☐ **3.** Poor family relationships
- ☐ **4.** Social isolation

2. To meet the criteria for a diagnosis of anorexia nervosa, a patient's weight must drop below what percentage of ideal body weight?

- ☐ **1.** 75%
- ☐ **2.** 80%
- ☐ **3.** 85%
- ☐ **4.** 90%

3. The nurse is caring for a patient with anorexia nervosa who engages in purging behavior. The nurse understands that purging behavior is usually triggered by:

- ☐ **1.** sensations of fullness or bloating.
- ☐ **2.** guilt, humiliation, and self-condemnation.
- ☐ **3.** fear of being discovered as a binge-eater.
- ☐ **4.** feelings of nausea.

4. Which medication would the nurse least likely expect to be ordered for a patient with bulimia nervosa?

- ☐ **1.** Paroxetine (Paxil)
- ☐ **2.** Amitriptyline (Elavil)
- ☐ **3.** Diazepam (Valium)
- ☐ **4.** Imipramine (Tofranil)

5. Which finding would the nurse least likely expect in a patient with anorexia nervosa?

- ☐ **1.** Amenorrhea
- ☐ **2.** Weight within normal range
- ☐ **3.** Bowel distention
- ☐ **4.** Lanugo

6. The nurse is reviewing the laboratory test results of a patient with anorexia nervosa. Which results would the nurse correctly correlate with the patient's diagnosis? Select all that apply:

- ☐ **1.** Elevated platelet count
- ☐ **2.** Prolonged bleeding time
- ☐ **3.** Low serum calcium
- ☐ **4.** Elevated serum amylase
- ☐ **5.** Elevated follicle-stimulating hormone
- ☐ **6.** Low serum uric acid

7. The nurse has just assessed a patient with anorexia in the outpatient clinic. Which finding would prompt the nurse to anticipate the need for hospitalization for this patient?

- ☐ **1.** Persistent tachycardia
- ☐ **2.** Hyperthermia
- ☐ **3.** Blood pressure of 84/50 mm Hg
- ☐ **4.** Amenorrhea

8. When monitoring the weight of a patient with anorexia nervosa, it would be most important for the nurse to:

- ☐ **1.** obtain the patient's weight twice per day.
- ☐ **2.** check the patient's pockets or other clothing for added objects.
- ☐ **3.** expect the patient's weight to increase at a rate of approximately 2 lb (0.9 kg) per week.
- ☐ **4.** use the same scale each time, keeping it in the patient's room.

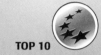

TOP 10

Items to study for your next test on eating disorders

1. Common characteristics of patients with eating disorders

2. Types of eating disorders

3. Factors contributing to the development of eating disorders

4. Signs and symptoms of anorexia nervosa

5. Signs and symptoms of bulimia nervosa

6. Psychological assessment of eating disorders

7. Physiological assessment of eating disorders

8. Treatment options for patients with eating disorders

9. Nursing interventions for patients with eating disorders

10. Appropriate medications used for patients with eating disorders

9. When evaluating the food intake of a patient with bulimia, the nurse knows that the patient is least likely to report her consumption of:

☐ **1.** sugar.
☐ **2.** calories.
☐ **3.** carbohydrates.
☐ **4.** protein.

10. A patient with anorexia nervosa is hospitalized and is receiving I.V. therapy. The physician orders 1,000 ml of dextrose 5% and half normal saline to run over 10 hours. Using I.V. tubing that delivers 10 drops per milliliter, the nurse would set the I.V. rate at how many drops per minute?

ANSWERS AND RATIONALES

1. CORRECT ANSWER: 1
Anorexia nervosa has a mortality rate of about 5%, with approximately one-third of those deaths due to suicide. Coexisting depression, poor family relationships, and social isolation all may occur with anorexia; however, these aren't the most serious complications.

2. CORRECT ANSWER: 3
The patient's weight must drop below 85% of ideal body weight to meet the diagnostic criteria for anorexia nervosa.

3. CORRECT ANSWER: 2
Guilt, humiliation, and self-condemnation usually trigger the desire to purge. Physical sensations, such as fullness, bloating, or nausea, aren't related to this behavior; nor is the fear of being discovered.

4. CORRECT ANSWER: 3
TCAs, such as amitriptyline and imipramine, and SSRIs, such as paroxetine, are commonly used to treat bulimia nervosa. A mild tranquilizer, such as diazepam, is rarely indicated. Additionally, if the patient is experiencing suicidal ideation, diazepam, a benzodiazepine, would be avoided.

5. CORRECT ANSWER: 2
The patient with anorexia nervosa typically appears emaciated with a loss of fatty tissue; her weight loss is 15% or more of her ideal body weight. Amenorrhea, bowel distention, and lanugo are findings associated with anorexia nervosa.

6. CORRECT ANSWER: 2, 3, 4, 6
Laboratory findings correlating with anorexia nervosa include prolonged bleeding time, low serum calcium levels, elevated serum amylase levels, and low serum uric acid levels. Platelet count and follicle-stimulating hormone levels would be low.

7. CORRECT ANSWER: 3
A systolic blood pressure that's less than 90 mm Hg is among the criteria for hospitalization, along with persistent bradycardia (not tachycardia) and hypothermia (not hyperthermia). Although amenorrhea is one of many physical findings associated with anorexia, it doesn't indicate a need for hospitalization.

8. CORRECT ANSWER: 2

The nurse should check the patient's pockets or other clothing for added articles that may falsely add to the patient's weight. The patient is weighed daily using the same scale each time, with the patient wearing the same clothing. The anticipated weight gain is 1 lb (0.5 kg) per week. Although the same scale should be used, it shouldn't be kept in the patient's room because doing so would overfocus on weight and create power struggles.

9. CORRECT ANSWER: 4

Most patients with bulimia prefer foods that are sweet, soft, and high in calories and carbohydrates. Therefore, the nurse wouldn't expect the patient to report her sugar intake.

10. CORRECT ANSWER: 17

First, determine the number of milliliters to infuse in 1 hour:

$$1{,}000 \text{ ml divided by 10 hours} = \frac{X \text{ ml}}{1 \text{ hour}}$$

Then solve for X:

$$X = 100 \text{ ml/hour, or } 100 \text{ ml/60 minutes}$$

Using the formula: volume/time (in min) × (drop factor), set the problem up as follows:

$$\frac{100 \text{ ml}}{60 \text{ minutes}} \times 10 \text{ gtt/ml}$$

Then solve:

$$1.67 \times 10 \text{ gtt/min} = 16.7 \text{ gtt/min, or } 17 \text{ gtt/min.}$$

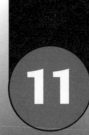

Substance abuse disorders

LEARNING OBJECTIVES

After studying this chapter, you should be able to:

● List the types of substance abuse disorders.

● State the street names for commonly abused substances.

● Describe the proposed causes of substance abuse and dependence.

● Describe the assessment process for substance abuse and dependence.

● Discuss the major treatment methods for substance abuse.

● Describe the nursing interventions for patients experiencing substance withdrawal.

CHAPTER OVERVIEW

Substance abuse affects males and females of all ages, cultures, and socioeconomic groups. People have used alcohol and other psychoactive substances — those that affect the central nervous system (CNS) — for centuries to induce changes in perception, mood, cognition, or behavior. These substances produce a state of consciousness that the user deems pleasant, positive, or euphoric.

Substance abuse commonly coexists with, and complicates the treatment of, other psychiatric disorders. Likewise, many people with emotional disorders or mental illness turn to drugs and alcohol to self-medicate and to make their feelings more tolerable.

UNDERSTANDING SUBSTANCE ABUSE DISORDERS

● **General information**
- A substance of abuse may be any chemical substance or preparation (normally used for therapeutic or recreational purposes) that's used in a maladaptive manner
- Commonly abused substances include alcohol; amphetamines and amphetamine-like drugs; barbiturates; caffeine; cannabis; cocaine and crack; hallucinogens; inhalants; nicotine; sedatives, hypnotics, and anxiolytics (primarily benzodiazepines); and opioids
- Many people abuse a combination of substances; drug mixing is the most dangerous form of substance abuse

● **Consequences of substance abuse**
- Substance abuse commonly leads to physical dependence, psychological dependence, or both
- It may cause unhealthy lifestyles and behaviors such as a poor diet
- Chronic substance abuse impairs social and occupational functioning, creating personal, professional, financial, and legal problems (drug seeking is commonly associated with illegal activities, such as robbery or assault)
- Drug use beginning in early adolescence may lead to emotional and behavioral problems, including depression, problems with family relationships, problems with or failure to complete school, and chronic substance abuse problems
- In pregnant women, substance abuse jeopardizes fetal well-being
- I.V. drug abuse may lead to life-threatening complications
  - Increased risk of infections, such as human immunodeficiency virus (HIV), viral hepatitis (especially hepatitis B and C), and bacterial infections
  - Nephropathy secondary to heroin use
  - Talc granulomatosis (if drug is mixed with an inert substance such as talcum powder)
  - Skin lesions and abscesses
  - Thrombophlebitis, vasculitis, and gangrene
  - Cardiac and respiratory arrest
  - Intracranial hemorrhage
  - Subacute bacterial endocarditis
  - Septicemia
  - Pulmonary emboli and respiratory infections
  - Malnutrition and GI disturbances
  - Musculoskeletal dysfunction
  - Depression, psychosis, and increased risk of suicide
- Psychoactive substances produce negative outcomes in many patients, including maladaptive behavior, "bad trips," and even long-term psychosis
- Illicit street drugs pose added dangers; materials used to dilute them can cause toxic or allergic reactions

● **Differentiating terminology**
- According to the *Diagnostic and Statistical Manual of Mental Disorders,* Fourth Edition, Text Revision (*DSM-IV-TR*), substance-related disorders encompass both substance-use disorders and substance-induced disorders

Characteristics of substance abuse

- May be any chemical substance or preparation that's used in a maladaptive manner
- Many people abuse a combination of substances
- Drug mixing is most dangerous form of substance abuse

Consequences of substance abuse

- Commonly leads to physical dependence, psychological dependence, or both
- May cause unhealthy lifestyles and behaviors
- Chronic substance abuse impairs social and occupational functioning, creating personal, professional, financial, and legal problems
- In pregnant women, substance abuse jeopardizes fetal well-being

Terminology of substance abuse

- Substance abuse
- Substance dependence
- Tolerance
- Physical dependence
- Addiction
- Withdrawal
- Intoxication

Defining substance abuse and substance dependence

Substance abuse
- The repeated use of alcohol or other psychoactive drugs that leads to problems

Substance dependence
- The persistent use of alcohol or other psychoactive drugs despite problems caused by such use
- Involves compulsive use or addiction
- Can cause significant withdrawal symptoms when drug use is reduced or stopped completely

Scope of substance abuse

- Major public health problem
- Alcohol is most commonly abused substance overall; among illicit drugs, marijuana ranks first

---

The language of substance abuse

Here are some important definitions you'll need to know to fully understand this chapter.

- *Substance abuse:* repeated use of a psychoactive drug that doesn't result in compulsive use or addiction and doesn't lead to withdrawal symptoms when the drug's use is terminated.
- *Substance dependence:* compulsive, repetitive use of a psychoactive substance resulting in tolerance to the drug's effects and withdrawal symptoms when drug use is decreased or stopped.
- *Tolerance:* decreased response to a drug that occurs with repeated use. A user who develops a tolerance to the rewarding properties of the abused drug must take increasingly higher amounts to get the desired effect.
- *Physical dependence:* an adaptive state that occurs as a normal physiologic response to repeated drug exposure; physical dependence doesn't necessarily indicate drug abuse or addiction.
- *Addiction:* state of chronic or recurrent drug intoxication in which a person experiences severe psychological and behavioral dependence on the drug and tolerance.
- *Withdrawal:* an uncomfortable syndrome that occurs when tissue and blood levels of the abused substance decrease in a person who has used that substance heavily over a prolonged period. Withdrawal symptoms may cause the person to resume taking the substance to relieve the symptoms, thereby contributing to repeated drug use.
- *Intoxication:* a reversible, substance-specific syndrome caused by ingestion of or exposure to that substance.

- *Substance abuse* is the repeated use of alcohol or other psychoactive drugs that leads to problems
  - Doesn't involve compulsive use or addiction
  - Doesn't cause significant withdrawal symptoms when drug use is reduced or stopped completely
- *Substance dependence* refers to the persistent use of alcohol or other psychoactive drugs despite problems caused by such use
  - Involves compulsive use or addiction
  - Can cause significant withdrawal symptoms when drug use is reduced or stopped completely
- *Tolerance* is the result of compulsive and repetitive substance use (the user becomes increasingly tolerant to the drug's effects, needing higher doses to get the same therapeutic or recreational effect)
- *Withdrawal symptoms* occur when drug use is decreased or stopped (see *The language of substance abuse*)

● Scope of the problem
- Substance abuse is a major public health problem; according to recent statistics, roughly 7% of the total U.S. population abuse or are dependent on alcohol or illicit drugs
- Alcohol is the most commonly abused substance overall; among illicit drugs, marijuana ranks first (used by approximately 76% of illicit drug users)
- Experimentation with drugs commonly begins during adolescence, although recent statistics show a trend toward drug use among preadolescents

CAUSES OF SUBSTANCE ABUSE

● General information
- The exact causes of substance abuse and addiction aren't known
- Probable influences include genetic predisposition, pharmacologic properties of the particular drug, peer pressure, emotional distress, and environmental factors

● Genetic theories
- Genetic theories propose that inherited mechanisms cause or predispose a person to drug addiction
- Genetic factors have been explored most extensively in alcoholism
  - Studies showing that many Asians carry a gene that confers reduced risk of alcoholism
  - Possible increased risk conferred by other genetic factors
  - Chromosomes 1 and 7 linked to susceptibility to alcohol dependence
- Most likely, both heredity and environment influence whether a person will become a substance abuser
- Researchers continue to debate which of the two factors is more important, and research findings have been confusing
  - Many suffer alcoholism with no known alcoholic relatives; many alcoholic parents have children who don't become alcoholics themselves (suggesting environmental influence)
  - Biological children of alcoholics adopted into nonalcoholic homes at early age more likely to become alcoholics than children of nonalcoholics adopted into alcoholic homes (suggesting hereditary influence)

● Neurobiological theories
- According to neurobiological theories, chronic exposure to drugs leads to biological and cellular adaptation
- Drug addicts may have an inborn deficiency of endorphins (peptide hormones that bind to opiate receptors, reducing pain sensations and exerting a calming effect)
  - Deficiency may heighten sensitivity to pain and confer a greater susceptibility to opioid abuse
- Regular opiate use may reduce the body's natural endorphin production, causing a reliance on the drug for ordinary pain relief
- According to another neurobiological theory, enzymes produced by a given gene might influence hormones and neurotransmitters, contributing to the development of a personality that's more sensitive to peer pressure—including the pressure to use illicit drugs

● Psychobiological theories
- Introducing an opiate into the body may cause metabolic adjustments that require continued and increasing dosages to prevent withdrawal
- Studies haven't yet identified cell metabolism changes that are linked to addiction

● Behavioral theories
- Behavioral scientists view drug abuse as the result of conditioning, or cumulative reinforcement from drug use

---

Common causes of substance abuse

- *Genetic theories:* inherited mechanisms cause or predispose a person to drug addiction
- *Neurobiological theories:* chronic exposure to drugs leads to biological and cellular adaptation
- *Psychobiological theories:* introducing an opiate into the body may cause metabolic adjustments that require continued and increasing dosages to prevent withdrawal
- *Behavioral theories:* drug abuse is result of conditioning, or cumulative reinforcement from drug use
- *Social and psychological theories:* adolescents and young adults take drugs to preserve childhood and avoid dealing with adult conflicts and responsibilities

– Drug use: causes euphoric experience perceived as rewarding, thereby motivating user to keep taking the drug (which then serves as a biological reward)
– Stimuli and settings associated with drug use: may themselves become reinforcing or may trigger drug craving that can lead to relapse (many recovering addicts change their environment to eliminate cues that could promote drug use)

● **Social and psychological theories**
• According to some theories, adolescents and young adults take drugs to preserve childhood and avoid dealing with adult conflicts and responsibilities
• Many users see drugs as a way to cope with their personal and social needs and changing situational demands
• In some cultures, drugs may be more available and socially acceptable, or social pressures for drug use may be stronger
• Social ritual may also play a role by affecting the meaning and style of drug use adopted by a person in a given setting

ALCOHOL DEPENDENCE

● **Defining characteristics**
• Alcohol (ethanol) is a CNS depressant that reduces the activity of neurons in the brain
• Chronic, uncontrolled alcohol intake is the greatest substance abuse problem in the United States
• Alcohol dependence is characterized by three main symptom clusters
– Biological adaptation: adaptation to or physical dependence on alcohol, which manifests as tolerance or withdrawal
– Loss of control: inability to limit alcohol intake to moderate amount; repeated but unsuccessful attempts to cut down on or stop drinking; compulsive thoughts and actions, with much of day spent thinking about drinking or recovering from alcohol binge
– Maladaptive consequences: continued use despite reduced occupational functioning and negative psychological, social, and health consequences
• Alcohol abuse cuts across all socioeconomic boundaries and life stages, sometimes starting as early as elementary school age
– Abuse or dependence suffered by about 13% of U.S. residents older than age 18 at some time in their lives
– Alcohol use peaks between ages 21 and 34, but nearly 20% of adolescents have serious drinking problem (current statistics)
– Alcohol abuse two to five times more likely in males than in females
• Alcohol abuse decreases the life span by roughly 15 years
– Accounts for nearly 25% of premature deaths in men, 15% in women
– Most body tissues adversely affected by heavy intake, especially those of the liver, kidney, and brain (see *Complications of alcohol abuse*)

● **Causes**
• Possible genetic influences
– Higher incidence among identical twins than among fraternal twins
– Fourfold increased risk of alcoholism among biological children of alcoholics (even if adopted at birth)

Characteristics of alcohol dependence

• Three main symptom clusters — biological adaptation, loss of control, and maladaptive consequences
• *Biological adaptation:* adaptation to or physical dependence on alcohol, which manifests as tolerance or withdrawal
• *Loss of control:* inability to limit alcohol intake to moderate amount; repeated but unsuccessful attempts to cut down on or stop drinking; compulsive thoughts and actions
• *Maladaptive consequences:* continued use despite reduced occupational functioning and negative psychological, social, and health consequences

Common causes of alcohol dependence

• Possible genetic influences
• Biochemical abnormalities
• Urge to drink to reduce anxiety or symptoms of mental illness
• Desire to avoid responsibility in family, social, and work relationships
• Low self-esteem
• Easy access
• Group or peer pressure
• Stressful lifestyle
• Social attitudes accepting of frequent alcohol consumption

Complications of alcohol abuse

Alcohol damages body tissues by irritating them directly, through changes that occur during its metabolism, by interacting with other drugs, by aggravating existing disease, or through accidents brought on by intoxication. Tissue damage can lead to a host of complications.

CARDIOPULMONARY COMPLICATIONS
- Arrhythmias
- Cardiomyopathy
- Essential hypertension
- Chronic obstructive pulmonary disease
- Pneumonia
- Increased risk of tuberculosis

GI COMPLICATIONS
- Chronic diarrhea
- Esophagitis
- Esophageal cancer
- Esophageal varices
- Gastric ulcers
- Gastritis
- GI bleeding
- Malabsorption
- Pancreatitis

HEPATIC COMPLICATIONS
- Alcoholic hepatitis
- Cirrhosis
- Fatty liver

NEUROLOGIC COMPLICATIONS
- Alcoholic dementia
- Alcoholic hallucinosis
- Alcohol withdrawal delirium
- Korsakoff's syndrome
- Peripheral neuropathy
- Seizure disorders
- Subdural hematoma
- Wernicke's encephalopathy

PSYCHIATRIC COMPLICATIONS
- Amotivational syndrome
- Depression
- Impaired social and occupational functioning
- Multiple substance abuse
- Suicide

OTHER COMPLICATIONS
- Beriberi
- Fetal alcohol syndrome
- Hypoglycemia
- Leg and foot ulcers
- Prostatitis

Complications of alcohol abuse
- Cardiopulmonary
- GI
- Hepatic
- Neurologic
- Psychiatric
- Beriberi
- Fetal alcohol syndrome
- Hypoglycemia
- Leg and foot ulcers
- Prostatitis

Key signs and symptoms of alcohol dependence

Alcohol dependency
- Minor complaints
- Poor personal hygiene
- Untreated injuries
- Unusually high tolerance for sedatives and opioids
- Nutritional deficiency
- Secretive behavior
- Denial of problem
- Tendency to blame others and rationalize problems

Excessive alcohol use
- Episodes of anesthesia or amnesia during intoxication
- Violent behavior
- Need for daily or episodic alcohol to function adequately
- Inability to stop or reduce alcohol intake

Alcohol withdrawal
- Anorexia, nausea
- Anxiety, agitation
- Fever
- Insomnia
- Diaphoresis
- Tremor progressing to severe tremulousness
- Possible hallucinations and violent behavior
- Severe agitation
- Withdrawal delirium

– Irish-Americans up to seven times more likely than Italian-Americans to become alcohol-dependent
– Predisposition to impulsivity and sensation seeking
- Biochemical abnormalities: nutritional deficiencies, endocrine imbalances, and alterations in molecular and cellular components in the brain
- Psychological factors: urge to drink to reduce anxiety or symptoms of mental illness; desire to avoid responsibility in family, social, and work relationships; low self-esteem
- Sociocultural factors: easy access, group or peer pressure, stressful lifestyle, social attitudes accepting of frequent alcohol consumption

Signs and symptoms
- Alcohol dependency
  – Minor complaints: malaise, dyspepsia, mood swings or depression, increased incidence of infection
  – Poor personal hygiene, untreated injuries (cigarette burns, fractures, bruises that can't be fully explained)
  – Unusually high tolerance for sedatives and opioids

– Nutritional deficiency (vitamins and minerals)
– Secretive behavior (may attempt to hide disorder or alcohol supply)
– Consumption of alcohol-containing products (mouthwash, aftershave lotion, hair spray, lighter fluid)
– Denial of problem
– Tendency to blame others and rationalize problems (possibly displacing anger, guilt, or inadequacy onto others to avoid confronting illness)
• Excessive alcohol use (overt indications)
– Episodes of anesthesia or amnesia during intoxication (blackouts)
– Violent behavior when intoxicated
– Need for daily or episodic alcohol to function adequately
– Inability to stop or reduce alcohol intake
• Alcohol withdrawal (initial signs and symptoms)
– Anorexia, nausea
– Anxiety, agitation
– Fever
– Insomnia
– Diaphoresis
– Tremor progressing to severe tremulousness
– Possible hallucinations and violent behavior
– Possible major motor seizures (sometimes called *rum fits*)
– Severe agitation
– Autonomic overactivity (dramatic increases in pulse, respirations, and blood pressure)
– Symptoms beginning shortly after drinking stops and lasting up to 10 days
– Withdrawal delirium (life-threatening complication formerly called *delirium tremens*) in about 5% to 10% of patients (see *Assessing for alcohol withdrawal*)

● **Diagnosis**
• Centers on pattern of difficulties associated with alcohol use (not on amount and frequency of consumption)
• Blood alcohol level to indicate intoxication (0.10% weight/volume [200 mg/dl]); doesn't confirm alcoholism but can reveal how recently person has been drinking and when to expect withdrawal symptoms in heavy drinker
• Urine toxicology to reveal use of other drugs
• Serum electrolyte analysis revealing electrolyte abnormalities associated with alcohol use
• Blood testing revealing elevated blood urea nitrogen (BUN), increased plasma ammonia level (severe liver disease, cirrhosis), and decreased serum glucose level (severe liver disease)
• Liver function studies demonstrating alcohol-related liver damage
• Hematologic workup possibly revealing anemia, thrombocytopenia, and increased prothrombin and partial thromboplastin times
• Echocardiography and electrocardiography (ECG) demonstrating cardiac problems (cardiomegaly)
• Diagnosis of alcohol dependence or alcohol abuse confirmed when *DSM-IV-TR* criteria met

Diagnosing alcohol dependence

● Blood alcohol level to indicate intoxication
● Urine toxicology to reveal use of other drugs
● Serum electrolyte analysis revealing electrolyte abnormalities associated with alcohol use
● Blood testing revealing elevated BUN, increased plasma ammonia level, and decreased serum glucose level
● Liver function studies demonstrating alcohol-related liver damage
● Confirmed if *DSM-IV-TR* criteria met

Assessing for alcohol withdrawal

Alcohol withdrawal symptoms may vary from mild (morning hangover) to severe (alcohol withdrawal delirium). Formerly known as *delirium tremens* or *DTs*, alcohol withdrawal delirium is marked by acute distress brought on by drinking cessation in a person who's physically dependent on alcohol.

SIGNS AND SYMPTOMS	MILD WITHDRAWAL	MODERATE WITHDRAWAL	SEVERE WITHDRAWAL
Motor impairment	Inner tremulousness with hand tremor	Visible tremors; obvious motor restlessness and painful anxiety	Gross, uncontrollable shaking; extreme restlessness and agitation with intense fearfulness
Sleep disturbance	Restless sleep or insomnia	Marked insomnia and nightmares	Total wakefulness
Appetite	Impaired appetite	Marked anorexia	Rejection of all food and fluid except alcohol
GI symptoms	Nausea	Nausea and vomiting	Dry heaves and vomiting
Confusion	None	Variable	Marked confusion and disorientation
Hallucinations	None	Vague, transient visual and auditory hallucinations and illusions (commonly nocturnal)	Visual and, occasionally, auditory hallucinations, usually with fearful or threatening content; misidentification of people and frightening delusions related to hallucinatory experiences
Pulse rate	Tachycardia	100 to 120 beats/minute	120 to 140 beats/minute
Blood pressure	Normal or slightly elevated systolic	Usually elevated systolic	Elevated systolic and diastolic
Sweating	Slight	Obvious	Marked hyperhidrosis
Seizures	None	Possible	Common

Treatment
* Symptomatic treatment; may involve respiratory support, fluid replacement, I.V. glucose to prevent hypoglycemia, correction of hypothermia or acidosis, and emergency measures for trauma, infection, or GI bleeding
* Withdrawal in a monitored, therapeutic setting (to avoid serious complications such as death)
* I.V. glucose administration and administration of fluids containing thiamine and other B-complex vitamins to correct nutritional deficiencies and aid in glucose metabolism
* Various medications
  – Furosemide (Lasix) to reduce overhydration

Key signs and symptoms of alcohol withdrawal

Mild withdrawal
* Inner tremulousness with hand tremor
* Impaired appetite
* Nausea
* Tachycardia

Moderate withdrawal
* Visible tremors
* Obvious motor restlessness and painful anxiety
* Marked insomnia and nightmares
* Marked anorexia
* Vague, transient visual and auditory hallucinations
* Pulse 100 to 120 beats/minute
* Usually elevated systolic pressure
* Obvious sweating
* Possible seizures

Severe withdrawal
* Gross, uncontrollable shaking
* Extreme restlessness and agitation; intense fearfulness
* Total wakefulness
* Dry heaves and vomiting
* Marked confusion and disorientation
* Visual and, occasionally, auditory hallucinations
* Pulse 120 to 140 beats/minute
* Elevated systolic and diastolic pressure
* Marked hyperhidrosis
* Seizures

Key treatment options for alcohol dependence

- Symptomatic treatment
- Withdrawal in a monitored, therapeutic setting
- Multifaceted management
- Medications that deter alcohol use
- Measures to relieve associated physical problems
- Psychotherapy
- Counseling and ongoing support groups
- Aversion therapy (with disulfiram)
- Antagonist therapy
- Counseling and psychotherapy for long-term rehabilitation

Key signs and symptoms of disulfiram reaction

- Flushing
- Throbbing of neck and head
- Nausea and vomiting
- Headache
- Sweating
- Thirst
- Shortness of breath or other respiratory difficulties
- Chest pain, palpitations, tachycardia, hyperventilation, hypotension, or syncope
- Weakness
- Vertigo
- Blurred vision
- Confusion

– Magnesium sulfate to reduce CNS irritability
– Chlordiazepoxide (Librium), diazepam (Valium), anticonvulsants, antiemetics, or antidiarrheals as needed to ease withdrawal symptoms
– Antipsychotics to control hyperactivity and psychosis
– Phenobarbital (Bellatal) for sedation
- No known cure; total abstinence is the only effective treatment
- Multifaceted management
    – Medications that deter alcohol use (as in aversion, emetic, or antagonist therapy) and treat withdrawal symptoms
    – Measures to relieve associated physical problems
    – Psychotherapy, usually involving behavior modification, group therapy, and family therapy
    – Counseling and ongoing support groups to help the patient overcome alcohol dependence
- Aversion therapy: involves the use of a daily oral dose of disulfiram (Antabuse) to prevent compulsive drinking
    – Impedes alcohol metabolism and increases blood acetaldehyde levels
    – Can cause an immediate unpleasant reaction resembling a hangover if alcohol is consumed within 2 weeks of taking drug
    – Reaction may be induced even by alcohol in food sauces and cough medicines, or inhaled traces from shaving lotion or furniture varnish
    – Signs and symptoms of disulfiram reaction
        • Flushing
        • Throbbing of the neck and head
        • Nausea and vomiting
        • Headache
        • Sweating
        • Thirst
        • Shortness of breath or other respiratory difficulties
        • Chest pain, palpitations, tachycardia, hyperventilation, hypotension, or syncope
        • Weakness
        • Vertigo
        • Blurred vision
        • Confusion
- Aversion therapy by administering alcohol along with an emetic agent
- Antagonist therapy: uses the opioid antagonist naltrexone (ReVia) to reduce alcohol craving and help prevent an alcoholic from relapsing to heavy drinking (when it's combined with counseling)
    – Blocks the brain's pleasure centers, reducing the urge to drink
    – Patient addicted to opioids must stop taking all such drugs 7 to 10 days before starting naltrexone therapy
    – Therapy usually lasts at least 12 weeks
- Counseling and psychotherapy for long-term rehabilitation
    – Long-term abstinence: supportive programs offering detoxification, rehabilitation, and aftercare—including continued involvement in Alcoholics Anonymous (AA)—offer best results
    – Rehabilitation: may involve job training, sheltered workshops, halfway houses, or other supervised facilities for alcoholics who have lost contact with family and friends and have a long history of problems related to alcohol abuse, such as unemployment or legal problems

General interventions for acute drug intoxication

Care for a substance-abusing patient starts with an assessment to determine which substance he's abusing. Signs and symptoms vary with the substance and dosage.

During the acute phase of drug intoxication and detoxification, care focuses on maintaining the patient's vital functions, ensuring his safety, and easing discomfort.

During rehabilitation, caregivers help the patient acknowledge his substance abuse problem and find alternative ways to cope with stress. Health care professionals can play an important role in helping patients achieve recovery and stay drug-free.

These general nursing interventions are appropriate for patients during and after acute intoxication with most types of psychoactive drugs.

DURING AN ACUTE EPISODE

- Continuously monitor the patient's vital signs and urine output; watch for complications of overdose and withdrawal, such as cardiopulmonary arrest, seizures, and aspiration.
- Maintain a quiet, safe environment.
- Take appropriate measures to prevent suicide attempts and assaults, according to facility policy; remove harmful objects from the room, and use restraints only if you suspect the patient might harm himself or others.
- Approach the patient in a nonthreatening way; limit sustained eye contact, which he may perceive as threatening.
- Institute seizure precautions.

- Administer I.V. fluids to increase circulatory volume.
- Give medications as ordered; monitor and record their effectiveness.

DURING DRUG WITHDRAWAL

- Administer medications, as ordered, to decrease withdrawal symptoms; monitor and record their effectiveness.
- Maintain a quiet, safe environment because excessive noise may agitate the patient.

WHEN THE ACUTE EPISODE HAS RESOLVED

- Carefully monitor and promote adequate nutrition.
- Administer drugs carefully to prevent hoarding; check the patient's mouth to ensure that he has swallowed oral medication, and closely monitor visitors who might supply him with drugs.
- Refer the patient for rehabilitation as appropriate; give him a list of available resources.
- Encourage family members to seek help regardless of whether the abuser seeks it; suggest private therapy or community mental health clinics.
- Use the episode to develop personal self-awareness and an understanding and positive attitude toward the patient; control your reactions to his undesirable behaviors—commonly, psychological dependency, manipulation, anger, frustration, and alienation.
- Set limits when dealing with demanding, manipulative behavior.

General nursing interventions for a patient with acute drug intoxication

- Continuously monitor patient's vital signs and urine output.
- Watch for complications of overdose and withdrawal.
- Maintain quiet, safe environment.
- Take appropriate measures to prevent suicide attempts and assaults.
- Approach patient in a nonthreatening way; limit sustained eye contact.
- Institute seizure precautions.
- Administer I.V. fluids to increase circulatory volume.
- Give medications as ordered; monitor and record their effectiveness.

Key nursing interventions for a patient with alcohol dependence

- Warn patient taking disulfiram that even a small amount of alcohol will induce an adverse reaction.
- Arrange visit with patient's religious or spiritual advisor, if desired, to help provide motivation for commitment to sobriety.
- Recommend that patient join AA, and arrange a visit from an AA member.
- Tell patient's family about Al-Anon and Alateen.
- Refer adult children of alcoholics to the National Association for Children of Alcoholics.

● Nursing interventions

- Assess the patient for signs and symptoms of acute alcohol intoxication or withdrawal
- Assist with specific measures, as needed, to treat intoxication or withdrawal (see *General interventions for acute drug intoxication*)
- Warn the patient taking disulfiram that even a small amount of alcohol will induce an adverse reaction

Characteristics of amphetamines

- Increase arousal, reduce fatigue, and can make a person feel stronger, more alert, and more decisive
- Most abusers take them for their stimulant or euphoric effects or to counteract the "down" feeling from alcohol or tranquilizers
- May be taken orally or by injection, snorting, or smoking
- Intensely pleasurable sensation immediately after methamphetamine is injected or smoked
- Long-lasting high – rather than a rush – after snorting
- Users can become addicted quickly, with rapid dose escalation
- Use is highest among white males between ages 20 and 35

Types of amphetamines

- Amphetamine sulfate
- Methamphetamine
- Dextroamphetamine

Effects of amphetamine abuse on the body

- Increases release of the neurotransmitters dopamine, norepinephrine, and serotonin into brain synapses
- "Rush" or "high" results from high levels of dopamine in brain areas that regulate feelings of pleasure
- May also have neurotoxic effect, damaging brain cells that contain dopamine and serotonin

---

- Alcohol sensitivity increasing with duration of disulfiram use
- Disulfiram reaction possible with paraldehyde (sedative that's chemically similar to alcohol)
- Arrange a visit with the patient's religious or spiritual advisor, if desired, to help provide the motivation for a commitment to sobriety
- Recommend that the patient join AA, and arrange a visit from an AA member (advise female patients that women's AA groups are available, and advise nonsmokers that nonsmoking groups are available)
- Tell the patient's family about Al-Anon and Alateen
  - Can teach family members to relinquish responsibility for the alcoholic's drinking so they can live meaningful and productive lives
  - Can help reduce family tensions when involved in the patient's rehabilitation
- Refer adult children of alcoholics to the National Association for Children of Alcoholics for support in understanding and coping with the past

AMPHETAMINE ABUSE

● Defining characteristics

- Amphetamines increase arousal, reduce fatigue, and can make a person feel stronger, more alert, and more decisive; most abusers take them for their stimulant or euphoric effects or to counteract the "down" feeling from alcohol or tranquilizers
- There are three types of amphetamines
  - Amphetamine sulfate (also known by the common street names *bennies, grannies,* and *cartwheels*)
  - Methamphetamine (also called *speed, meth, crank,* or *crystal;* has a high potential for abuse and dependence)
  - Dextroamphetamine (also called *dexies, hearts,* and *oranges*)
- Amphetamines may be taken orally or by injection, snorting, or smoking
  - Intensely pleasurable sensation ("rush") immediately after methamphetamine is injected or smoked (lasts a few minutes)
  - Long-lasting high — rather than a rush — after snorting (may last up to half a day)
- Users can become addicted quickly, with rapid dose escalation; higher doses may lead to increasing toxicity and complications
- According to a recent survey, an estimated 8.8 million people in the United States have tried methamphetamine; use of this drug is highest among white males between ages 20 and 35

● Drug effects

- Increase the release of the neurotransmitters dopamine, norepinephrine, and serotonin into brain synapses
- "Rush" or "high" experienced resulting from high levels of dopamine in the brain areas that regulate feelings of pleasure
- May also have a neurotoxic effect, damaging brain cells that contain dopamine and serotonin; studies suggesting that over time, methamphetamine reduces dopamine levels, possibly leading to parkinsonian-like symptoms

● **Health hazards and impairments**
  - Adverse physiologic effects of methamphetamine abuse: headache, poor concentration, poor appetite, abdominal pain, vomiting or diarrhea, sleep difficulties, paranoid or aggressive behavior, and psychosis
  - Chronic methamphetamine abuse: can cause inflammation of the heart lining
  - Injection: may damage blood vessels and cause skin abscesses
  - May have episodes of violent behavior, paranoia, anxiety, confusion, and insomnia
  - With heavy use: progressive social and occupational deterioration may occur
  - Users who become drug tolerant: must take higher or more frequent doses or change their method of drug intake; users may even forgo food and sleep while on a "run" (binge-injecting as much as 1 g of methamphetamine every 2 to 3 hours over several days until the supply runs out or the user becomes too disorganized to continue)
  - Chronic methamphetamine abuse: may damage the brain's frontal areas and basal ganglia
  - May experience a toxic psychosis that resembles paranoid schizophrenia — intense paranoia, rages, auditory hallucinations, mood disturbances, and delusions (some may experience *formication* — the sensation of insects creeping on the skin); psychotic symptoms may last months or years after drug use ceases

● **Causes**
  - Exact cause hard to identify
  - May be an effort to relieve fatigue, induce euphoria, or ease depression or other uncomfortable feelings

● **Signs and symptoms**
  - Amphetamine influence
    – Euphoria
    – Hyperactivity and increased alertness
    – Diaphoresis
    – Shallow respirations
    – Dilated pupils
    – Dry mouth
    – Exhaustion
    – Anorexia and weight loss
    – Nausea or vomiting
    – Tachycardia
    – Hypertension
    – Hyperthermia
    – Tremors
    – Seizures
    – Altered mental status (confusion, agitation, paranoia)
    – Psychotic behavior (with prolonged use)
  - Amphetamine intoxication
    – Signs and symptoms of amphetamine influence
    – Arrhythmias
    – Heart failure
    – Subarachnoid hemorrhage
    – Stroke
    – Cerebral hemorrhage

Adverse effects of amphetamine abuse

- Headache
- Poor concentration
- Poor appetite
- Abdominal pain
- Vomiting or diarrhea
- Sleep difficulties
- Paranoid or aggressive behavior
- Psychosis
- Inflammation of the heart lining (with chronic methamphetamine abuse)
- Damage to blood vessels; skin abscesses (with injection)

Common causes of amphetamine abuse

- Hard to identify
- Possible effort to relieve fatigue, induce euphoria, or ease depression

Key signs and symptoms of amphetamine abuse

Amphetamine influence
- Euphoria
- Hyperactivity and increased alertness
- Dilated pupils
- Dry mouth
- Tachycardia
- Hypertension
- Seizures
- Altered mental status
- Psychotic behavior (with prolonged use)

Amphetamine withdrawal
- CNS depression
- Hallucinations
- Abdominal tenderness
- Disorientation
- Irritability
- Suicide attempts (after sudden withdrawal)

Diagnosing amphetamine abuse

- Urine drug screening to confirm or rule out abuse
- Other diagnostic tests, such as blood alcohol level tests, liver function studies, or X-rays
- Confirmed if *DSM-IV-TR* criteria met

Key treatment options for amphetamine abuse

- Airway management, fluid resuscitation, or vigorous cooling measures
- Close monitoring of vital signs
- Arrhythmia treatment
- Vomiting or gastric lavage, if drug was ingested
- Ammonium or ascorbic acid added to I.V. solution to acidify urine to pH of 5
- Mannitol to induce diuresis
- Sedatives to induce sleep
- Anticholinergics and antidiarrheal agents to relieve GI distress
- Antianxiety drugs for severe agitation and symptomatic treatment of complications
- Cognitive-behavioral therapy to treat methamphetamine dependence
- Antidepressants to help combat the depression commonly seen in methamphetamine users

---

- Coma
- Death
- Amphetamine withdrawal
  - CNS depression (ranges from lethargy to coma)
  - Hallucinations
  - Overstimulation (includes euphoria, violent behavior)
  - Abdominal tenderness
  - Muscle aches
  - Disorientation
  - Irritability
  - Long periods of sleep
  - Apathy and depression
  - Suicide attempts (after sudden withdrawal)

● **Diagnosis**
- Urine drug screening to confirm or rule out abuse
- Other diagnostic tests, such as blood alcohol level tests, liver function studies, or X-rays (if trauma is noted), depending on patient's symptoms
- Diagnosis of amphetamine abuse or dependence confirmed if *DSM-IV-TR* criteria met

● **Treatment**
- Airway management, fluid resuscitation, or vigorous cooling measures as well as close monitoring of vital signs
- Arrhythmia treatment (may warrant cardioversion, defibrillation, and antiarrhythmic drugs)
- Vomiting or gastric lavage, if drug was ingested; activated charcoal and a saline or magnesium cathartic may be given
- Symptom-specific treatments
  - Ammonium or ascorbic acid added to I.V. solution to acidify urine to a pH of 5
  - Mannitol (Osmitrol) to induce diuresis
  - Sedatives to induce sleep
  - Anticholinergics and antidiarrheal agents to relieve GI distress
  - Antianxiety drugs for severe agitation and symptomatic treatment of complications
- Cognitive-behavioral therapy to treat methamphetamine dependence; helps modify the patient's thinking, expectations, and behaviors, and increases his ability to cope with stress
- Antidepressants to help combat the depression commonly seen in methamphetamine users who have recently stopped taking the drug
- After withdrawal, rehabilitation to prevent relapse
  - Inpatient and outpatient programs available
  - Usually last 1 month or longer
  - May include individual, group, and family psychotherapy
  - May include participation in a drug-oriented, self-help group; serves as adjunct to behavioral interventions and promotes long-term recovery
  - Requires lifetime of abstinence, usually aided by participation in Narcotics Anonymous (NA) or a similar group

Nursing interventions
- Assess the patient for signs and symptoms of acute amphetamine intoxication
- Assist with measures to treat intoxication or withdrawal, as needed (see *General interventions for acute drug intoxication,* page 281)

CAFFEINE INTOXICATION

Defining characteristics
- A mild CNS stimulant, caffeine may be used to restore mental alertness when a person feels tired, weak, or drowsy; however, used in excess, it causes uncomfortable symptoms of stimulation
- Caffeine intoxication can occur with consumption of more than 250 mg of caffeine (equivalent to about 2½ cups of coffee)
- Dietary sources of caffeine include coffee, tea, chocolate, and cola drinks; other sources include some prescription and over-the-counter (OTC) drugs such as those for headache (for example, aspirin, acetaminophen, and caffeine tablets [Excedrin])
- Age and body size influence caffeine effects
  - Child or small adult: may feel effects more strongly than a large adult does
  - People with caffeine sensitivities: feel effects at smaller doses
- Caffeine can be habit-forming; most experts agree that some heavy caffeine users may develop caffeine tolerance or dependence
- Someone who abruptly stops using caffeine may experience headache, fatigue, or drowsiness

Drug effects
- Unclear how caffeine exerts its effects
- May antagonize adenosine, an inhibitory brain chemical that affects norepinephrine, dopamine, and serotonin activity, thereby increasing neurotransmitter levels and causing psychostimulation

Causes
- Exact causes and risk factors for caffeine dependence or sensitivity to caffeine withdrawal unknown
  - Coffee and caffeine-containing drinks as beverages of choice
  - Perceived need for stimulant to "get going" in the morning, relieve fatigue, or stay awake
- Possible genetic influence (differences in metabolism, history of substance abuse, or mood disorders)

Signs and symptoms
- Caffeine intoxication
  - Tachycardia
  - Palpitations
  - Arrhythmias
  - Fatigue that worsens during the day
  - Anxiety, nervousness, irritability, and easy excitability
  - Exaggerated startle response
  - Disorganized thoughts and speech
  - Facial flushing

Key nursing interventions for a patient with amphetamine abuse
- Assess patient for signs and symptoms of acute amphetamine intoxication.

Characteristics of caffeine intoxification
- Can occur with consumption of 250 mg of caffeine
- Age and body size influence effects
- Can be habit-forming

Common causes of caffeine intoxication
- Exact cause unknown
- Possible genetic influence

Key signs and symptoms of caffeine intoxication
- Tachycardia
- Palpitations
- Arrhythmias
- Fatigue that worsens during the day
- Exaggerated startle response
- Disorganized thoughts and speech
- Dehydration
- Restless leg syndrome

   – Dehydration (from caffeine's diuretic effect)
   – Hyperactivity
   – Gross muscle tremors
   – Restless leg syndrome (muscle cramping and twitching)
   – Sleep disturbances, such as insomnia or decreased sleep quality (with grogginess in the morning caused by symptoms occurring overnight)

- Caffeine withdrawal
  – May occur with abrupt cessation or reduction after long period of daily use
  – Tend to be worse in heavy caffeine users (500 mg/day or more), although discomfort possible with as little as 100 mg/day (about one cup of coffee)
  – May start within a few hours after the time of normal caffeine consumption, peak within 1 or 2 days, and persist for up to 2 weeks
    - Headache
    - Nausea or vomiting
    - Jitteriness, irritability, and anxiety
    - Fatigue
    - Drowsiness
    - Depression
    - Poor concentration or poor performance on mental tasks
    - Caffeine craving

Diagnosis

- Blood testing to determine serum caffeine levels (limited use as a screening tool)
- Urine toxicology studies to reveal illicit drug use (if suspected)
- Thyroid studies to rule out hyperthyroidism
- ECG to investigate cardiac irregularities
- Diagnosis of caffeine intoxication confirmed if *DSM-IV-TR* criteria met

Treatment

- Avoidance of caffeine in all forms (as symptoms resolve when the caffeine use stops)
- Monitoring for caffeine withdrawal; treatment based on individual symptoms

Nursing interventions

- Advise the patient about the expected symptoms of caffeine withdrawal and the duration of those symptoms; reassure him that they're benign and will subside
- Assess the patient for other disorders, such as hyperthyroidism or use of other illicit drugs, that cause similar symptoms (if discomfort lasts longer than 2 weeks)
- Teach the patient about common sources of caffeine (see *Caffeine-containing products*)
- Encourage the use of stress-reduction techniques (such as deep breathing, meditation) and healthy lifestyle choices (such as regular exercise) to help relieve stress associated with withdrawal and stress that might have played a role in the patient's need for excessive caffeine intake

TIME-OUT FOR TEACHING

Caffeine-containing products

Caffeine intoxication can occur with consumption of more than 250 mg of caffeine. A patient with caffeine dependency or intoxication may be unaware of the amount of caffeine he consumes each day. Common sources of caffeine are listed below.

- Coffee, brewed – 40 to 180 mg per cup
- Coffee, instant – 30 to 120 mg per cup
- Coffee, decaffeinated – 3 to 5 mg per cup
- Tea, brewed (American) – 20 to 90 mg per cup
- Tea, brewed (imported) – 25 to 110 mg per cup
- Tea, instant – 28 mg per cup
- Tea, canned iced – 22 to 36 mg per 12 ounces
- Cola and other soft drinks – 36 to 90 mg per 12 ounces

- Cola and other soft drinks, decaffeinated – none
- Cocoa – 4 mg per cup
- Chocolate milk – 3 to 6 mg per ounce
- Chocolate, bittersweet – 25 mg per ounce

Over-the-counter preparations that contain caffeine include Caffedrine Caplets, Enerjets, NoDoz Maximum Strength Caplets, and Vivarin. Some pain relievers, such as Excedrin and Midol, also contain caffeine.

CANNABIS ABUSE

● Defining characteristics

- Cannabis is a hemp plant from which marijuana (a tobacco-like substance) and hashish (the plant's resinous secretions) are produced
- In the United States and most other Western countries, cannabis is the most widely used illicit drug; common street names include *pot, grass, weed, Mary Jane, MJ, roach, reefer, joints, THC, blunt, herb, sinsemilla, smoke, boo, broccoli, ace,* and *Colombian*
- Cannabis can be smoked, consumed as a tea, or mixed into foods
  - Most smoke in hand-rolled cigarettes; some use pipes or bongs (water pipes)
  - Marijuana cigars (blunts) also popular; users slice open cigars and replace tobacco with marijuana (may be combined with crack cocaine or another drug)
- Duration of action is 6 to 12 hours, with symptoms most pronounced during the first 1 to 2 hours
- Medicinal use of cannabis—mainly as an antiemetic in patients undergoing cancer chemotherapy and other types of drug therapy—has been the subject of intense legal and medical debate
- More than 83 million people in the United States age 12 and older have tried marijuana at least once
  - Used equally among all races
  - Used by more males than females

Common sources of caffeine
- Coffee
- Tea
- Cola
- Cocoa
- Chocolate milk
- Chocolate, bittersweet
- Caffedrine Caplets
- Enerjets
- NoDoz Maximum Strength Caplets
- Vivarin
- Pain relievers, such as Excedrin and Midol

Characteristics of cannabis
- Most widely used illicit drug
- Can be smoked, consumed as a tea, or mixed into foods
- Duration of action is 6 to 12 hours, with symptoms most pronounced during the first 1 to 2 hours

Common street names for cannabis
- Pot
- Grass
- Weed
- Mary Jane
- MJ
- Roach
- Reefer
- Joints
- THC
- Blunt
- Herb
- Sinsemilla
- Smoke
- Boo
- Broccoli
- Ace
- Colombian

Effects of delta-1-THC on the body

- Delta-1-THC is most powerful psychoactive substance in cannabis.
- When marijuana is smoked, delta-1-THC rapidly passes from the lungs into the bloodstream, which carries it to the brain and other organs.
- Delta-1-THC connects to cannabinoid receptors on neurons, influencing their activity.

Adverse effects of cannabis abuse

- Acute intoxication may trigger tachycardia and orthostatic hypotension
- May adversely affect reproductive system
- May weaken immune system, having a profoundly negative effect on development in very young teens
- Can result in perceptual distortions and impairments in short-term memory, learning ability, judgment, and verbal skills
- Can be harmful to the lungs
- Has adverse impact on learning and memory
- Creates problems at work
- Associated with anxiety, depression, and personality disturbances
- Combinations with other substances can compound the known risks

- – Abused by all age-groups; adolescents and young adults most common abusers
- – Among arrested adults: about 40% of males and 25% of females test positive for marijuana
- – Among arrested juveniles: marijuana is most commonly used drug

Drug effects
- Most powerful psychoactive substance in cannabis: delta-l-tetrahydro-cannabinol (delta-1-THC)
- When marijuana is smoked: delta-1-THC rapidly passes from the lungs into the bloodstream, which carries it to the brain and other organs
- Brain effects: delta-1-THC connects to cannabinoid receptors on neurons, influencing their activity

Health hazards and impairments
- Cannabis: can be addictive and may cause various adverse physiologic effects
  - – Acute cannabis intoxication: may trigger tachycardia and orthostatic hypotension
  - – May adversely affect the reproductive system
    - • In females, may increase number of anovulatory cycles
    - • In males, may reduce levels of follicle-stimulating hormone, leading to decreased testosterone production and testicular atrophy; also decreases sperm counts (exact effect on fertility is unclear)
  - – May weaken the immune system, having a profoundly negative effect on development in very young teens
  - – Can result in perceptual distortions and impairments in short-term memory, learning ability, judgment, and verbal skills
- Marijuana: harmful alone or in combination with other drugs
  - – Marijuana smoke: can harm the lungs
    - • Contains carcinogens similar to those found in tobacco smoke
    - • May increase the risk of chronic obstructive pulmonary disease (with chronic and heavy use)
    - • Increases risk of respiratory tumors (with habitual use)
  - – Adverse impact on learning and memory: can last for days or weeks after the acute drug effects wear off
    - • Trouble with sustaining and shifting attention, and in registering, organizing, and using information
    - • Lower scores on standardized tests of verbal and mathematical skills
  - – Commonly causes problems at work; use has been linked with increased absences, tardiness, accidents, workers' compensation claims, and job turnover
  - – Associated with anxiety, depression, and personality disturbances
  - – Combined with other substances: combinations with crack cocaine, phencyclidine (PCP), formaldehyde, and codeine-containing cough syrup (sometimes without the user's knowledge) can compound the known risks

Causes
- Exact cause of dependency unknown

Risk factors
- Young age

- Drug availability (influenced by geographic and cultural factors)
- Coexisting alcohol abuse or dependence
- Coexisting abuse of other drugs

● **Signs and symptoms**
- Cannabis influence
  - Relaxation
  - Euphoria; feeling of well-being or grandiosity
  - Spontaneous laughter
  - Visual distortions and other perceptual changes
  - Subjective sense that time is passing more slowly than normal
  - Tachycardia
  - Dry mouth
  - Conjunctival redness
  - Drowsiness and sluggishness (or paradoxical hyperalertness)
  - Decreased muscle strength
  - Poor coordination
  - Increased hunger (the "munchies")
- Chronic cannabis use
  - Appetite changes
  - Lack of ambition and energy
  - Reduced social and occupational drive
- Cannabis intoxication (dysphoric effects)
  - Panic and disorientation
  - Paranoia
  - Mood swings
  - Altered perceptions (illusions or frank hallucinations)
  - Depersonalization
  - Psychotic episodes
- Cannabis overdose
  - Pulmonary edema
  - Respiratory depression
  - Aspiration pneumonia
  - Hypotension
- Cannabis withdrawal (typically less severe than with that of other drugs)
  - Restlessness
  - Irritability
  - Appetite loss
  - Sleep difficulties

● **Diagnosis**
- Urine toxicology screening to identify chronic use (cannabis present in urine up to 21 days after use)
- Diagnosis of cannabis abuse or dependence confirmed when *DSM-IV-TR* criteria met

● **Treatment**
- Acute cannabis intoxication: usually resolves within 4 to 6 hours; symptom-based treatment (patient should be moved to a quiet room with minimal stimulation)

Key signs and symptoms of cannabis abuse

Cannabis influence
- Relaxation
- Euphoria; feeling of well-being or grandiosity
- Spontaneous laughter
- Visual distortions and other perceptual changes
- Subjective sense that time is passing more slowly than normal
- Tachycardia
- Dry mouth
- Drowsiness and sluggishness (or paradoxical hyperalertness)
- Increased hunger

Cannabis intoxication
- Panic and disorientation
- Paranoia
- Mood swings
- Altered perceptions
- Depersonalization
- Psychotic episodes

Diagnosing cannabis abuse

- Urine toxicology screening to identify chronic use
- Confirmed if *DSM-IV-TR* criteria met

Treatment options for cannabis abuse

- For acute cannabis intoxication (usually resolves within 4 to 6 hours): treat symptoms
- Short course of sedatives or tranquilizers
- Psychotherapy
- Exercise
- Relaxation techniques
- Nutritional support

General nursing interventions for a patient with cannabis abuse

- Continuously monitor patient's vital signs and urine output.
- Watch for complications of overdose and withdrawal.
- Maintain quiet, safe environment.
- Take appropriate measures to prevent suicide attempts and assaults.
- Approach patient in a nonthreatening way; limit sustained eye contact.
- Institute seizure precautions.
- Administer I.V. fluids to increase circulatory volume.
- Give medications as ordered; monitor and record their effectiveness.

Characteristics of cocaine

- Powerfully addictive opioid and stimulant, and one of the oldest known drugs
- Effects occur almost immediately after single dose, disappear within minutes or hours
- Two chemical forms: Cocaine hydrochloride salt, and crack or freebase
- Can be snorted, injected, smoked, or rubbed onto mucous membrane tissues

- A short course of sedatives or tranquilizers to ease withdrawal symptoms, insomnia, anxiety, and depression; nonpharmacologic measures may include psychotherapy, exercise, relaxation techniques, and nutritional support
- Follows the general principles of substance abuse treatment
  - Goal of total abstinence from all psychoactive substances
  - May include psychiatric evaluation and counseling, individual or group psychotherapy, occupational and family assessment, self-help groups, and lifestyle changes (such as avoiding drug-related situations)
- Few treatment programs focused solely on marijuana abuse (possibly because many marijuana users also use other drugs); however, with more people seeking help to control marijuana abuse, alternative treatment approaches being explored

● Nursing interventions

- Assess the patient for signs and symptoms of cannabis dependency, intoxication, or abuse
- Assist with measures for management of intoxication or withdrawal, as needed (see *General interventions for acute drug intoxication,* page 281)

COCAINE ABUSE

● Defining characteristics

- Cocaine is a powerfully addictive opioid and stimulant, and one of the oldest known drugs
  - Source is coca leaves; have been ingested for thousands of years
  - Pure drug is cocaine hydrochloride salt; has been abused for more than 100 years
- Cocaine use can range from occasional to repeated or compulsive abuse
- Its effects occur almost immediately after a single dose and disappear within a few minutes or hours
  - Taken in small amounts (up to 100 mg), makes user feel euphoric, energetic, talkative, and mentally alert (especially to sensations of sight, sound, and touch)
  - May temporarily reduce the need for food and sleep
  - May allow for quicker performance of simple physical and intellectual tasks (may also have opposite effect on some users)
- Cocaine exists in two chemical forms
  - Cocaine hydrochloride salt: fine, white, crystallized powder that's generally snorted or dissolved in water and injected; effects last 15 minutes to 2 hours
  - Crack or freebase: chunky, off-white compound that hasn't been neutralized by an acid; smoked after being processed with ammonia or sodium bicarbonate salt and water and then heated to remove the hydrochloride; produces an immediate euphoric high followed by a "down" feeling
- On the street, cocaine is commonly known as *coke, C, snow, snowball, blow, flake, nose candy, hits, tornado, wicky stick, rock,* and *crank*
  - Usually diluted by street dealers with inert substances (cornstarch, talcum powder, or sugar) or cut with procaine or amphetamines
  - May be combined with heroin in a "speedball"
- Cocaine can be taken by various routes

- Snorted (absorbed into the bloodstream through the nasal tissues)
- Injected (released directly into the bloodstream, intensifying its effects)
- Smoked (inhaled into the lungs as a vapor, where it's absorbed into the bloodstream as rapidly as by injection)
- Rubbed onto mucous membrane tissues
- Cocaine may be used medically — as a local anesthetic for nasal surgeries or for cuts in children and to stop nosebleeds
- Cocaine is the second most commonly used illicit drug in the United States (about 10% of those over age 12 have tried cocaine at least once; about 3.6 million are chronic cocaine users)
  - Highest usage rate in adults ages 18 to 25
  - Used by more men than women

Drug effects

- Produces pleasurable effects through its action on structures deep within the brain — most notably, a region called the *ventral tegmental area (VTA)*
- Neurons originating in the VTA extend to the nucleus accumbens, one of the brain's key pleasure centers
- Pleasurable events accompanied by a significant rise in the amount of dopamine released in the nucleus accumbens by neurons arising from the VTA

Health hazards and impairments

- Possibly devastating medical consequences, made even worse by absorption of toxic amounts of the drug
  - Sudden death
  - Acute cardiovascular problems, including arrhythmias (particularly ventricular fibrillation), tachycardia, chest pain, and myocardial infarction (MI)
  - Stroke
  - Seizures
  - Respiratory failure
  - Bowel gangrene (with cocaine ingestion)
- Combining cocaine with alcohol: causes the conversion of the two drugs to cocaethylene, which has a longer duration of action in the brain and is more toxic than either drug alone
  - Most common two-drug mixture resulting in drug-related death
- A cocaine binge (taking the drug repeatedly and at increasingly high doses): may cause increasing irritability, restlessness, and paranoia
  - Possible resultant full-blown paranoid psychosis
  - Loss of touch with reality, auditory hallucinations
- Regular cocaine snorting: can lead to the loss of the sense of smell and to nosebleeds, swallowing difficulty, hoarseness, and nasal septum irritation (which may cause a chronically inflamed, runny nose)
- Cocaine injection: can cause an allergic reaction (to cocaine or to an additive in street cocaine)
  - Death in severe cases
  - Increased risk for such infections as HIV and hepatitis (shared needles)
- Sudden death occurring with first use of cocaine or thereafter (rare cases)

Effects of cocaine on the body

- Acts on structures deep within the brain – most notably, the VTA
- Pleasurable events are accompanied by significant rise in amount of dopamine released in the nucleus accumbens by neurons arising from the VTA

Adverse effects of cocaine abuse

- Possibly devastating medical consequences made even worse by absorption of toxic amounts
- Sudden death
- Acute cardiovascular problems
- Stroke
- Seizures
- Respiratory failure
- Bowel gangrene (with cocaine ingestion)
- Possible increasing irritability, restlessness, and paranoia (with cocaine binge); possible resultant full-blown paranoid psychosis and loss of touch with reality; auditory hallucinations
- Powerfully addictive
- Tolerance with continued use

- Commonly a result of cardiac arrest or seizures followed by respiratory arrest
- May result from increased sensitivity to cocaine's anesthetic and convulsant effects, even without increasing the dose
- Powerfully addictive
  - Progression to heavy use in about 10% of those who try it
  - After trying it, person may have trouble predicting or controlling extent to which he'll keep using it
- Tolerance with continued use; the user needs higher doses at more frequent intervals to obtain the same level of pleasure experienced with initial use

Causes
- Family history of substance abuse (may be risk factor for early use and rapid dependence)
- Excess dopamine production (may account for susceptibility to cocaine's addictive properties, including positive reinforcement gained by repeated use)
- Genetic changes (involving alteration of specific brain protein that regulates dopamine's action) with repeated cocaine exposure

Signs and symptoms
- Cocaine influence
  - Euphoria, increased energy, excitement
  - Sociability, good humor, laughing
  - Reduced appetite
  - Grandiosity, sense of increased physical and mental strength
  - Decreased pain sensation
  - Talkativeness or pressured speech
  - Dilated pupils
  - Runny nose, nasal congestion
  - Nausea and vomiting
  - Headache
  - Vertigo
  - Increased or decreased blood pressure
  - Chest pain, tachycardia, ventricular fibrillation, cardiac arrest
  - Tachypnea; deep, rapid, or labored respirations; respiratory arrest
- Pronounced effects with high doses (some users)
  - Flightiness, emotional instability
  - Restlessness, irritability, inability to sit still
  - Apprehension
  - Teeth grinding
  - Cold sweats
  - Tremors, muscle twitching
  - Seizures
  - Hallucinations (cocaine "bugs" or "snow lights" as well as voices, sounds, and smells)
  - Violent, bizarre behavior
  - Cocaine psychosis (resembles paranoid schizophrenia)
- Cocaine withdrawal
  - Anxiety, agitation, irritability
  - Depression
  - Fatigue

Common causes of cocaine abuse
- Family history
- Excess dopamine production
- Genetic changes

Key signs and symptoms of cocaine abuse

Cocaine influence
- Euphoria, increased energy, excitement
- Reduced appetite
- Grandiosity, sense of increased physical and mental strength
- Decreased pain sensation
- Dilated pupils
- Runny nose, nasal congestion
- Chest pain, tachycardia, ventricular fibrillation, cardiac arrest

Pronounced effects with high doses
- Restlessness, irritability, inability to sit still
- Apprehension
- Cold sweats
- Hallucinations
- Violent, bizarre behavior
- Cocaine psychosis

- Angry outbursts
- Lack of motivation
- Nausea and vomiting
- Muscle pain
- Sleep disturbances
- Intense drug craving
- Episodes of ST-segment elevation (on ECG)

● Diagnosis

- May include blood studies and other diagnostic tests to rule out underlying medical causes for signs and symptoms
- Based on *DSM-IV-TR* criteria

● Treatment

- Acute cocaine intoxication: symptomatic treatment
  - Cardiopulmonary resuscitation for ventricular fibrillation and cardiac arrest
  - Vital signs monitoring
  - Propranolol (Inderal) for tachycardia
  - Anticonvulsant medications for seizures
  - Sedatives to induce sleep
  - Anticholinergics and antidiarrheal agents to relieve GI distress
  - Antianxiety agents for severe agitation
  - I.V. fluid replacement and nutritional and vitamin supplements
- Forced diuresis and hemoperfusion or hemodialysis (depending on the amount of cocaine taken and the duration between drug use and medical care)
- Detoxification and management of withdrawal
  - Detoxification: method depends on route by which it was taken
    - If ingested, induced vomiting or gastric lavage
    - If snorted, removal from mucous membranes
  - Easing withdrawal: may include nonpharmacologic measures, such as psychotherapy, exercise, relaxation techniques, and nutritional support
  - Pharmacologic approaches
    - Currently no medications for treating cocaine addiction; agents, such as selegiline (Carbex) and disulfiram (used to treat alcoholism), currently being studied (may also be effective in reducing cocaine abuse)
    - Antidepressants for mood changes that may occur during early stages of cocaine abstinence
    - Sedatives and tranquilizers (short-term) to help relieve insomnia and anxiety
- Rehabilitation: includes lifetime of abstinence, usually aided by participation in NA or similar self-help group
- Long-term treatment (rehabilitation); must address a variety of problems, including psychobiological, cultural, social, and pharmacologic aspects of the patient's drug abuse
- Behavioral treatments (outpatient and residential)
  - Regimen must be tailored to patient's cultural needs
  - Positive results for many who undergo treatment called *contingency management*

- Voucher-based system that gives positive rewards for staying in treatment and remaining cocaine-free (maintaining drug-free urine tests)
  - Vouchers exchanged for rewards that promote healthy living such as gym membership
- Cognitive-behavioral coping skills therapy; short-term, focused approach that helps cocaine addicts become abstinent
  - Helps patient recognize and avoid situations in which he's most likely to use cocaine
  - Helps him cope more effectively with problems and drug-related behaviors
- Therapeutic communities; may benefit patients with more severe problems, such as coexisting mental health problems and criminal involvement
  - Requires 6- to 12-month stay
  - Focus is on resocializing patient to society; some include on-site job rehabilitation and other supportive services

● **Nursing interventions**
- Assess for signs and symptoms of acute cocaine intoxication
- Assist with specific measures to treat toxicity or withdrawal (see *General interventions for acute drug intoxication,* page 281)

HALLUCINOGEN ABUSE

● **Defining characteristics**
- Hallucinogens (sometimes called *psychedelic drugs*) produce hallucinations or profound distortions in the perception of reality as well as dramatic behavioral changes
  - May see images, hear sounds, and feel sensations that seem real but don't actually exist
  - May cause rapid, intense emotional swings
- Most hallucinogens have no known medical use; however, naturally occurring hallucinogens have been used in religious and cultural rites for centuries
- Use of hallucinogens is less common than that of alcohol, amphetamines, and cocaine; fewer than 5% of the U.S. population have tried these drugs (commonly used only experimentally)
- These agents include a wide range of substances; most are taken orally, but some may be injected

● **Classification**
- Lysergic acid diethylamide (LSD) is the most potent mood- and perception-altering drug known (street names include *acid, green dragon* or *red dragon, microdot, sugar,* and *big D*)
  - Synthetic substance first developed by a pharmaceutical company in 1938
  - Potency much greater than that of other hallucinogens (100 to 200 times more so than psilocybin, and 4,000 times more so than mescaline); oral doses as small as 30 mcg can produce effects lasting 6 to 12 hours
  - Produced in crystalline form
  - Pure crystal crushed into powder and mixed with binding agents
    - Produces tablets known as *microdots* or thin gelatin squares called *windowpanes*

Key nursing interventions for a patient with cocaine abuse

- Assess for signs and symptoms of acute cocaine intoxication.
- Assist with specific measures to treat toxicity or withdrawal.

Characteristics of hallucinogens

- Sometimes called *psychedelic drugs*
- Produce hallucinations or profound distortions in the perception of reality as well as dramatic behavioral changes
- Most hallucinogens have no known medical use
- Most are taken orally, but some may be injected

Key facts about LSD

- Most potent mood- and perception-altering drug known
- Synthetic substance first developed by a pharmaceutical company in 1938
- Potency much greater than that of other hallucinogens
- Produced in crystalline form
- Pure crystal crushed into powder and mixed with binding agents
- Has dramatic effects on senses, causing highly intensified perception of colors, smells, sounds, and other sensations

- More commonly, dissolved, diluted, and applied to paper (called *blotter acid*)
  - Has dramatic effects on senses, causing highly intensified perception of colors, smells, sounds, and other sensations
    - May cause blending of sensory perceptions (person may "see" sounds or "hear" or "feel" colors)
    - Also can distort or transform shapes and movements (person may feel that time is moving very slowly or that his body is changing shape)
- Ecstasy, or 3,4-methylenedioxymethamphetamine (MDMA), is a potentially addictive, synthetic drug with both stimulant and hallucinogenic properties
  - Available as capsules or tablets (tablets commonly contain other harmful drugs in addition to MDMA)
  - Taken orally or, rarely, injected or snorted
  - Previously used mainly at dance clubs and raves; now seen in other social settings
  - Street names include *XTC, clarify, essence*, and *Adam*; Ecstasy experience is sometimes called *rolling*
  - Effects include distortions of time and perception, and an amphetamine-like hyperactivity; depending on dosage, acute drug effects last 3 to 6 hours
- Ketamine is used therapeutically in veterinary medicine as an anesthetic
  - Induces amnesia, distorts perceptions of sight and sound, and produces dissociative effects (feelings of detachment from self and the environment)
  - Increasingly used as a club drug and distributed at raves and parties
  - Common street names: *K, special K, Ket, vitamin K*, and *Kit*
  - Usually evaporated to form powder that's snorted, smoked, or compressed into tablets; liquid form can be injected I.V. or I.M.
  - Odorless and tasteless
    - Can be added to beverages without being detected
    - Sometimes given to unsuspecting victims to aid in the commission of sexual assault ("drug rape" or date rape)
- Dextromethorphan, sometimes called *DXM* or *robo*, is a cough-suppressing ingredient found in some OTC cold and cough medications
  - Most common source of abused dextromethorphan is extra-strength cough syrup
  - At low doses, has mild stimulant effect and causes distorted visual perceptions; at much higher doses, causes dissociative effects similar to those of ketamine
  - Effects typically lasting 6 hours
- Mescaline, which is found in several cactus species (Peyote, San Pedro), causes hallucinations and alters spatial perception
  - Mescaline "buttons" or "discs": cut, dried, and usually swallowed; also may be processed into powdered form and taken by capsule, injection, or smoking
  - Causes dizziness, vomiting, tachycardia, increased blood pressure, increased pulse and respiratory rates, sensations of warmth and cold, and headache; effects last approximately 12 hours
- Psilocybin, a compound obtained from the *Psilocybe mexicana* mushroom and some types of European mushrooms, is traditionally used by Mexican healers

Key facts about psilocybin

- Compound obtained from the *Psilocybe mexicana* mushroom and some types of European mushrooms
- Produces effects similar to those of LSD
- In small amounts, induces relaxation and sensation of being detached from the body; users may also see brilliant arrangements of color and light
- In larger doses, may cause nausea, anxiety, light-headedness, sweating, chills, and numbness of the mouth, lips, and tongue

Effects of hallucinogens on the body

- Disrupt interaction of nerve cells
- Affect functioning of serotonin, a neurotransmitter crucial to the regulation of mood, sleep, pain, emotion, and appetite

Adverse effects of LSD use

- Causes unpleasant and potentially dangerous flashbacks long after drug is used
- Vivid sensory experience of a past hallucinogen "trip"
- User believes he's currently experiencing the drug's effects and may respond or behave accordingly

– Can be eaten in the dried mushroom form or consumed as a white powder
– Produces effects similar to those of LSD
– In small amounts, induces relaxation and sensation of being detached from the body; users may also see brilliant arrangements of color and light
– In larger doses, may cause nausea, anxiety, light-headedness, sweating, chills, and numbness of the mouth, lips, and tongue

Drug effects

- Disruption of interaction of nerve cells by hallucinogens; affect the functioning of serotonin, a neurotransmitter crucial to the regulation of mood, sleep, pain, emotion, and appetite
- LSD binding to and activating serotonin receptors in the brain; effects most prominent in two brain regions
  – Cerebral cortex: involved in mood, cognition, and perception
  – Locus ceruleus: receives sensory signals from all areas of the body and is sometimes called the brain's *novelty detector*
- Mescaline and psilocybin structured similar to serotonin and produce their effects by disrupting normal functioning of the serotonin system
- Increased levels of at least three neurotransmitters—serotonin, dopamine, and norepinephrine—by Ecstasy
- Ketamine alters the distribution of glutamate, which is involved in memory, pain perception, and responses to the environment

Health hazards and impairments

- LSD: Causes unpleasant and potentially dangerous flashbacks long after the drug is used
  – Vivid sensory experience of a past hallucinogen "trip" (commonly an unpleasant one)
  – User believes he's currently experiencing the drug's effects and may respond or behave accordingly
- Large doses: seizures, ruptured blood vessels in the brain, and irreversible brain damage
- LSD intoxication: seizures and fatal accidents
- Ketamine: respiratory depression, heart rate abnormalities, heart failure, inability to move muscles, and insensitivity to pain (can lead to serious injury)
  – Possible sexual assault (rape) in victims incapacitated by ketamine
- Ecstasy: increases the blood pressure and pulse rate; may cause confusion, depression, sleep problems, drug craving, severe anxiety, and paranoia (during and sometimes weeks after taking the drug)
  – Possible physical symptoms: muscle tension, involuntary teeth clenching, nausea, blurred vision, rapid eye movements, faintness, chills or sweating
  – Consequences of stimulant properties: may enable users to perform activities, such as dancing, for extended periods
    • In some, leads to malignant hyperthermia, dehydration, hypertension, and even heart or kidney failure
    • Other potential complications: headache, vomiting, panic, anxiety, seizures, MI, exhaustion, dehydration, heat stroke, and death (if dehydration and elevated body temperature aren't controlled)

Psychological impairments associated with hallucinogen use

In addition to the serious, sometimes life-threatening medical problems that result from use of hallucinogenic substances, psychological impairment may occur as well. The type and degree of impairment vary with the specific drug and length of time used.

LSD-RELATED IMPAIRMENTS
- LSD psychosis
  - Causes persistent psychotic state (including dramatic mood swings from mania to profound depression, visual disturbances, and hallucinations)
  - May last for years after user stops taking drug
- "Bad trips"
  - Panic attacks at the height of the drug experience, characterized by terrifying thoughts and nightmarish feelings of anxiety and despair
  - Perception of real-world sensations as unreal, even frightening
- Flashbacks
  - Spontaneous, repeated, and sometimes continuous recurrences of the sensory distortions originally produced by LSD
  - Occur suddenly, often without warning; may begin a few days (sometimes more than a year) after user stops taking drug
  - Typically include visual disturbances, such as seeing false motion on the edges of the field of vision, bright or colored flashes, and halos or trails attached to moving objects
  - Most common in people who have used hallucinogens chronically or have an underlying personality problem (although otherwise healthy people occasionally have them)

ECSTASY-RELATED IMPAIRMENTS
- Heavy and prolonged use
  - Confusion
  - Depression
  - Sleep problems
  - Persistent anxiety
  - Aggressive and impulsive behavior
  - Selective impairment of working memory and attention
- Long-term use
  - Possible damage to brain's serotonin system
  - May lead to various cognitive and behavioral disturbances, including memory impairment

KETAMINE-RELATED IMPAIRMENTS
- Feeling disconnected and out of control
- Terrifying feeling of nearly total sensory detachment (commonly described as a near-death experience)

- Possible sexual assault (rape) in women
- Hallucinogens: short-term impairments in cognition, perception, mood, and communication; they may even prevent a person from recognizing reality, sometimes resulting in bizarre or dangerous behavior
- Overuse: can trigger psychosis in a person with a history of psychosis (see *Psychological impairments associated with hallucinogen use*)

● **Causes**
- Exact cause unknown
- Traditional use as part of religious rites and spiritual (healing) practices

Diagnosing hallucinogen abuse

- Urine toxicology screening
- Laboratory studies rarely useful in diagnosing intoxication
- Other blood studies or diagnostic testing to rule out possible underlying medical conditions
- Confirmed if *DSM-IV-TR* criteria met

Key treatment options for hallucinogen abuse

- Based on patient's status
- Pharmacologic treatments to help ease symptoms
- Psychotherapy to help patient adjust to visual distractions associated with hallucinogens
- Long-term treatment and rehabilitation

Key nursing interventions for a patient with hallucinogen abuse

- Assess for signs and symptoms of acute hallucinogen intoxication.
- Assess for signs of sexual assault in patient who may have knowingly or unknowingly taken ketamine or Ecstasy.
- Assist with specific measures to treat toxicity or withdrawal.

- Experimental use (by some) to enhance bodily sensations and induce sensory gratification; also used in attempt to transcend bodily limits and time-space continuum

● **Signs and symptoms**
- Vary depending on drug used (see *Assessing for hallucinogen use*)

● **Diagnosis**
- Urine toxicology screening can identify Ecstasy intoxication (only hallucinogen that shows up on standard toxicology screens)
- Laboratory studies rarely useful in diagnosing intoxication with other hallucinogens
- Other blood studies or diagnostic testing to rule out possible underlying medical conditions for the signs and symptoms
- Diagnosis of hallucinogen abuse or dependence confirmed when *DSM-IV-TR* criteria met

● **Treatment**
- Based on the patient's status
  - Patient who experiences a "bad trip" or acute panic reaction: placement in quiet room with minimal stimuli; shouldn't be left alone; should be reassured that drug's effects will wear off in several hours
  - Patient who poses a danger to himself or others: may require physical or chemical restraints; always following facility protocol and avoiding prolonged or excessive physical restraint (can contribute to hyperthermia and rhabdomyolysis and can exacerbate paranoia)
  - Patient who ingested massive quantity of drug: supportive care usually needed (gastric emptying rarely proves successful because drug is absorbed quickly)
  - Patient with marked hyperthermia: aggressive cooling measures
- Pharmacologic treatments to help ease symptoms
  - Benzodiazepines (typically) for anxiety or agitation or for mild hypertension or tachycardia
  - Nifedipine (Procardia) or nitroprusside (Nitropress) for severe hypertension or tachycardia
  - Diazepam for seizures
  - Antidepressants for LSD flashbacks (sometimes)
- Psychotherapy to help the patient adjust to visual distractions associated with hallucinogens; may ease fears of suffering from brain damage or other psychiatric disorders
- Long-term treatment and rehabilitation to address wide-ranging effects of patient's drug abuse

● **Nursing interventions**
- Assess for signs and symptoms of acute hallucinogen intoxication (see *Assessing for hallucinogen use*)
- Assess for signs of sexual assault in a patient who may have knowingly or unknowingly taken ketamine or Ecstasy
  - Assist with rape kit, if indicated; carry out ordered sexually transmitted disease screenings and pregnancy testing

Assessing for hallucinogen use

Suspect hallucinogen use if your patient has these signs and symptoms.

LSD OR MESCALINE

A patient under the influence of lysergic acid diethylamide (LSD) or mescaline may report a sense of depersonalization, grandiosity, hallucinations, illusions, distorted perception of time and space, or mystical experiences.

GI findings include nausea, vomiting, diarrhea, and abdominal cramps. Cardiovascular findings may include arrhythmias, palpitations, tachycardia, and hypertension.

Other signs and symptoms may include:
- Chills
- Dizziness
- Dry mouth
- Fever
- Sweating
- Appetite loss
- Hyperpnea
- Increased salivation
- Muscle aches

PSILOCYBIN

Signs and symptom of psilocybin use include:
- Euphoria
- Color distortions
- Vivid hallucinations
- "Seeing" music or "hearing" color
- Dramatic mood swings and personality changes
- Increases in blood pressure and body temperature

ECSTASY

A patient under the influence of Ecstasy may report or exhibit:
- Distractibility
- Heightened alertness
- Irritability or confusion
- Euphoria
- Enhanced emotional and mental clarity
- Increased sensitivity to touch
- Enhanced sexuality
- Increased energy and motor activity
- Increased pulse rate
- Elevated blood pressure
- Dilated pupils
- Perceptual changes
- Tightened jaw muscles or jaw grinding or clenching
- Increased body temperature, heavy perspiration, and dehydration

At high doses, Ecstasy may cause hallucinations, depression, paranoia, and irrational behavior (including violence).

KETAMINE

Ketamine causes dissociative effects and alters visual and auditory perception. At low doses, it causes impairments in attention, learning ability, and memory. At higher doses, it may produce delirium, amnesia, impaired motor function, high blood pressure, depression, and potentially fatal respiratory problems.

DEXTROMETHORPHAN

Dextromethorphan use may cause euphoria and a floating sensation, along with increased perceptual awareness and altered time perception. The patient may report tactile, auditory, or visual hallucinations. Some users experience paranoia and disorientation.

Assessing for hallucinogen abuse

LSD or mescaline
- Sense of depersonalization
- Grandiosity
- Hallucinations, illusions
- Distorted perception of time and space
- Mystical experiences
- Nausea, vomiting, diarrhea, abdominal cramps
- Possible arrhythmias, palpitations, tachycardia, hypertension

Ecstasy
- Distractibility
- Heightened alertness
- Irritability or confusion
- Euphoria
- Enhanced emotional and mental clarity
- Increased sensitivity to touch
- Enhanced sexuality
- Increased energy and motor activity

Ketamine
- Dissociative effects
- Altered visual and auditory perception
- Impaired attention, learning ability, and memory (with low doses)
- Delirium, amnesia, impaired motor function, hypertension, depression, potentially fatal respiratory problems (with higher doses)

– If results indicate an assault, notify social services and law enforcement according to facility protocols
- Assist with specific measures to treat toxicity or withdrawal (see *General interventions for acute drug intoxication,* page 281)

Characteristics of inhalant abuse

- Commonly called *huffing* or *bagging*
- Deliberate inhalation of chemical vapors to attain an altered mental or physical state

General categories of inhalants

- Aerosols
- Gases
- Nitrites
- Volatile solvents

Effects of inhalants on the body

- Possibly change solubility of cell membranes of neurons
- May potentiate effects of GABA, the most important inhibitory neurotransmitter

Adverse effects of inhalant abuse

- Possible psychological dependence and physical addiction
- Possible serious and irreversible damage to brain, heart, liver, kidneys, and lungs (with chronic use)
- Death within minutes of inhalant use, usually from arrhythmias leading to heart failure
- Death from asphyxiation, aspiration, or suffocation

INHALANT ABUSE

● Defining characteristics

- Inhalant abuse, commonly called *huffing* or *bagging*, is the deliberate inhalation of chemical vapors to attain an altered mental or physical state (usually a quick "buzz")
- Users inhale vapors from a wide range of substances found in more than 1,000 common household products
- Inhalants fall into several general categories
  - Aerosols: sprays containing propellants and solvents (deodorant, hair products, cooking sprays, fabric protectors)
  - Gases: such as those found in refrigerants, medical anesthetics, propane tanks, butane lighters, whipped cream (nitrous oxide gas)
  - Nitrites: chemicals found in amyl nitrite, butyl nitrite, and cyclohexylnitrite (primarily used to enhance sexual experiences)
  - Volatile solvents: liquids that vaporize at room temperature when unsealed (paint thinner, gasoline, correction fluid, nail polish and polish remover, felt-tip markers, and glue)
- Street names for inhalants include *bang, bolt, boppers, bullet, climax, glading, gluey, hardware, head cleaner, hippie crack, kick, locker room, poor man's pot, poppers, rush,* and *snappers*
- Inhalants are breathed in through the nose or mouth in various ways
  - Inhaling chemical vapors directly from open containers, or huffing fumes from rags soaked in a chemical substance held to the face or stuffed in the mouth
  - Spraying aerosol directly into the nose or mouth
  - Pouring chemical onto collar, sleeves, or cuffs and then sniffing repeatedly
  - Inhaling (bagging) fumes from substances that are sprayed or deposited inside a paper or plastic bag or that are discharged into a small container or device (soda can, balloon)
- Inhalant abuse has been increasing steadily (almost 17 million people in the United States have experimented with inhalants at some time in their lives); currently, about 140,000 people in the United States abuse or are dependent on inhalants
  - Most users between ages 12 and 17; about 20% attempt before eighth grade
  - Roughly equal among males and females

● Drug effects

- Scientists unsure how inhalants produce their effects
- Possibly a change in the solubility of cell membranes of neurons by inhaled substance; may potentiate the effects of gamma-aminobutyric acid (GABA), the most important inhibitory neurotransmitter

● Health hazards and impairments

- Can produce both psychological dependence and physical addiction
- May lead to serious and possibly irreversible damage to the brain, heart, liver, kidneys, and lungs (chronic abuse)
- Death within minutes of inhalant use, usually from arrhythmias leading to heart failure; death from asphyxiation, aspiration, or suffocation

- Brain damage causing personality changes, diminished cognitive functioning, memory impairment, slurred speech, relationship problems, and long-term problems related to education and employment
- Impaired judgment leading to fatal injuries from motor vehicle accidents or sudden falls

Causes

- Desire for rapid, euphoric effect similar to alcohol intoxication, along with loss of inhibitions; after initial excitation, causes drowsiness, light-headedness, and agitation
- Desire for enhanced sexual experience (common with nitrite abusers, who tend to be adults rather than adolescents); causes dilation of blood vessels, increased pulse rate, and production of a sensation of heat and excitement that can last several minutes

Signs and symptoms

- Loss of muscle control
- Slurred speech
- Dizziness, drowsiness, or loss of consciousness
- Hallucinations and delusions
- Belligerence
- Apathy
- Impaired judgment, drunk or disoriented demeanor
- Double vision
- Seizures
- Nausea, appetite loss
- Red or runny nose; watery eyes; sores or rash around the nose or mouth
- Arrhythmias
- Strong chemical odors on the breath or clothing
- Paint or other stains on the hands, face, or clothing
- Long-term inhalant use
  - Inflammation, atrophy, or perforation of nasal mucosa
  - Weight loss
  - Disorientation
  - Inattentiveness
  - Irritability
  - Depression
  - Muscle weakness, permanent ataxia (staggering gait or incoordination)
  - Peripheral neuropathies
  - Possible cognitive impairment
- Inhalant withdrawal
  - Excessive sweating
  - Headache
  - Rapid pulse
  - Hand tremors
  - Muscle cramps
  - Insomnia
  - Hallucinations
  - Nausea and vomiting

Common causes of inhalant abuse

- Desire for rapid, euphoric effect similar to alcohol intoxication, along with loss of inhibitions
- Desire for enhanced sexual experience (common with nitrite abusers, who tend to be adults rather than adolescents)

Key signs and symptoms of inhalant abuse

Inhalant influence
- Loss of muscle control
- Slurred speech
- Dizziness, drowsiness, or loss of consciousness
- Hallucinations and delusions
- Belligerence
- Apathy
- Impaired judgment, drunk or disoriented demeanor
- Double vision
- Red or runny nose; watery eyes; sores or rash around nose or mouth
- Strong chemical odors on breath or clothing

Inhalant withdrawal
- Excessive sweating
- Headache
- Rapid pulse
- Hand tremors
- Muscle cramps
- Hallucinations
- Nausea and vomiting

Diagnosing inhalant abuse

- Laboratory tests necessary when patient is known to have used an inhalant
- CBC
- Serum electrolyte analysis
- Confirmed if *DSM-IV-TR* criteria met

Key treatment options for inhalant abuse

- Supportive and symptomatic (acute inhalant intoxication)
- Antianxiety drugs
- I.V. fluid replacement, sedatives, anticholinergics, antidiarrheals, continuous ECG monitoring
- Adequate detoxification
- Rehabilitation

Key nursing interventions for a patient with inhalant abuse

- Assess for signs and symptoms of acute inhalant toxicity.
- Assist with specific treatment measures.

Characteristics of nicotine dependence

- Nicotine considered one of the most commonly used addictive drugs
- Cigarette smoking is most prevalent form of nicotine dependence in United States
- Regular use can result in nicotine dependence
- Some rank nicotine higher than alcohol, cocaine, and heroin in terms of dependency risk

● **Diagnosis**
- Laboratory tests necessary when patient is known to have used an inhalant; includes testing for serum drug levels if particular inhalant is known
  - Complete blood count (CBC): may reveal leukocytosis, anemia, thrombocytopenia, thrombocytosis, or platelet defects
  - Serum electrolyte analysis: may show hyperchloremia, hypokalemia, and hypophosphatemia
- Diagnosis of inhalant abuse or dependence confirmed when *DSM-IV-TR* criteria met

● **Treatment**
- Supportive and symptomatic (acute inhalant intoxication)
- Antianxiety drugs (haloperidol [Haldol]) for severe agitation; combative patients may require restraint (follow facility protocol)
- I.V. fluid replacement, sedatives (to induce sleep), anticholinergics and antidiarrheals (to relieve GI distress), and continuous ECG monitoring (many inhalants can induce arrhythmia)
- Adequate detoxification; regular inhalant abusers may need 30 to 40 days to detoxify
  - Nonpharmacologic measures (psychotherapy, exercise, relaxation techniques, and nutritional support) to ease withdrawal
- Rehabilitation (aftercare and follow-up) to prevent relapse (inhalant abusers have high relapse rates)
  - Outpatient or residential treatment program (some patients)
  - Long-term (up to 2 years) rehabilitation (required by many patients)
  - Also may include family therapy (inhalant abuse prevalent among adolescents)

● **Nursing interventions**
- Assess for signs and symptoms of acute inhalant toxicity
- Assist with specific treatment measures (see *General interventions for acute drug intoxication*, page 281)

NICOTINE DEPENDENCE

● **Defining characteristics**
- Nicotine is one of the most commonly used addictive drugs
  - Main psychoactive component found in smoke from tobacco products (cigarettes, cigars, and pipes)
  - High nicotine levels also in smokeless tobacco products (snuff, chewing tobacco)
- Cigarette smoking is the most prevalent form of nicotine dependence in the United States (an estimated 57 million U.S. residents currently smoke cigarettes; 7.6 million use smokeless tobacco)
- Most cigarettes contain at least 10 mg of nicotine; the average smoker takes in 1 to 2 mg of nicotine with each cigarette
- Regular nicotine use can result in nicotine dependence; some experts rank nicotine higher than alcohol, cocaine, and heroin in terms of dependency risk
  - Adolescent who smokes as few as four cigarettes per day might develop lifelong addiction to nicotine

- Most regular tobacco use a result of nicotine addiction
- Although serious attempt to quit made by nearly 35 million smokers each year, fewer than 7% attempting on their own stay abstinent for more than 1 year (most relapse within few days of attempt)
- A nicotine-dependent person who stops using nicotine experiences a withdrawal syndrome that may last a month or longer; some have intense nicotine cravings for 6 months or longer
- The incidence of smoking is highest among blacks, blue-collar workers, less educated persons, and those in lower socioeconomic groups

Drug effects

- Absorbed through the skin and mucosal lining of the mouth and nose or by inhalation in the lungs
- Activates the brain circuitry that regulates feelings of pleasure (the so-called *reward pathways*), raising dopamine levels—a reaction that's thought to underlie the pleasurable sensations that many smokers experience
- Pharmacokinetic properties enhance abuse potential
  - Nicotine rapidly distributed to brain through cigarette smoking; drug levels peak within 10 seconds of inhalation
  - Acute effects dissipate in a few minutes; smoker must continue to dose throughout the day to maintain pleasurable drug effects and prevent withdrawal
  - Tolerance necessitates need to use progressively higher doses
- Can act as both a stimulant and a sedative
  - Small, rapid doses: produce alertness and arousal
  - Long, drawn-out doses: induce relaxation and sedation
- Stimulates hypothalamic corticotropin-releasing factor and increases levels of endorphins, adrenocorticotropic hormone, and arginine vasopressin
  - "Kick" that occurs immediately after exposure results partly from adrenal stimulation and subsequent epinephrine discharge
  - Epinephrine "rush" triggers glucose release, raises blood pressure, and speeds pulse and respiratory rates

Health hazards and impairments

- Impacts morbidity and mortality, and economic costs to society
- The leading preventable cause of death in the United States, killing more than 430,000 U.S. residents each year (more than alcohol, cocaine, heroin, homicide, suicide, car accidents, fire, and acquired immunodeficiency syndrome combined) (see *Nicotine's ugly aftermath,* page 304)
- Illnesses related to smoking: lead to missed work days, increased medical expenses, and adverse effects on quality of life for the individual

Causes

- Possible genetic susceptibility to nicotine addiction
  - Twin studies suggesting that genetic predisposition accounts for 50% to 70% of the risk of becoming a smoker
  - Possibly as many as 50 genes involved in nicotine addiction

Risk factors (smoking among adolescents)

- Use of alcohol and other drugs
- Attention-deficit disorder
- Depression

Effects of nicotine on the body

- Activates the brain circuitry that regulates feelings of pleasure, raising dopamine levels
- Pharmacokinetic properties enhance abuse potential
- Can act as both a stimulant and a sedative
- Stimulates hypothalamic corticotropin-releasing factor
- Increases levels of endorphins, adrenocorticotropic hormone, and arginine vasopressin

Common causes of nicotine dependence

- Possible genetic susceptibility to nicotine addiction
- May involve as many as 50 genes

Adverse effects of nicotine dependence

- Linked to nearly 90% of all lung cancers
- Associated with cancers of mouth, pharynx, larynx, esophagus, stomach, pancreas, cervix, kidney, ureter, and bladder
- Causes lung diseases
- Can exacerbate asthma symptoms
- May heighten risk of peptic ulcers, GI disorders, maternal and fetal complications, and other disorders
- Increasing risk of cardiovascular disease
- Secondhand smoke causes lung cancer deaths and deaths from cardiovascular disease

Key signs and symptoms of nicotine withdrawal

- Depressed mood
- Insomnia
- Irritability, frustration, or anger
- Difficulty concentrating
- Nicotine craving, weight gain (may last for months)
- Increased appetite, desire for sweets
- Increased coughing

Diagnosing nicotine dependence

- Blood studies and other diagnostic tests to rule out possible underlying medical conditions
- Confirmed if *DSM-IV-TR* criteria met

Nicotine's ugly aftermath

Tobacco use accounts for approximately one-third of all cancers. Cigarette smoking is linked to nearly 90% of all lung cancers—the leading cause of cancer deaths in both men and women. Additionally, it's associated with cancers of the mouth, pharynx, larynx, esophagus, stomach, pancreas, cervix, kidney, ureter, and bladder. Overall death rates from cancer are twice as high among smokers as that of nonsmokers.

Smoking also causes lung diseases, such as chronic bronchitis and emphysema, and can exacerbate asthma symptoms. It may also heighten the risk of peptic ulcers, GI disorders, maternal and fetal complications, and other disorders.

CARDIOVASCULAR DISEASE
Smoking dramatically increases the risk of cardiovascular disease, including coronary artery disease, myocardial infarction, stroke, vascular problems, and aneurysms. Smoking accounts for nearly 20% of deaths from heart disease.

PASSIVE SMOKING AND ITS CONSEQUENCES
Secondhand smoke (passive smoking) causes approximately 3,000 lung cancer deaths yearly in nonsmokers, and contributes to as many as 40,000 deaths from cardiovascular disease.

Exposure to tobacco smoke in the home contributes to childhood asthma and increases its severity.

- Peer influences
- Urge to experiment
- Disruptive behavior
- Failing to perceive the risks of smoking
- Having friends who abuse substances
- Having family members who smoke
- Divorce or family conflict

● **Signs and symptoms (withdrawal)**
- May begin a few hours after the last cigarette and can quickly drive smoker back to tobacco use
- Usually peaks within first few days of not smoking and subsides within a few weeks
  - Depressed mood
  - Insomnia
  - Irritability, frustration, anger
  - Anxiety
  - Difficulty concentrating
  - Restlessness
  - Nicotine craving, weight gain (may last for months)
  - Increased appetite, desire for sweets
  - Increased coughing

● **Diagnosis**
- Blood studies and other diagnostic tests to rule out possible underlying medical conditions causing signs and symptoms
- Diagnosis of dependence confirmed if *DSM-IV-TR* criteria met

Treatment

- Various behavioral and pharmacologic treatments proven effective in treating nicotine dependence
- For motivated patients, a combination of behavioral and pharmacologic treatments (such as using a behavioral technique along with a nicotine patch) to double success rates (versus placebo in studies)
- Pharmacologic therapies, including nicotine replacement, antagonist therapy, aversion therapy, nicotine-mimicking agents, and nonnicotine medication
  - Nicotine replacement: used to relieve withdrawal symptoms and nicotine craving
    - Includes nicotine gum, transdermal patches, nasal spray, and inhalers (all seem equally effective)
    - Cause milder physiologic changes than tobacco-based cessation systems; generally provide lower overall nicotine levels than tobacco does
    - Little abuse potential (don't cause pleasurable effects of tobacco); also, don't contain carcinogens and gases found in tobacco smoke
  - Antagonist therapy: used to prevent positive reinforcing and subjective effects of cigarette smoking
    - Includes mecamylamine (Inversine), a noncompetitive blocker of CNS and peripheral nicotinic receptors, and naltrexone (long-acting form of the opioid antagonist naloxone [Narcan])
  - Aversion therapy: typically involves use of silver acetate (produces bad taste when combined with sulfides in tobacco smoke)
  - Nicotine-mimicking agents: mimic effects of nicotine (include clonidine [Catapres] and anxiolytics [such as diazepam], antidepressants, stimulants, and anorectic agents
  - Bupropion (Zyban): first nonnicotine medication for smoking cessation; taken in pill form to aid in decreasing nicotine cravings
- Nonpharmacologic therapies, including sensory replacement and acupuncture
  - Sensory replacement agents: used to decrease nicotine cravings or withdrawal or to substitute for satisfaction from cigarettes (include black pepper extract, capsaicin, denicotinized tobacco, flavorings, and regenerated [denicotinized] smoke)
  - Acupuncture: may be helpful in smoking cessation and nicotine withdrawal (studies don't support claims of efficacy equal to other treatments)
- Behavioral interventions
  - Help patients identify high-risk relapse situations, create aversion to smoking, self-monitor smoking behavior, and establish alternative coping responses
  - Involves identifying and removing environmental cues that influence patient to smoke (such as cigarettes, lighters, and ashtrays)
  - Includes such techniques as smoking rapidly without inhaling, and nicotine fading (patient smokes same number of cigarettes, but amount of nicotine is reduced)
- Adjunctive measures
  - Learning and using coping skills (considered the single most important factor in nicotine abstinence)
  - Social supports (ideally, patient should avoid smokers and smoking environments and receive support from family and friends)

Key treatment options for nicotine dependence

- Nicotine replacement
- Antagonist therapy
- Aversion therapy
- Sensory replacement agents
- Acupuncture
- Behavioral interventions
- Learning and using coping skills
- Social supports
- Self-help materials

Enhancing a patient's coping skills

- Spend uninterrupted periods of time with patient.
- Try to identify factors that cause, exacerbate, or reduce patient's inability to cope.
- Encourage patient to make decisions about his care.
- Praise patient for making decisions and performing activities.
- Encourage patient to use support systems.
- Help patient evaluate his current situation and coping behaviors.
- Encourage patient to try alternative coping behaviors.
- Ask patient for feedback about behaviors.

Key nursing interventions for a patient with nicotine dependence

- Teach patient about dangers of smoking and ways to stop.
- Provide emotional support and encouragement for patient's attempts to stop smoking.
- Explain how to use nicotine replacement devices, antagonist or aversive medications, or other prescribed drugs.
- Provide referrals for appropriate smoking cessation programs.

Characteristics of opioids

- Narcotics that can produce euphoria and have a high potential for abuse and dependence
- Produce relaxation with an immediate "rush"
- Can have initial unpleasant effects, such as restlessness and nausea
- With a typical dose, effects last 3 to 6 hours

Improving the patient's coping skills

Many patients who abuse drugs exhibit ineffective coping and need help in identifying and using available support systems. To enhance your patient's coping skills, use these nursing interventions.

- Spend uninterrupted periods of time with the patient; encourage him to express his feelings, and accept what he says.
- Try to identify factors that cause, exacerbate, or reduce the patient's inability to cope, such as the fear of health problems or losing his job.
- Encourage the patient to make decisions about his care to increase his sense of self-worth and mastery over his current situation.
- Praise him for making decisions and performing activities to reinforce coping behaviors.

- Encourage him to use support systems that can help him cope.
- Help him evaluate his current situation and coping behaviors to encourage a realistic view of his crisis.
- Encourage the patient to try alternative coping behaviors; a patient in crisis tends to accept interventions and develop new coping behaviors more easily.
- Ask the patient for feedback about behaviors that seem to work; this encourages him to evaluate the effect of these behaviors.

  – Self-help materials, educational and support groups, exercise, hypnosis, 12-step programs, biofeedback, family therapy, interpersonal therapy, and psychodynamic therapies

● **Nursing interventions**
- Teach the patient about the dangers of smoking and ways to stop
- Provide emotional support and encouragement for the patient's attempts to stop smoking
- Explain how to use nicotine replacement devices, antagonist or aversive medications, or other prescribed drugs
- Provide referrals for appropriate smoking cessation programs
- Assist the patient with developing and improving coping skills (see *Improving the patient's coping skills*)

OPIOID ABUSE

● **Defining characteristics**
- Opioids are narcotics that can produce euphoria and that have a high potential for abuse and dependence
  – Naturally occurring opioids include morphine (Duramorph) and codeine
  – Partially synthetic morphine derivatives include heroin, oxycodone (Percocet, OxyContin), oxymorphone (Numorphan), and hydrocodone (Vicodin)
  – Synthetic opioids include fentanyl (Sublimaze), alfentanil (Alfenta), meperidine (Demerol), methadone (Dolophine), and propoxyphene (Darvocet)

- Opioids are used medically as analgesics; some have additional uses such as codeine's use as an antitussive
- Opioids produce relaxation with an immediate "rush"; they can also have initial unpleasant effects, such as restlessness and nausea
- With a typical dose, effects last 3 to 6 hours
- Codeine, meperidine, and morphine may be ingested, injected, or smoked; oxycodone, oxymorphone, and hydrocodone are ingested
- Heroin (street names include *junk, horse,* and *H*) may be injected, inhaled, or smoked
- Opium (known as *O, ope,* or *OP*) may be ingested or smoked
- According to recent statistics, 3.1 million U.S. residents reported having used heroin at least once during their lifetime (in 2000, there were 146,000 new heroin users, most under age 26); lifetime prevalence of opioid use is over 2% in adolescents and slightly higher in middle-age people because of peak heroin use during the 1960s and 1970s

Drug effects
- Stimulate opioid receptors in the CNS and surrounding tissues
- CNS effects, including euphoria and sedation, followed by elation, relaxation and, then, sedation or sleep

Health hazards and impairments
- Prolonged abuse possibly leading to criminal behavior related to seeking money to buy drugs
- Increased risk of infection with injected forms
- Respiratory depression, stupor, and coma with overdose

Causes
- Strong reinforcement mechanisms that perpetuate addictive behavior (produced by drug's euphoric and anxiolytic effects and reward-punishment mechanism)
- Rapid development of physical dependence and a prolonged withdrawal syndrome (can make abstinence difficult)
- Genetic, social, cultural, and psychological factors
  - Genetic vulnerability (supported by identical twin studies)
  - Easy drug access (now made easier — especially for adolescents — by on-line "pharmacies" offering mail-order opioids without a prescription)
  - Social acceptance of drug use
  - Higher drug use rates in urban areas with poor parental functioning, greater drug exposure, and higher crime and unemployment rates
  - Incidence of abuse following use of opioids prescribed for pain relief
  - Self-medication to manage uncomfortable emotions (anxiety, guilt, and anger)

Signs and symptoms
- Opioid use
  - Suspicious behaviors and attempts to hide drug use from family, friends, coworkers, and health care professionals (may include drug-seeking behavior such as "doctor shopping," when person goes to multiple medical facilities or physicians with the same pain-related complaint) (see *When to suspect drug abuse,* page 308)

Types of opioids
- Naturally occurring opioids: morphine, codeine
- Partially synthetic morphine derivatives: heroin, oxycodone, oxymorphone, hydrocodone
- Synthetic opioids: fentanyl, alfentanil, meperidine, methadone, propoxyphene

Effects of opioids on the body
- Stimulate opioid receptors in the CNS and surrounding tissues
- CNS effects, including euphoria and sedation, followed by elation, relaxation and, then, sedation or sleep

Common causes of opioid abuse
- Strong reinforcement mechanisms that perpetuate addictive behavior
- Rapid development of physical dependence and a prolonged withdrawal syndrome
- Genetic, social, cultural, and psychological factors

Assessing for drug abuse

- Use of fictitious name and address
- Reluctance to discuss previous hospitalizations
- Seeking treatment at medical facility not near own home
- History of drug overdose
- Complaints of painful injury or chronic illness but refusal of diagnostic workup
- Feigned illnesses
- Fever
- Needle marks or tracks
- Attempts to conceal or disguise injection sites with tattoos
- Cellulitis or abscess from self-injection
- Puffy hands
- Dental conditions
- Excoriated skin
- Uncooperativeness, disruptive behavior, violence (hospitalized abuser)
- Mood swings, anxiety, impaired memory, sleep disturbances, flashbacks, slurred speech, depression, thought disorders (hospitalized abuser)

Key signs and symptoms of opioid abuse

Opioid influence

- Suspicious behaviors and attempts to hide drug use
- Constricted pupils, bloodshot eyes, drooping eyelids, nystagmus
- Slurred speech
- Sweating; clammy skin
- Visible needle marks, skin lesions or abscesses, soft-tissue infection, and thrombosed veins (with I.V. use)
- Respiratory depression
- Hypotension, arrhythmias
- Drowsiness, decreased LOC

When to suspect drug abuse

Many patients try to hide their drug abuse – especially if they inject drugs. If you suspect your patient is abusing drugs, carefully review his medical history and perform a physical assessment.

HISTORY FINDINGS

History findings that suggest drug abuse include:

- Use of a fictitious name and address
- Reluctance to discuss previous hospitalizations
- Seeking treatment at a medical facility across town rather than near his own home
- History of a drug overdose
- High tolerance for potentially addictive drugs
- History of hepatitis or human immunodeficiency virus infection
- Amenorrhea
- Complaints of a painful injury or chronic illness – but refusal of a diagnostic workup
- Feigned illnesses, such as migraine headache, myocardial infarction, or renal colic, in an attempt to obtain drugs
- Claims of an allergy to over-the-counter analgesics
- Requests for a specific medication

PHYSICAL FINDINGS

Physical findings that hint at drug abuse include:

- Fever (from stimulant intoxication, withdrawal, or infection caused by I.V. drug use)
- Needle marks or tracks (from I.V. drug use)
- Attempts to conceal or disguise injection sites with tattoos
- Use of inconspicuous injection sites, such as under the nails or tongue
- Cellulitis or abscess from self-injection
- Puffy hands (a late sign of thrombophlebitis or of fascial infection caused by self-injection on the hands or arms)
- Dental conditions (from poor oral hygiene associated with chronic drug use)
- Excoriated skin (from scratching induced by formication, a sensation of bugs crawling on the skin)
- Refractory, acute onset hypertension or cardiac arrhythmias (from stimulant use)
- Liver enlargement, with or without tenderness (from hepatitis caused by sharing contaminated needles)

BEHAVIORAL CLUES

A hospitalized drug abuser is likely to be uncooperative, disruptive, or even violent. He may experience mood swings, anxiety, impaired memory, sleep disturbances, flashbacks, slurred speech, depression, and thought disorders.

To obtain drugs, some patients resort to eliciting unwarranted sympathy or to bribery or threats. They may try to manipulate caregivers by pitting one staff member against another.

– Constricted pupils, bloodshot eyes, drooping eyelids, nystagmus
– Slurred speech
– Sweating; clammy skin
– Visible needle marks, skin lesions or abscesses, soft-tissue infection, and thrombosed veins (with I.V. use)
– Anorexia, nausea and vomiting, constipation, hemorrhoids
– Respiratory depression

- Hypotension, arrhythmias
- Seizures
- Drowsiness, decreased level of consciousness (LOC) (possible delirium and coma with severe intoxication)
- Impaired judgment, indifference to pain, apathy
- Euphoria, sense of tranquillity, detachment from reality
- Opioid overdose
  - Bilateral crackles and rhonchi
  - Pulmonary edema, respiratory depression, aspiration pneumonia, and hypotension
- Opioid withdrawal
  - Abdominal cramps, nausea or vomiting, anorexia, hyperactive bowel sounds
  - Fever or chills, profuse sweating
  - Dilated pupils
  - Runny nose, watery eyes
  - Tremors
  - Yawning
  - Irritability, panic state
  - Bone pain or diffuse muscle aches
  - Piloerection
  - Drug craving
- Opioid withdrawal (heroin)
  - Resembles bad case of flu
  - Generally begins 12 to 14 hours after last dose; peaks within 36 to 72 hours
  - May last 7 to 14 days

Diagnosis
- Urine drug screen (when opioid abuse or dependence is suspected)
- Tests when I.V. drug abuse is known or suspected
  - Liver function tests
  - Rapid plasma reagin test for syphilis
  - Blood testing for hepatitis
  - HIV testing
  - Lung X-rays to check for pulmonary fibrosis
  - Naloxone challenge test before starting an opioid antagonist for maintenance therapy; positive result indicated by typical withdrawal signs and symptoms (usually lasting 30 to 60 minutes) after I.V. or I.M. naloxone administration
- Serum electrolyte studies and CBC when withdrawal is suspected
- Diagnosis of opioid abuse or dependence confirmed if *DSM-IV-TR* criteria met

Treatment
- For intoxication or overdose: general supportive measures include ensuring an adequate airway and ventilation (with ventilatory support, if needed) and supporting cardiovascular function; other treatments depend on symptoms, the specific opioid, and the administration route
  - Vomiting induced or gastric lavage performed if drug was ingested
  - Possible I.V. fluids and nutritional and vitamin supplements

Key signs and symptoms of opioid abuse

Opioid withdrawal
- Abdominal cramps, nausea or vomiting, anorexia, hyperactive bowel sounds
- Dilated pupils
- Runny nose, watery eyes
- Yawning
- Irritability, panic state
- Piloerection
- Drug craving

Heroin withdrawal
- Symptoms resembling bad case of flu
- Generally begins 12 to 14 hours after last dose; peaks within 36 to 72 hours
- May last 7 to 14 days

Diagnosing opioid abuse
- Urine drug screen
- Liver function tests
- Rapid plasma reagin test for syphilis
- Blood testing for hepatitis
- HIV testing
- Naloxone challenge test
- Serum electrolyte studies and CBC
- Confirmed if *DSM-IV-TR* criteria met

Key treatment options for opioid abuse

- For intoxification or overdose: general supportive measures
- For withdrawal: patient should receive sufficient amount of opioid on first day to decrease symptoms, followed by gradual withdrawal of abused drug over 5 to 10 days
- For detoxification: abused opioid usually replaced with drug that has similar action but longer duration
- For maintenance: patient typically receives opioid agonist as substitute for abused drug
- Acupuncture
- Psychotherapy

Key facts about naloxone therapy

- Used to reverse effects of opioids
- Displaces opioids from their receptors in the CNS
- Administered I.V., I.M., or subcutaneously every 2 to 3 minutes
- Rapidly reverses opioid-induced CNS depression and increases respiratory rate within 1 to 2 minutes

Common drugs used for maintenance therapy

- Methadone
- ORLAAM
- Naltrexone

Naloxone for opioid reversal

Naloxone (Narcan) is an opioid antagonist used to reverse the effects of opioids. It works by displacing opioids from their receptors in the central nervous system (CNS).

Naloxone is administered I.V., I.M., or subcutaneously every 2 to 3 minutes as needed. It rapidly reverses opioid-induced CNS depression and increases the respiratory rate within 1 to 2 minutes. Adverse effects include nausea, vomiting, diaphoresis, tachycardia, CNS excitement, and increased blood pressure.

RELAPSE AND RESPIRATORY PERIL

Because the opioid's duration of action may exceed that of naloxone, the patient may relapse into respiratory depression. Be sure to monitor respiratory rate and depth. Be prepared to provide oxygen, ventilation, and other resuscitation measures.

- – Possible opioid antagonist such as naloxone (see *Naloxone for opioid reversal*)
- – Sedatives (to induce sleep), anticholinergics and antidiarrheal agents (to relieve GI distress), and antianxiety agents (for severe agitation)
- – Possible forced diuresis and hemoperfusion or hemodialysis (depending on opioid dosage and time elapsed before admission)
- For withdrawal: the patient should receive a sufficient amount of opioid on the first day to decrease symptoms, followed by gradual withdrawal of the abused drug over 5 to 10 days
  - – May include antidiarrheals, decongestants for runny nose, and nonopioid analgesics for pain
  - – May include giving clonidine (alpha-2 adrenergic agonist that decreases sympathetic nervous system overactivity and produces sedation) or buprenorphine (Buprenex) (partial opioid agonist and potent antagonist to block withdrawal symptoms)
- For detoxification: the abused opioid usually is replaced with a drug that has a similar action but a longer duration (gradual substitution controls withdrawal effects, reducing discomfort and associated risks)
  - – May be managed on an inpatient or outpatient basis, depending on drug of abuse
  - – May involve ultrarapid (1-day) detoxification program (patient is placed under heavy sedation or general anesthesia and given I.V. naloxone or oral naltrexone; acute withdrawal takes place during unconscious state)
- For maintenance: the patient typically receives an opioid agonist as a substitute for the abused drug; the goal is to replace the abused drug with one that's available legally, can be taken orally, and requires only a once-daily dose
  - – Methadone is most commonly used opioid agonist in opioid detoxification; reduces drug cravings, improves the patient's functioning, promotes stability, reduces illicit drug use and other criminal behavior, and improves productive social behavior
    - · Given once per day as an oral liquid; has nearly all the physiologic properties of heroin
    - · Three-quarters of patients who take methadone for maintenance typically remain heroin-free for 6 months or longer

– Levomethadyl acetate (ORLAAM): a methadone derivative, may also be used
  • Longer acting than methadone; can be taken just two or three times per week
  • As effective as methadone
– For some patients, opioid antagonist (typically naltrexone) therapy preferred to methadone or ORLAAM
  • Naltrexone: blocks the "high" produced by opioids; patient must be opioid-free for at least 5 days before starting
  • Mixed success; only 10% to 20% of patients who try naltrexone take it for 6 months or longer
– Acupuncture technique called *auriculotherapy* gaining popularity in treating opioid abuse (needles inserted into each ear and connected to a constant-current electrical stimulator)
• Psychotherapy and self-help for long-term management of opioid dependence (abstinence)
  – Detoxification alone (without ongoing psychotherapy) not sufficient for long-term management
  – Standard drug counseling required for abstinence, along with cognitive-behavioral, dynamic, or group therapy; some patients may even prefer aversion therapy
  – Cognitive-behavioral therapy: focuses on patient's thoughts and behaviors, helping him learn specific skills for resisting drug abuse and coping skills to reduce problems related to drug use
  – Dynamic psychotherapy: based on concept that all symptoms arise from underlying unconscious psychological conflicts; goal is to make patient aware of conflicts and develop better coping mechanisms to resolve them
  – Group therapy: targets social stigma attached to drug abuse; acknowledgment of abuse problem by other users is therapeutic and helps patient develop alternative methods of staying sober
  – NA: based on 12-step recovery method similar to AA, helps many substance abusers attempting abstinence

● **Nursing interventions**
• Assess for signs and symptoms of opioid abuse, and provide treatment as needed (see *General interventions for acute drug intoxication,* page 281)
• Provide extra blankets or a hypothermia blanket for hypothermia
• Reorient the patient to time, place, and person
• Monitor breath sounds for evidence of pulmonary edema
• Frequently monitor vital signs and cardiopulmonary status until opioids have cleared from the system
• Monitor for withdrawal symptoms
• Help the patient improve social interaction skills
  – Avoid focus on delusion or hallucinations; provide reality-based information, reassure safety
  – Provide additional interaction with patient on each shift; begin with one-to-one interaction and increase to group interaction when ready
  – Positive reinforcement for appropriate and effective interaction behaviors
  – Assist patient and family in progressive participation in care and therapies (family therapy may be needed)

Types of psychotherapy for opioid dependence

● Standard drug counseling
● Cognitive-behavioral therapy
● Dynamic psychotherapy
● Group therapy
● NA

Key nursing interventions for a patient with opioid abuse

● Assess for signs and symptoms of opioid abuse, and provide treatment as needed.
● Reorient patient to time, place, and person.
● Frequently monitor vital signs and cardiopulmonary status until opioids have cleared from the system.
● Monitor for withdrawal symptoms.

Characteristics of PCP

- A dissociative drug
- Makes user feel disconnected and out of control
- Has numbing effect on the mind
- Can cause unpredictable and even violent behavior in many users
- Many users have bad reactions
- May cause flashbacks long after user stops drug
- Can result in memory loss and depression (up to 1 year after chronic user stops taking drug)

Common names for PCP

- Angel dust
- Wack
- Ozone
- Love boat
- Superweed
- Hog
- Peace pill
- Embalming fluid
- Elephant tranquilizer
- Rocket fuel

Effects of PCP on the body

- Increases levels of GABA; increased GABA levels probably explain decreased awareness of pain seen in PCP users
- Alters action of dopamine, which is responsible for the euphoria and "rush" associated with many psychoactive drugs

PHENCYCLIDINE ABUSE

● Defining characteristics

- A dissociative drug, PCP was developed in the 1950s as an I.V. anesthetic; it was used in veterinary medicine but never approved for human use
- Today, PCP is manufactured illegally in laboratories; on the street, it's available as tablets, capsules, and powders
  - Street names include *angel dust, wack, ozone, love boat, superweed, hog, peace pill, embalming fluid, elephant tranquilizer,* and *rocket fuel*
  - Combination of PCP and marijuana: called *killer joint* or *crystal supergrass*
- PCP can be snorted (as powder), smoked (usually applied to leafy material, such as parsley, oregano, or marijuana), or swallowed (tablets)
- PCP makes the user feel disconnected and out of control
  - Has numbing effect on the mind and can cause unpredictable and even violent behavior in many patients
  - May cause psychological dependence and craving with repeated use
- Many people have bad reactions to PCP
  - May cause flashbacks long after stopping drug
  - Can result in memory loss and depression (up to 1 year after a chronic user stops taking drug)
- PCP use isn't widespread; it's most common among older teenagers and young adults

● Drug effects

- Primary sites of action: glutamate receptors known as *N-methyl-D-aspartate (NMDA) receptors;* acts as an NMDA antagonist, lowering the glutamate levels in the brain
- Increases levels of GABA, an inhibitory neurotransmitter; increased GABA levels probably explain the decreased awareness of pain seen in PCP users
- Alters the action of dopamine, which is responsible for the euphoria and "rush" associated with many psychoactive drugs

● Health hazards and impairments

- At low to moderate doses: physiologic effects include increased body temperature, marked rises in blood pressure and pulse, shallow respirations, flushing, and profuse sweating
- At high doses: decreases blood pressure and slows the pulse and respiratory rates; cardiac arrest, hypertensive crisis, renal failure, and seizures may occur
- Violent or suicidal behavior, seizures, decreased awareness of pain, coma, and death; death more commonly results from accidental injury or suicide during PCP intoxication
- In adolescents, may interfere with the learning process and with hormones related to normal growth and development
- Rhabdomyolysis, a life-threatening condition marked by breakdown of muscle fibers and leakage of potentially toxic cellular contents into the systemic circulation, with various complications
  - Compartment syndrome (causing vessel and nerve compressions)
  - Hypovolemia, hyperkalemia, and metabolic acidosis
  - Cardiac arrest and arrhythmias
  - Disseminated intravascular coagulation
  - Acute renal failure

Causes

- Precise causes unknown
- Possible desire for feeling of strength, power, and invulnerability
- In young people, commonly involves peer pressure
- Associated risk factors: male gender and young adulthood

Signs and symptoms

- Physical findings
  - Numbness of the arms and legs, poor muscle coordination, loss of balance, dizziness, diminished deep tendon reflexes, gait ataxia
  - Sparse, garbled speech
  - Blurred vision, blank stare, nystagmus
  - Drooling
  - Nausea and vomiting
  - Fever
  - Hyperactivity
  - Increased vital signs
  - Tachycardia
- Psychological effects
  - Euphoria, excitation
  - Amnesia, disordered thinking
  - Poor perception of time and distance; distorted sense of sight, hearing, and touch
  - Decreased awareness of pain
  - Distorted body image
  - Sudden behavioral changes (may include delusions and hallucinations, panic, violent behavior, paranoia)
  - Stupor or coma
- PCP withdrawal
  - Dysphoria
  - Intense drug craving

Diagnosis

- Urine drug screen (may be done if PCP use is suspected)
- Serum enzyme levels, especially creatine kinase (may be done because PCP can cause rhabdomyolysis)
- Diagnosis of abuse or dependence confirmed when *DSM-IV-TR* criteria met

Treatment

- Acute PCP intoxication: placing patient in a quiet room with minimal stimulation; restraining if violent (following facility protocol)
- Inducing vomiting or gastric lavage, administering activated charcoal
- Drug therapy according to symptoms
  - Benzodiazepines (such as diazepam) to ease seizures, agitation, aggressiveness, psychotic symptoms, hypertension, and tachycardia
  - Haloperidol for agitation or psychotic behavior
  - Diuretics to force diuresis
  - Anticholinergics and antidiarrheal agents to relieve GI distress
  - Propranolol for hypertension or tachycardia
  - Nitroprusside for severe hypertensive crisis
  - I.V. fluids

Key nursing interventions for a patient with PCP abuse

- Assess for signs and symptoms of PCP intoxication.
- Assist with treatment measures as needed.

Characteristics of sedatives, hypnotics, or anxiolytics

- Most are classified as benzodiazepines
- Typically act as hypnotics in high doses, anxiolytics in moderate doses, and sedatives in low doses
- May be used to prevent seizures or help patients withdraw from alcohol
- In United States, benzodiazepines are most widely prescribed CNS medications

Common names for benzodiazepines

- Dolls
- Green and whites
- Roaches
- Yellow jackets

- PCP overdose: treating with physostigmine (Eserine), an acetylcholinesterase inhibitor used as a partial antidote (PCP has anticholinergic properties)
  - Given I.M. or I.V.
  - Doses repeated as needed until desired response or adverse cholinergic effects occur
- Inducing emesis, gastric lavage, or activated charcoal with large overdose to support respiratory function and decrease drug absorption
- Addressing high risk of violence for a patient with PCP-induced psychosis
  - May require seclusion or restraint; suicide and assault precautions should be instituted
  - If psychosis persists, may require antipsychotic, such as haloperidol or risperidone (Risperdal); most patients weaned from antipsychotics within 6 months
  - Psychiatric follow-up care and chemical dependency treatment usually needed

- **Nursing interventions**
  - Assess for signs and symptoms of PCP intoxication
  - Assist with treatment measures as needed (see *General interventions for acute drug intoxication,* page 281)

SEDATIVE, HYPNOTIC, OR ANXIOLYTIC ABUSE

- **Defining characteristics**
  - Sedative, hypnotic, and anxiolytic drugs produce sedation, ease anxiety, and relax muscles
  - Most of these drugs are classified as benzodiazepines
    - Typically act as hypnotics in high doses, anxiolytics in moderate doses, and sedatives in low doses
    - Also may be used to prevent seizures or help patients withdraw from alcohol
  - In the United States, benzodiazepines are the most widely prescribed CNS medications
    - Widespread availability contributes to common abuse
    - Abusers maintain supply by getting prescriptions from several physicians, forging prescriptions, or buying drugs on the street (street names include *dolls, green and whites, roaches,* and *yellow jackets*)
  - Benzodiazepines are ingested or injected, with a duration of action ranging from 4 to 8 hours
  - Some people use benzodiazepines to get intoxicated; others take intentional or accidental overdoses
    - May be used by heroin users when heroin is unavailable, to enhance heroin's effects, or when trying to stop using heroin
    - May be taken by amphetamine and Ecstasy users when "coming down" from a high or to induce sleep
  - Adult males and females have similar rates of nonmedical use of prescription drugs, yet females are almost two times more likely than males to become addicted to sedatives, hypnotics, and anxiolytics

- **Drug effects**
  - Slow CNS activity

- Potentiate the activity of GABA, causing sedation, relaxing muscles, easing anxiety, and demonstrating anticonvulsant properties
- Peripheral nervous system: stimulation of GABA receptors may decrease cardiac contractility and enhance perfusion

Health hazards and impairments

- Cause tolerance and physical dependence
- Repeated use: can lead to amnesia, hostility, irritability, and vivid or disturbing dreams
- Concurrent use with alcohol or other depressants: can be life-threatening
- When used to enhance the "high" of other drugs: can lead to severe health effects, such as collapsed veins; red, swollen, infected skin; necessity for limb amputation (because of poor circulation); stroke; cardiac and respiratory arrest; death; and increased risk of contracting hepatitis and HIV by sharing needles, syringes, and other injecting equipment
- At low to moderate doses: can produce drowsiness, fatigue, lethargy, dizziness, vertigo, blurred or double vision, slurred speech, stuttering, mild impairment of memory and thought processes, feelings of isolation, and depression
- At high doses: may induce oversedation, sleep, or effects similar to alcohol intoxication (confusion, poor coordination, impaired memory and judgment, difficulty thinking clearly, blurred or double vision, and dizziness); mood swings and aggressive outbursts may also occur; as the high dose wears off, the user may feel jittery and excitable
- Overdose: can cause coma; when combined with alcohol, death may occur

Causes

- Genetic tendency toward drug dependence or addiction in some patients
- Environmental factors, including drug availability and prescriber dispensing practices

Signs and symptoms

- Benzodiazepine use
  - Headache
  - Sweating
  - Dizziness
  - Hypertension, hypotension
  - Poor appetite, nausea and vomiting, abdominal pain
  - Sleep disturbances
  - Relaxation, drowsiness
  - Confusion
  - Seizures
  - Nervousness, tension, anxiety, panic attacks
  - Depression
  - Feelings of isolation and unreality
  - Delirium and paranoia
  - Ataxia (poor muscle coordination)
  - Slurred speech
  - Increased self-confidence
- Chronic benzodiazepine abuse
  - Drowsiness
  - Lack of motivation

Effects of benzodiazepines on the body

- Slow CNS activity
- Sedation, muscle relaxation, easing anxiety, and anticonvulsant properties
- Peripheral nervous system: stimulation of GABA receptors may decrease cardiac contractility and enhance perfusion

Adverse effects of benzodiazepine abuse

- Tolerance and physical dependence
- Amnesia, hostility, irritability, and vivid or disturbing dreams
- Concurrent use with alcohol or other depressants: possibly life-threatening

Common causes of benzodiazepine abuse

- Genetic tendency
- Environmental factors

Key signs and symptoms of benzodiazepine abuse

Benzodiazepine influence
- Sweating
- Dizziness
- Hypertension, hypotension
- Poor appetite, nausea and vomiting, abdominal pain
- Sleep disturbances
- Nervousness, tension, anxiety, panic attacks
- Ataxia

Chronic abuse
- Drowsiness
- Lack of motivation
- Clouded thinking, memory loss
- Personality, emotional change
- Disturbing dreams
- Increased risk of accidents

Key signs and symptoms of benzodiazepine overdose

- Dizziness, weakness, ataxia, hypotonia
- Altered mental status
- Slurred speech
- Blurred vision, nystagmus
- Respiratory depression
- Hallucinations
- Impaired cognition, amnesia

Key signs and symptoms of benzodiazepine withdrawal

- Similar to those of alcohol withdrawal (possibly severe, requiring hospitalization)
- Symptoms usually developing 3 to 4 days after drug stopped; possibly earlier with shorter-acting agents or later with longer-acting agents
- Symptoms lasting a few weeks or months (in some cases, up to 1 year or longer)

Diagnosing benzodiazepine abuse

- Urine drug screen
- Other blood studies and diagnostic tests to rule out possible underlying medical conditions
- Confirmed if *DSM-IV-TR* criteria met

- Clouded thinking, memory loss
- Changes in personality and emotional responses
- Anxiety, irritability, aggression
- Insomnia
- Disturbing dreams
- Nausea, increased appetite, weight gain
- Headache
- Skin rash
- Menstrual problems
- Sexual problems
- Increased risk of accidents (including falls in older adults)
- Benzodiazepine overdose
  - Dizziness, weakness, ataxia, hypotonia (reduced skeletal muscle tone)
  - Altered mental status, ranging from confusion and drowsiness to unresponsiveness or coma
  - Slurred speech
  - Blurred vision, nystagmus
  - Respiratory depression
  - Hypotension
  - Anxiety and agitation
  - Hallucinations
  - Impaired cognition, amnesia
- Benzodiazepine withdrawal
  - Similar to that of alcohol withdrawal (possibly severe, requiring hospitalization)
  - Symptoms usually developing 3 to 4 days after drug stopped; possibly earlier with shorter-acting agents or later with longer-acting agents
  - Symptoms lasting a few weeks or months (in some cases, up to 1 year or longer)

Diagnosis
- Urine drug screen to identify possible drug
- Other blood studies and diagnostic tests to rule out possible underlying medical conditions as cause of signs and symptoms
- Benzodiazepine dependence confirmed if *DSM-IV-TR* criteria met

Treatment
- Depends on which drug was taken, how much, and when
- Supportive care and monitoring, including cardiac monitoring, I.V. fluid administration, pulse oximetry, and vital signs monitoring
- Assisted ventilation for respiratory depression
- Single-dose activated charcoal (detoxification) if the patient ingested the drug within the past 4 hours; alternatively, gastric lavage (ipecac is contraindicated because of the risk of CNS depression and subsequent aspiration of emesis)
- Antidote is flumazenil (Romazicon), a GABA antagonist
  - Given I.V., reverses sedation, benzodiazepine-induced memory and psychomotor impairments, and respiratory depression
  - Usually reserved for severe poisoning because it can cause withdrawal and seizures in chronic benzodiazepine abusers (see *Drug detoxification programs*)

Drug detoxification programs

Designed to help patients achieve abstinence, drug detoxification programs offer a relatively safe alternative to self-withdrawal after prolonged dependence on alcohol or drugs. These programs, offered in outpatient centers or in special units, provide symptomatic treatment as well as counseling or psychotherapy on an individual, group, or family basis.

Be aware that deeply motivated patients with strong support systems are most likely to overcome their substance abuse.

WITHDRAWAL AND REHABILITATION

To help the patient through withdrawal, the physician gradually lowers the dosage of the abused drug or substitutes a drug with similar action. For example, he may substitute methadone for heroin, or treat cocaine addiction with bromocriptine or naltrexone. If these options aren't available, treatment is supportive and symptomatic.

Urine and blood samples are obtained for alcohol and drug screening to provide information on the most recent ingestion. Medical and psychosocial evaluations help determine appropriate treatment as well as whether it should be provided on an inpatient or outpatient basis.

After withdrawal from alcohol or drugs, the patient needs rehabilitation to prevent recurrence of abuse. Rehabilitation may include supportive counseling or individual, group, or family psychotherapy. For the drug abuser, rehabilitation may include psychotherapy.

NURSING ACTIONS

Caring for patients undergoing detoxification requires skill, compassion, and commitment.
- Because substance abusers have low self-esteem and commonly try to manipulate people, be prepared to control your natural feelings of anger and frustration.

- If the patient is undergoing opioid withdrawal, detoxify him by administering methadone as ordered.
- To ease withdrawal from opioids, depressants, and other drugs, provide nutritional support, suggest mild exercise, and teach relaxation techniques; if appropriate, administer sedatives or tranquilizers to help the patient cope with anxiety, depression, or insomnia.
- Encourage the patient's participation in rehabilitation programs and self-help groups; be alert for continued substance abuse after admission to the detoxification program; carefully administer prescribed medications to prevent hoarding by the patient, and closely monitor visitors (who might bring the patient drugs or alcohol).
- Be aware that a patient who returns to a social setting in which others are abusing drugs will probably have a relapse; encourage professional and family support after the patient leaves the detoxification program.
- Emphasize the benefits of joining an appropriate self-help group, such as Alcoholics Anonymous or Narcotics Anonymous, and recommend that the patient's spouse or mature children accompany him to group meetings.
- Stress to the patient that he ultimately must accept responsibility for avoiding abused substances.
- Refer his family to a support group, if necessary.

Treatment options for benzodiazepine abuse

- Supportive care and monitoring
- Assisted ventilation for respiratory depression
- Single-dose activated charcoal
- Antidote: flumazenil, a GABA antagonist
- Outpatient treatment or drug rehabilitation center treatment
- Prolonged recovery and rehabilitation phase

General nursing interventions for a patient undergoing detoxification

- Be prepared to control your natural feelings of anger and frustration.
- Detoxify patient by administering methadone as ordered.
- Provide nutritional support, suggest mild exercise, and teach relaxation techniques.
- Encourage patient's participation in rehabilitation programs and self-help groups.
- Encourage professional and family support after patient leaves detoxification program.
- Emphasize benefits of joining appropriate self-help group.
- Stress to patient that he ultimately must accept responsibility for avoiding abused substances.
- Refer patient's family to support group, if necessary.

Diagnosing drug overdose

- Arterial blood gas analysis
- Blood and urine screening tests

Treatment options for drug overdose

- Oxygen administration
- Intubation and mechanical ventilation
- Cardiac monitoring (12-lead ECG)
- Toxicology screening of urine, blood, and vomitus
- Possible use of restraints

Dealing with drug overdose

Whether intentional or accidental, a drug overdose is life-threatening. In very high doses, some drugs cause central nervous system (CNS) depression, ranging from lethargy to coma. Others cause CNS stimulation, ranging from euphoria to violent behavior.

Depending on the specific drug and the extent of damage, other symptoms of overdose may include hallucinations, respiratory depression, seizures, abnormal pupil size and response, or nausea and vomiting.

DIAGNOSING OVERDOSE

Arterial blood gas analysis and blood and urine screening tests help detect drug use and guide treatment.

TREATMENT

A patient with signs of respiratory depression receives oxygen, or intubation and mechanical ventilation. He's attached to a cardiac monitor, and a 12-lead electrocardiogram is taken. Urine, blood, and vomitus specimens are obtained for toxicology screening. Restraints may be applied to prevent him from harming himself or others.

EMERGENCY NURSING INTERVENTIONS

- Take appropriate steps to stop further drug absorption; if the patient ingested the drug, induce vomiting or use gastric lavage, as ordered (activated charcoal may be administered to help adsorb the substance, and a saline cathartic may be used to speed its elimination).
- Frequently reassess your patient's airway, breathing, and circulation; keep oxygen, suction equipment, and emergency airway equipment nearby; be prepared to perform cardiopulmonary resuscitation, if necessary.
- When possible, find out which drug the patient took, how much, and when. (Did he combine several drugs or take a drug along with alcohol?) Question the patient's family, friends, or rescue personnel thoroughly.
- Watch for complications.
  —Stay alert for shock, indicated by decreased blood pressure and a faint, rapid pulse; reassess respiratory rate and depth.
  —Auscultate breath sounds frequently.
  —Be aware that dyspnea and tachypnea may warn of impending respiratory complications, such as pulmonary edema or aspiration pneumonia. (A patient with crackles who's pale, diaphoretic, and gasping for air may have pulmonary edema; a patient with rhonchi or decreased breath sounds probably has aspiration pneumonia.)
- Carefully monitor heart rate and rhythm.
- Frequently assess neurologic function; the patient's neurologic status may change as his body metabolizes the drug.
- Anticipate possible hypothermia or hyperthermia; expect to use either extra blankets and a hyperthermia mattress or an antipyretic and a hypothermia mattress, as ordered.
- If the overdose was accidental, recommend a rehabilitation program for substance abuse; if it was intentional, refer the patient to crisis intervention for psychological counseling.

- Outpatient treatment or drug rehabilitation center treatment
  - Inpatient setting indicated for patients who have been using high doses of sedatives or hypnotics, have a history of withdrawal seizures or delirium tremens (also called *DTs*) or have concurrent medical illnesses
  - First step involves gradual reduction of the drug to prevent withdrawal and seizures (gradual replacement of benzodiazepine with other drug with similar actions)
  - Long-term abuser with severe withdrawal symptoms (such as elevated vital signs or delirium) should receive agent with rapid onset, in doses sufficient to suppress withdrawal symptoms (I.V. lorazepam (Ativan) or diazepam commonly given for their immediate results)
  - When stabilized, patient is switched to equivalent dose of long-acting agent (such as phenobarbital) to ease withdrawal symptoms; gradually weaned off new agent over 2 to 6 months
  - For mild withdrawal symptoms: anticonvulsants not cross-dependent with sedative-hypnotics (such as carbamazepine [Tegretol] and valproate [Depacon]) have been used successfully
- Prolonged recovery and rehabilitation phase
  - Needs social support and involvement of family and friends during this difficult stage
  - Inpatient and outpatient programs available; usually last 1 month or longer and may include individual, group, and family psychotherapy
  - During and after rehabilitation, participation in drug-oriented self-help group may be helpful

- **Nursing interventions**
  - Assess for signs and symptoms of acute intoxication (see *Dealing with drug overdose*)
  - Assist with specific treatment for intoxication or withdrawal as needed (see *General interventions for acute drug intoxication,* page 281)

NCLEX CHECKS

It's never too soon to begin your NCLEX preparation. Now that you've reviewed this chapter, carefully read each of the following questions and choose the best answer. Then compare your responses to the correct answers.

1. Which finding would the nurse expect to assess in a patient who ingests alcohol and is also taking disulfiram? Select all that apply:
- ☐ **1.** Chest pain
- ☐ **2.** Hypervolemia
- ☐ **3.** Bradycardia
- ☐ **4.** Blurred vision
- ☐ **5.** Headache
- ☐ **6.** Hypotension

2. A patient admits to taking "crystal." The nurse correctly identifies the substance as belonging to which drug group?
- ☐ **1.** Sedatives
- ☐ **2.** Stimulants
- ☐ **3.** Hallucinogens
- ☐ **4.** Antidepressants

Key nursing interventions for a patient with benzodiazepine abuse

- Assess for signs and symptoms of acute intoxication.
- Assist with specific treatment for intoxication or withdrawal as needed.

TOP 10

Items to study for your next test on substance abuse disorders

1. Terminology related to substance use and abuse
2. Types of substances commonly abused
3. Theories related to possible causes of substance abuse
4. Effects and health-related hazards for commonly abused substances
5. Major treatment methods for alcohol abuse
6. Nursing interventions for acute drug intoxication
7. Characteristics of withdrawal for commonly abused substances
8. Six major hallucinogens that are abused
9. Nursing interventions for opioid abuse: Intoxication or overdose, withdrawal, detoxification, and maintenance
10. Nursing interventions in detoxification programs

3. Which assessment finding of a patient with a substance abuse problem would most strongly suggest I.V. drug abuse?
- ☐ **1.** Skin lesions
- ☐ **2.** Gastritis
- ☐ **3.** Tachycardia
- ☐ **4.** Tachypnea

4. A patient is experiencing tachycardia induced by cocaine. The nurse would expect to administer which drug?
- ☐ **1.** Buprenorphine (Buprenex)
- ☐ **2.** Diazepam (Valium)
- ☐ **3.** Nifedipine (Procardia)
- ☐ **4.** Propranolol (Inderal)

5. A patient admits to LSD use. How long would the nurse expect the drug effects to last?
- ☐ **1.** 2 to 4 hours
- ☐ **2.** 4 to 6 hours
- ☐ **3.** 6 to 12 hours
- ☐ **4.** 14 to 18 hours

6. A patient who overdosed on codeine is admitted to the emergency department. The nurse would expect the physician to order which agent to reverse the effects of the overdose?
- ☐ **1.** Disulfiram (Antabuse)
- ☐ **2.** Naloxone (Narcan)
- ☐ **3.** Diazepam (Valium)
- ☐ **4.** Bupropion (Wellbutrin)

7. A patient is experiencing moderate alcohol withdrawal. Which finding would the nurse expect to assess?
- ☐ **1.** Marked confusion and disorientation
- ☐ **2.** Restlessness
- ☐ **3.** Slight sweating
- ☐ **4.** Vague transient hallucinations

8. The community nurse teaches a group of students about common sources of caffeine. The nurse knows that further teaching is needed when the group includes which product as a source of caffeine in a list they're compiling?
- ☐ **1.** Iced tea
- ☐ **2.** Cola
- ☐ **3.** Excedrin
- ☐ **4.** Whole milk

9. A patient is prescribed physostigmine (Eserine) as treatment for a drug overdose. The nurse understands that this drug is used to treat overdose of which agent?
- ☐ **1.** Heroin
- ☐ **2.** PCP
- ☐ **3.** Cannabis
- ☐ **4.** LSD

10. Which findings are signs and symptoms of severe alcohol withdrawal? Select all that apply:

- ☐ **1.** Restless sleep
- ☐ **2.** Dry heaves
- ☐ **3.** Total wakefulness
- ☐ **4.** Marked anorexia
- ☐ **5.** Elevated diastolic and systolic blood pressures
- ☐ **6.** Marked hyperhidrosis

ANSWERS AND RATIONALES

1. CORRECT ANSWER: 1, 3, 4, 5, 6

A patient who consumes alcohol up to 2 weeks after taking disulfiram will experience a reaction that includes shortness of breath, chest pain, nausea, vomiting, facial flushing, headache, red eyes, blurred vision, sweating, tachycardia, hypotension, and fainting.

2. CORRECT ANSWER: 2

"Crystal" is a street name for methamphetamine, a stimulant. Other amphetamines include amphetamine sulfate and dextroamphetamine. Benzodiazepines are examples of sedatives. LSD, Ecstasy, and ketamine are examples of hallucinogens. Examples of antidepressants include amitriptyline and fluoxetine.

3. CORRECT ANSWER: 1

A patient who abuses I.V. drugs is likely to have visible needle marks or tracks, skin lesions or abscesses, soft-tissue infection, and thrombosed veins. Gastritis, tachycardia, and tachypnea aren't specifically found in I.V. drug use.

4. CORRECT ANSWER: 4

Propranolol is typically given to treat tachycardia caused by cocaine use. Buprenorphine would be used to treat withdrawal symptoms associated with opioid use. Diazepam is typically administered to treat seizures associated with drug use. Nifedipine or nitroprusside would be used to treat severe hypertension or tachycardia associated with hallucinogens.

5. CORRECT ANSWER: 3

The duration of effect of LSD and most other hallucinogens is 6 to 12 hours.

6. CORRECT ANSWER: 2

Naloxone is an opioid antagonist that displaces previously administered opioid analgesics from CNS receptors; it's used to treat opioid overdose. Disulfiram is used to prevent compulsive drinking of alcohol. Diazepam is a benzodiazepine used to treat seizures associated with drug use. Bupropion is used for smoking cessation.

7. CORRECT ANSWER: 4

With moderate alcohol withdrawal, the patient typically experiences vague transient visual and auditory hallucinations and illusions, variable levels of confusion, marked insomnia and nightmares, and obvious sweating. Marked confusion and disorientation is characteristic of severe alcohol withdrawal. Restlessness and slight sweating are associated with mild withdrawal.

8. CORRECT ANSWER: 4

Whole milk isn't a source of caffeine; however, chocolate milk is. Iced tea, cola, and Excedrin are all sources of caffeine.

9. CORRECT ANSWER: 2

Physostigmine is an anticholinesterase inhibitor used to reverse the CNS toxicity associated with PCP overdose. Naloxone would be used to treat heroin (an opioid) overdose. Cannabis intoxication may require the use of benzodiazepines, but it usually resolves in 4 to 6 hours. Drug treatment for LSD is symptomatic and supportive.

10. CORRECT ANSWER: 2, 3, 5, 6

Total wakefulness, dry heaves, elevated systolic and diastolic blood pressure, and marked hyperhidrosis are all associated with severe alcohol withdrawal.

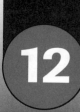

12

Sexual disorders

LEARNING OBJECTIVES

After studying this chapter, you should be able to:

- Identify the components of sexual identity.
- Describe the stages of sexual development.
- Explain the phases of the sexual response cycle.
- List the categories of sexual disorders.
- Define the various types of sexual disorders.
- Discuss the causes, diagnosis, and treatment of sexual disorders.
- Describe common nursing interventions for patients with sexual disorders.

CHAPTER OVERVIEW

A sexual disorder can cause distress and anxiety as well as strife in intimate relationships. Such disorders range from organic (physical) dysfunctions to problems with the psychological and behavioral aspects of sexual identity, arousal, and gratification.

UNDERSTANDING SEXUAL DISORDERS

● General information

- Sexuality is expressed not just in a person's appearance but also in his attitude, behaviors, and relationships
  - Influenced by ongoing biophysical and psychosocial factors
  - Starts to take shape during early childhood and is reshaped throughout life

● Sexual identity

- Sexual identity encompasses four components: biosexual identity, gender role, gender identity, and sexual orientation or preference
- Biosexual identity is the physical state of being either male or female, resulting from genetic and hormonal influences
- Gender role is the outward expression of one's own gender
  - Includes behaviors, feelings, and attitudes appropriate for either a male or female
  - Labels include "masculine" or "feminine," "traditional" or "conforming," and "gender-neutral"
  - Learned by the individual and influenced by culture, religion, schools, peers, and social messages
- Gender identity is a person's private experience of gender — the sense of being male, female, or ambivalent — and is usually based on physical features, parental attitudes and expectations, and psychological and social pressures
  - Biological theory: develops in utero and contributes to the fetus's anatomic development
  - Psychodynamic theory: evolves from role modeling, during which the child learns to identify with the same-sex parent
  - Social learning theory: learned and reinforced by the environment and social expectations
  - Cognitive theory: child can mentally construct male or female behavior and can tell these behaviors apart
- Sexual orientation or preference refers to a person's feelings about his or her sexual attraction and erotic potential
  - Heterosexuality: marked by sexual arousal from or sexual activity with people of the opposite sex
  - Homosexuality: refers to sexual arousal from or sexual activity with people of the same sex
  - Bisexuality: characterized by sexual arousal from or sexual activity with both sexes

● Abnormal sexual behavior

- The definition of "abnormal" sexual behavior depends largely on cultural and historical context
- Accepted norms of sexual behavior and attitudes vary greatly within and among different cultures
  - Historical belief that the only "normal" sexual behavior was intercourse between heterosexual partners for purpose of procreation

---

Key facts about sexual identity

- Four components: biosexual identity, gender role, gender identity, and sexual orientation or preference
- Biosexual identity: the physical state of being either male or female
- Gender role: the outward expression of one's own gender
- Gender identity: a person's private experience of gender; usually based on physical features, parental attitudes and expectations, and psychological and social pressures
- Sexual orientation or preference: a person's feelings about his or her sexual attraction and erotic potential

Key facts about abnormal sexual behavior

- The definition of "abnormal" sexual behavior depends largely on cultural and historical context
- Accepted norms of sexual behavior and attitudes vary greatly within and among different cultures

- Masturbation once widely seen as a perversion and a potential cause of mental disorders
- Until 1970s, homosexuality officially described as abnormal by psychiatrists and mental health professionals
- Currently, a much broader range of attitudes toward sexuality exists
  - Homosexuality now widely regarded as a normal variant of sexuality
  - Masturbation accepted as a normal sexual activity
- Some authorities classify abnormal sexual behavior as any behavior that causes personal distress; others view sexuality on a continuum from adaptive to maladaptive
  - Normal sexuality as adaptive
  - Abnormal sexuality as maladaptive
- Sexual disorders are described in the *Diagnostic and Statistical Manual of Mental Disorders*, Fourth Edition, Text Revision *(DSM-IV-TR)*
  - Paraphilias: group of complex psychosexual disorders, including exhibitionism and fetishism
  - Sexual dysfunctions: include such disorders as orgasmic disorder and premature ejaculation
  - Sexual pain disorders: include sexual dysfunction disorders such as dyspareunia
  - Gender identity disorder: characterized by marked discomfort with one's apparent or assigned gender

● Sexual dysfunctions

- Sexual dysfunctions are characterized by pain during sex or by a disturbance in one of the phases of the sexual response cycle
  - May cause marked distress and interpersonal problems
  - Can impair intimate relationships by reducing the enjoyment of normal sex or preventing the normal physiologic changes of the sexual response cycle
- In some people, a sexual dysfunction is present at the onset of sexual functioning and activity; in others, it follows a period of normal sexual functioning
- Sexual dysfunctions are commonly linked to psychological factors, medical conditions, substance use, or a combination of these factors
- Sexual dysfunctions fall into several categories (See *Types of sexual dysfunction,* page 326)
  - Sexual arousal disorders
  - Sexual desire disorders
  - Orgasmic disorders
  - Sexual pain disorders (see *Sexual pain disorders,* page 327)
  - Sexual dysfunction caused by a medical condition
- Sexual dysfunction may be generalized (occurs with all types of stimulation, situations, and partners) or situational (limited to certain types of stimulation, situations, or partners)
- The prognosis is good for temporary or mild sexual dysfunctions stemming from misinformation or situational stress and is guarded for dysfunctions that result from intense anxiety, chronically discordant relationships, psychological disturbances, or drug or alcohol abuse in either partner

(Text continues on page 328.)

Types of sexual disorders

- Paraphilias
- Sexual dysfunctions
- Sexual pain disorders
- Gender identity disorder

Categories of sexual dysfunction

- Sexual arousal disorders
- Sexual desire disorders
- Orgasmic disorders
- Sexual pain disorders

Classifying sexual dysfunction

- Sexual desire disorders: hypoactive sexual desire disorder, sexual aversion disorder
- Sexual arousal disorders: female sexual arousal disorder, male erectile disorder
- Orgasmic disorders: female orgasmic disorder, male orgasmic disorder, premature ejaculation
- Sexual dysfunction due to general medical condition
- Sexual pain disorders: dyspareunia, vaginismus

Types of sexual dysfunction

The *Diagnostic and Statistical Manual of Mental Disorders,* Fourth Edition, Text Revision, classifies sexual dysfunction (other than paraphilias and gender identity disorder) as described here.

SEXUAL DESIRE DISORDERS: HYPOACTIVE SEXUAL DESIRE DISORDER, SEXUAL AVERSION DISORDER

The key feature of hypoactive sexual desire disorder is a deficiency or absence of sexual fantasies or desire for sexual activity. The patient rarely initiates sexual activity but may engage in it reluctantly when the partner initiates it.

With sexual aversion disorder, the patient dislikes and avoids genital sexual contact with a sexual partner.

SEXUAL AROUSAL DISORDERS: FEMALE SEXUAL AROUSAL DISORDER, MALE ERECTILE DISORDER

With female sexual arousal disorder, the patient has a persistent or recurrent inability to attain or maintain (through the completion of sexual activity) an adequate lubrication-swelling response of sexual excitement.

With male erectile disorder, the patient has a persistent or recurrent inability to attain or maintain (through the completion of sexual activity) an adequate erection.

ORGASMIC DISORDERS: FEMALE ORGASMIC DISORDER, MALE ORGASMIC DISORDER, PREMATURE EJACULATION

With male and female orgasmic disorders, the patient experiences a persistent or recurrent delay in, or absence of, orgasm following a normal sexual excitement phase.

Premature ejaculation refers to a persistent and recurrent onset of orgasm and ejaculation with minimal sexual stimulation.

SEXUAL DYSFUNCTION DUE TO A GENERAL MEDICAL CONDITION

With sexual dysfunction due to a general medical condition, the patient's sexual dysfunction is fully explained by the direct physiologic effects of a general medical condition. This category includes sexual dysfunction caused by substance use (including alcohol, prescription drugs, and street drugs).

SEXUAL PAIN DISORDERS: DYSPAREUNIA, VAGINISMUS

The essential feature of dyspareunia is genital pain associated with sexual intercourse. Vaginismus refers to a recurrent or persistent involuntary contraction of the perineal muscles surrounding the outer third of the vagina when vaginal penetration is attempted. With some patients, even the anticipation of vaginal insertion may result in muscle spasm.

Sexual pain disorders

The two main types of sexual pain disorders are dyspareunia and vaginismus.

DYSPAREUNIA

With dyspareunia, which can occur in both males and females, unexplained genital pain occurs before, during, or after intercourse. The condition may be mild or may be severe enough to restrict the enjoyment of sex.

Causes

Physical conditions that can cause dyspareunia include:
- acute or chronic infections of the genitourinary tract
- allergic reactions (as from diaphragms, condoms, or other contraceptives)
- benign or malignant reproductive system growths or tumors
- deformities or lesions of the vagina or its opening
- disorders of the surrounding viscera (including the residual effects of pelvic inflammatory disease and disease of the adnexal and broad ligaments)
- endometriosis
- genital, rectal, or pelvic scar tissue
- insufficient lubrication (as from medications, estrogen loss, or radiation to the genital area)
- intact hymen
- local trauma (such as hymenal tears or bruising of the urethral meatus)
- retroversion of the uterus.

    Psychological causes of dyspareunia include a history of sexual abuse and problems in intimate relationships.

Treatment

When dyspareunia has a physical cause, treatment may include:
- creams and water-soluble jellies for inadequate lubrication
- medications for infections
- excision of hymenal scars

- gentle stretching of painful scars at the vaginal opening
- change in coital position to reduce pain on deep penetration.

    When the condition has a psychological cause, interventions may include psychotherapy or sensate focus exercises.

VAGINISMUS

With vaginismus, involuntary spasmodic muscle contractions occur at the entrance to the vagina when the male tries to insert his penis. Pain occurs if intercourse is attempted despite these contractions.

    This condition makes intercourse extremely painful or impossible. However, women with vaginismus are capable of becoming sexually aroused and achieving lubrication and orgasm through clitoral or other, alternative forms of stimulation.

    Vaginismus can be primary or secondary. With primary vaginismus, the patient has never been able to have intercourse with penetration (resulting, for example, in an unconsummated marriage). In secondary vaginismus, the patient previously experienced normal intercourse before developing the condition.

Causes

Most experts believe vaginismus is a learned response, commonly stemming from dyspareunia. Women who have had frightening, unsatisfying, or painful sexual experiences may fear that penetration and intercourse will cause pain. A strict cultural or religious background can have the same effect. This fear and anticipation of pain may lead to a pattern of sexual anxiety, causing vaginal dryness and tightness before intercourse.

(continued)

Key facts about dyspareunia

Causes
- Acute or chronic infections
- Allergic reactions
- Benign or malignant reproductive system growths or tumors
- Deformities or lesions of vagina or its opening
- Disorders of surrounding viscera
- Endometriosis
- Genital, rectal, or pelvic scar tissue
- Insufficient lubrication
- Intact hymen
- Local trauma
- History of sexual abuse or intimacy problems

Treatment
- Creams and water-soluble jellies
- Medications for infections
- Excision of hymenal scars
- Gentle stretching of scars at vaginal opening
- Change in coital position
- Psychotherapy, sensate focus exercises

Key facts about vaginismus

Causes
- Fear and anticipation of pain, leading to pattern of sexual anxiety resulting in vaginal dryness and tightness
- Fear of pregnancy, of being controlled by a man, or of losing control
- Vaginal infection
- Physical aftereffects of childbirth
- Fatigue

Key facts about vaginismus

Treatment
- Couples therapy
- Kegel exercises
- Sensate focus exercises
- Progressive use of plastic dilator or finger
- Medications for infection
- Comfort measures for childbirth and related effects
- Rest

Key facts about sexual development

Infancy to age 5
- Combination of mother's X chromosome and father's X or Y chromosome creates either male or female child
- Gender assignment is reinforced by family members' interactions with infant
- Children start to observe body differences and show an interest in bathroom habits
- By age 2, most have a clear sense of their gender identity
- Sexual discovery starts between ages 3 and 5
- Toward end of this stage, children pick up cues from others that sex is a "different" topic

Sexual pain disorders *(continued)*

Other psychological factors that may cause or contribute to vaginismus include fears of pregnancy, of being controlled by a man, or of losing control.

Physical causes of vaginismus include vaginal infection, physical after-effects of childbirth, and fatigue.

Treatment
Treatment for vaginismus stemming from psychological causes may include a combination of:
- couples therapy
- Kegel exercises to strengthen the pubococcygeal muscle
- sensate focus exercises for the couple
- progressive use of a plastic dilator or finger, which is inserted into the vaginal opening to progressively stretch the contracted muscles.

When treated by a professional using these or similar techniques, vaginismus has a cure rate of about 80% to 100%.

Treatment for vaginismus stemming from a physical cause may include pharmacotherapy for infection, comfort measures for childbirth-related effects, and rest.

STAGES OF SEXUAL DEVELOPMENT

● **General information**
- Beginning in infancy, humans progress through various phases of sexual and psychosexual development
- Characteristic physical attributes and feelings related to sex develop during each phase
- Crucial factors affecting sexual development include early role models, religious and cultural teachings, early sexual experiences, and parental attitudes toward sex
  - Parent's puritanical rejection of sexuality can produce guilt and shame in a child, subsequently inhibiting capacity to enjoy sex and develop healthy relationships as adult
  - Child treated with cruelty, hostility, or rejection may become sexually maladjusted

● **Infancy to age 5**
- The combination of the mother's X chromosome and the father's X or Y chromosome creates either a male or a female child
- Gender assignment of a healthy infant is reinforced by family members' interactions with the infant, which influence and reinforce either masculine or feminine behavior
- Between ages 1 and 3, children start to observe body differences and show an interest in bathroom habits
- By age 2, most children have a clear sense of their gender identity
- Sexual discovery starts between ages 3 and 5, when curious and explorative young children commonly ask where babies come from and what their sex organs are for
  - Are accepting and straightforward about sex and may comment on the differences between genders

– Learn that touching feels good

– Also may receive nonverbal messages about sex

- Toward the end of this stage, children pick up cues from others that sex is a "different" topic; they may become shy, ask fewer questions about sex, and show a desire for privacy related to their bodies

● **Ages 5 to 10**

- Children in this age-group may think in terms of "good" and "bad" parts of their bodies
- They're aware of bodily functions and how these relate to sex, and are same-sex oriented
- Outwardly, they may seem unconcerned about sex or uncomfortable or apprehensive about discussing it; however, they're actually quite interested in it
- Children receive verbal or nonverbal cues from the adults around them that they shouldn't talk about sex, so they may avoid the topic
  - Commonly exchange information about sex with peers
  - Masturbation and sexual exploration common at this stage

● **Ages 10 to 14**

- Puberty begins at about age 11 for girls and age 12 for boys
- Young adolescents may be confused, embarrassed, and self-conscious about their bodily changes and may be uncomfortable with, or unaware of, their social roles as they relate to their respective genders
- Sexual responsiveness develops during this stage, as does the ability to reproduce
- Some young adolescents become sexually active in response to peer pressure and other influences

● **Age 14 and older**

- From age 14 on, children become more adult—physically, emotionally, and socially
  - Easily influenced by peer pressure and media messages
  - Want to be in control of themselves and are forming their identities and self-concepts
- Approximately one-half of adolescents over age 14 are sexually active or experienced; however, they're still uncertain about sex and may perceive it as part of the "adult world"

● **Adulthood**

- By adulthood, sex and sexuality are normally part of a person's life
- An estimated 90% of adults are sexually active
- Adults hold views on sexuality that have been influenced by society and its standards of normal behavior; familial attitudes and cultural or religious beliefs also may have a strong influence

HUMAN SEXUAL RESPONSE CYCLE

● **General information**

- The sexual response cycle refers to the progressive mental, physical, and emotional changes that occur during sexual stimulation
- Sexual response is highly individualized; nearly everyone experiences certain basic physiologic changes

---

Key facts about sexual development

Ages 5 to 10

- Children may think in terms of "good" and "bad" parts of their bodies
- Are aware of bodily functions and how these relate to sex, and are same-sex oriented
- Outwardly, may seem unconcerned about sex or uncomfortable or apprehensive about discussing it
- Masturbation and sexual exploration common at this stage

Ages 10 to 14

- Puberty begins at about age 11 for girls and age 12 for boys
- May be confused, embarrassed, and self-conscious about their bodily changes
- Sexual responsiveness and ability to reproduce develop during this stage

14 to adulthood

- Children become more adult—physically, emotionally, and socially
- Easily influenced by peer pressure and media messages
- Want to be in control of themselves

Adulthood

- Sex and sexuality are normally part of a person's life
- Adults hold views on sexuality that have been influenced by society and its standards of normal behavior
- Familial attitudes and cultural or religious beliefs also may have strong influence on sexual views

5 phases of the sexual response cycle

- Desire phase: marked by strong urge for sexual stimulation and satisfaction, either by oneself or with another person
- Excitement phase or arousal phase: prepares both partners for intercourse
- Plateau phase: may be reached with continued stimulation during full arousal
- Orgasm phase: peak of sexual excitement
- Resolution phase: the body returns to its normal, unexcited state

● Phases of the sexual response cycle

- Different researchers have proposed various models of the sexual response cycle, describing three to five distinct phases; currently, many experts recognize a five-phase cycle that begins with desire
- The *desire phase* is marked by a strong urge for sexual stimulation and satisfaction, either by oneself or with another person
  - Range of stimulation that provokes sexual desire: affected by cultural and societal values
  - Behaviors meant to communicate sexual desire: may vary greatly along gender lines (in some cultures, disapproval of women's overt expression of sexual desire, while expecting such communication from men)
  - Potential sexual partners may communicate desire verbally; also may communicate through behavior and body language (for example, flirting), which may be subtle and easily misread
  - Desire is mental, not physical; without further mental or physical stimulation, desire phase may not progress to sexual excitement
  - Desire isn't necessary for sex to occur (such as couple trying to conceive a child by having intercourse even on days when they lack sexual desire); response to partner's advances possible even if recipient lacks initial desire
- The *excitement phase* or *arousal phase* prepares both partners for intercourse
  - Muscle tension increases, heart rate quickens, skin becomes flushed or blotchy (called *sexual flush*), and nipples grow hard or erect; vasoconstriction begins during this phase
  - In the female, clitoris, vagina, and labia minora swell; vaginal walls start to produce lubricating fluid; uterus and breasts enlarge; and the pubococcygeal muscle surrounding the vaginal opening tightens
  - In the male, penis becomes erect, testes become elevated and swollen, scrotal sac tightens, and Cowper's glands secrete lubricating fluid
- The *plateau phase* may be reached with continued stimulation (especially stroking and rubbing of the erogenous zones or sexual intercourse) during full arousal
  - Person may achieve, lose, and regain a plateau several times without orgasm occurring
  - Heart and respiratory rates and blood pressure rise further; sexual flush deepens, muscle tension increases
  - Person has sense of impending orgasm
    - Female: clitoris withdraws, vaginal lubrication increases, the labia continue to swell, the areolae enlarge, and the lower vagina narrows and tightens
    - Male: ridge of the glans penis becomes more prominent, Cowper's glands secrete pre-ejaculatory fluid, and the testes rise closer to the body
- The *orgasm phase* is the peak of sexual excitement
  - Shortest phase of the sexual response cycle, typically lasting just a few seconds (maybe slightly longer in women)
  - Physiologic changes: involuntary muscle contractions; elevated heart rate and blood pressure; rapid oxygen intake; sphincter muscle contraction; and sudden, forceful release of sexual tension
  - Male: orgasm usually climaxes with ejaculation of semen

– Female: orgasm involves rhythmic muscle contractions of the uterus; contractions put pressure on penis and promote male orgasm
– Intensely pleasurable for males and females unless sexual dysfunction is present
- During the *resolution phase*, the body returns to its normal, unexcited state; some changes occur rapidly, whereas others tend to take longer
  – Heart and respiratory rates slow; blood pressure decreases; muscle tone slackens
  – Swollen and erect body parts return to normal; skin flushing disappears
  – Phase marked by a general sense of well-being and enhanced intimacy
  – For male, resolution phase includes a refractory period (can't reach orgasm but may be able to maintain partial or full erection)
    · Lasts a few minutes to several days
    · Depends on such factors as age and frequency of sexual activity
  – For female, can return rapidly to orgasmic phase with minimal stimulation (may experience continued orgasms for up to 1 hour)

PARAPHILIAS

● **Defining characteristics**
- Paraphilias are complex psychosexual disorders marked by sexual urges, fantasies, or behaviors that center on inanimate objects (such as clothing); suffering or humiliation; or children or other nonconsenting persons
- Paraphilias involve an attraction to a nonsanctioned source of sexual satisfaction
  – Source may be a behavior, as with exhibitionism or sadism
  – Source may be a forbidden object of attraction, as with pedophilia or fetishism
- Paraphilias commonly involve sexual arousal and orgasm, usually achieved through masturbation and fantasy
  – Paraphiliac urge, fantasy, or behavior always present, although frequency and intensity may vary
  – Usually chronic and lifelong, although it may diminish with age
  – May worsen during times of increased psychological stress, when other mental disorders are present, or when opportunities to engage in paraphilia become more available
- *DSM-IV-TR* identifies eight specific paraphilias, three of the most commonly treated include exhibitionism, fetishism, and pedophilia (see *Five other paraphilias*, page 333)
- Certain unusual psychosexual behaviors are similar to paraphilias but aren't officially designated as such by the *DSM-IV-TR*
  – Compulsive masturbation: masturbation is the primary sexual outlet, even if the person has a stable, intimate relationship
  – Protracted promiscuity: pattern of repeated sexual conquests in which the person can't maintain a monogamous relationship despite a desire to do so
  – Pornography dependency: repetitive pattern involving use of pornographic materials, such as magazines, videos, and pornographic Web sites
  – Use of telephone sex: dependence on discussing sex over the telephone to achieve arousal

Characteristics of paraphilias
- Marked by sexual urges, fantasies, or behaviors that center on inanimate objects, suffering or humiliation, or children or other nonconsenting persons
- Involve an attraction to nonsanctioned source of sexual satisfaction
- Commonly involve sexual arousal and orgasm, usually achieved through masturbation and fantasy
- *DSM-IV-TR* identifies eight paraphilias
- Certain unusual psychosexual behaviors are similar to paraphilias but aren't officially designated as such by *DSM-IV-TR*

Psychosocial behaviors that resemble paraphilias
- Compulsive masturbation
- Protracted promiscuity
- Pornography dependency
- Use of telephone sex
- Severe sexual desire
- Use of sexual accessories

3 common types of paraphilias

- Exhibitionism
- Fetishism
- Pedophilia

Key facts about exhibitionism

- One of the most common paraphilias
- Most prominent sexual offense leading to arrest
- Accounts for approximately one-third of sexual crimes
- Marked by sexual fantasies, urges, or behaviors involving unexpected, unsolicited exposure of male genitals to strangers — primarily female passersby in public places
- Usually limited to genital exposure, with no harmful advances or assaults

Key facts about fetishism

- Marked by sexual fantasies, urges, or behaviors that involve use of a fetish to produce or enhance sexual arousal
- May involve a partner
- Can take one of two forms
- First form: involves partner and associates sexual activity with some object; relatively harmless if action is taken playfully and partner accepts it
- Second form (more extreme): person achieves orgasm when alone and fondling nonliving object, which completely replaces human partner

- Severe sexual desire: excessive sexual demands that burden the partner and interfere with intimate relationships
- Use of sexual accessories: repetitive use of sex "toys" or, in some cases, drugs for sexual arousal
- Some experts believe paraphilias are relatively rare; large commercial markets in paraphiliac pornography and paraphernalia suggest otherwise
  - In clinics specializing in paraphilia treatment, most commonly seen disorders include pedophilia, voyeurism, and exhibitionism (sexual masochism and sexual sadism much less common)
  - Majority of paraphiliacs are males; sexual masochists are exception (females outnumber males by 20 to 1)
- Some paraphilias are crimes in many jurisdictions
  - Those that involve or harm another person — particularly pedophilia, exhibitionism, voyeurism, frotteurism, and sexual sadism — commonly considered criminal acts, leading to arrest and possible incarceration
  - Exhibitionists, pedophiles, and voyeurs make up majority of apprehended sex offenders
  - Sex offenses against children, as in pedophilia, constitute significant portion of reported criminal sex acts

● Exhibitionism

- One of the most common paraphilias, exhibitionism is the most prominent sexual offense leading to arrest; it accounts for approximately one-third of sexual crimes
- Marked by sexual fantasies, urges, or behaviors involving unexpected, unsolicited exposure of male genitals to strangers — primarily female passersby in public places
- Usually limited to genital exposure, with no harmful advances or assaults (considered more of a nuisance than an actual danger)
- It has three characteristic features
  - Typically performed by men in presence of women with whom they're unacquainted
  - Occurs in places where sexual intercourse is impossible such as crowded shopping malls
  - Meant to be shocking; otherwise, loses its power to produce sexual arousal in the paraphiliac
- Usually begins during adolescence and continues into adulthood; commonly becomes less severe by about age 40 but can be a lifelong problem if untreated

● Fetishism

- Fetishism is characterized by sexual fantasies, urges, or behaviors that involve the use of a fetish (inanimate object or nonsexual part of the body) to produce or enhance sexual arousal
- It may involve a partner
- Sometimes it focuses on certain parts of the body, such as the feet, hair, or ears
- In some cases, the person can achieve sexual gratification only when using the fetish
- It usually begins during adolescence and persists into adulthood

Five other paraphilias

In addition to the three paraphilias described in this section, the *Diagnostic and Statistical Manual of Mental Disorders,* Fourth Edition, Text Revision (*DSM-IV-TR*), provides diagnostic criteria for five other paraphilias — frotteurism, sexual masochism, sexual sadism, voyeurism, and transvestic fetishism.

FROTTEURISM

A person with *frotteurism* becomes sexually aroused from touching or rubbing against a nonconsenting person. For example, he may rub his genitals against a woman's thigh or fondle her breasts. The behavior commonly occurs in crowded places, where it's easier to avoid detection. Frotteurism is most common between ages 15 and 25.

SEXUAL MASOCHISM

With *sexual masochism,* a person gets sexual gratification from being physically or emotionally abused. The term *masochism* comes from Leopold von Sacher-Masoch, a 19th-century writer whose novels describe a man who becomes a slave to a woman and encourages her to treat him in progressively more degrading ways.

Infantilism, another form of sexual masochism, is a desire to be treated as a helpless infant, including wearing diapers.

One dangerous form of sexual masochism, called *sexual hypoxyphilia*, relies on oxygen deprivation to induce sexual arousal. The person uses a noose, mask, plastic bag, or chemical to temporarily decrease brain oxygenation. Equipment malfunction or other mistakes can cause accidental death.

SEXUAL SADISM

With *sexual sadism*, a person achieves sexual gratification by inflicting pain, cruelty, or emotional abuse on others. The term dates back to 18th-century French writer and libertine Donatien Alphonse François. Known as the *Marquis de Sade,* he engaged in violent and scandalous behavior and published erotic writings.

The sexual sadist may verbally humiliate his partner and abuse her physically through torture, whipping, cutting, binding, beating, burning, stabbing, or rape.

Both sadism and masochism may start in adolescence or early adulthood. The behaviors are chronic and usually grow more severe over time.

VOYEURISM

The *voyeur* derives sexual pleasure from looking at sexual objects or sexually arousing situations such as an unsuspecting couple engaged in sex. He may experience an orgasm during the voyeuristic activity or later (in response to the memory of what he witnessed).

The onset of voyeurism occurs before age 15. The disorder tends to be chronic.

TRANSVESTIC FETISHISM

Seen only in heterosexual men, *transvestic fetishism* involves a person cross-dressing into women's clothing and becoming sexually aroused and gratified by imagining himself as a woman.

The man views women's garments as symbols of femininity and may choose to wear the garments under his male attire or to dress entirely as a female, fully attired in women's clothing and make-up.

A favorite article of clothing may be used during masturbation or intercourse.

Key facts about pedophilia

- Marked by sexual fantasies, urges, or activities involving child, usually age 13 or younger
- When pedophile is an adolescent, child is usually at least 5 years younger than he is
- Person is almost always a man, is erotically aroused by children, and seeks sexual gratification with them
- Some are also attracted to adults
- Urge is his preferred or exclusive sexual activity
- Prepubertal children are the most the common targets

Common causes of paraphilias

- Specific cause unknown
- Behavioral, psychoanalytical, biological, and learning theories
- Closed head injury
- CNS tumors
- Lack of knowledge about sex
- Neuroendocrine disorders
- Psychosocial stressors

- It can take one of two forms
  - First form: involves partner and associates sexual activity with some object such as a woman's panties; relatively harmless if the action is taken playfully and the partner accepts it
  - Second form (more extreme): person achieves orgasm when alone and fondling nonliving object, which completely replaces human partner; object may be underwear, boots, shoes, or a sumptuous fabric, such as velvet or silk

● **Pedophilia**
- Pedophilia is marked by sexual fantasies, urges, or activities involving a child, usually age 13 or younger (when the pedophile is an adolescent, the child is usually at least 5 years younger than he is)
- Person is almost always a man, is erotically aroused by children, and seeks sexual gratification with them
- Urge is his preferred or exclusive sexual activity, although some pedophiles are also attracted to adults
- During sexual activity, the person may undress the child, touch or fondle the child's genitals, encourage child to watch him masturbate, or forcefully perform sexual acts on the child
- Prepubertal children are the most common targets
  - Attraction to girls almost twice as common as attraction to boys
  - May sexually abuse own children or those of a friend or relative
- Many pedophiliacs probably never come to attention of authorities
  - Violent behavior by relatively few
  - Kidnapping or murdering victims even more rare; when done, probably to prevent victim from reporting predatory behavior
- More typically, the pedophile behaves seductively, showering the child with money, gifts, drugs, or alcohol
- He may be quite attentive to the child's needs to gain loyalty and prevent the child from reporting the encounters

● **Causes (all paraphilias)**
- Specific cause unknown
- Behavioral, psychoanalytical, biological, and learning theories
  - Behavioral models: child who was the victim or observer of inappropriate sexual behaviors learns to imitate such behavior and later gains reinforcement for it
  - Biological models: relationship among hormones, behavior, and the central nervous system (CNS) — especially the role of aggression and male sex hormones
- Other contributing factors
  - Closed head injury
  - CNS tumors
  - Lack of knowledge about sex
  - Neuroendocrine disorders
  - Psychosocial stressors

Risk factors

- Dysfunctional family life marked by isolation and sexual, emotional, or physical abuse
- Concurrent mental disorders, such as psychoactive substance use or personality disorders

Signs and symptoms

- History revealing particular pattern of abnormal sexual fantasies, urges, or behaviors associated with one of the eight recognized paraphilias
- Anxiety
- Depression
- Development of a hobby or an occupation change that makes the paraphilia more accessible
- Disturbance in body image
- Guilt or shame
- Ineffective coping
- Multiple paraphilias at same time
- Purchase of books, videos, or magazines related to the paraphilia or frequent visits to paraphilia-related Web sites
- Recurrent fantasies involving a paraphilia
- Sexual dysfunction
- Social isolation
- Troubled social or sexual relationships

Diagnosis

- Penile plethysmography (may be used to measure patient's sexual arousal in response to visual imagery; results can be unreliable)
- Diagnosis confirmed if *DSM-IV-TR* criteria met

Treatment

- Help seldom sought because of guilt, shame, and fear of social ostracism and legal problems
  - Usually sought only at behest of family or when forced by legal authorities
  - Treatment mandatory if sexual behavior is harmful to others
- Depending on the specific paraphilia, may involve a combination of psychotherapy, cognitive therapy, behavioral therapy, pharmacotherapy, and surgery
- Aversive stimuli (bad odors or electric shocks when engaging in the paraphiliac behavior) in behavioral therapy
- Teaching alternatives to the forbidden behaviors
- Effectiveness varies; in most cases, long-term treatment needed
- Social skills training for some patients with paraphilias (especially pedophilia) because of deficient social skills; effective social skills are needed to obtain sexual satisfaction with consenting adults
- Multifaceted for paraphiliacs who are sex offenders
  - Specialized sex offender program
  - Group therapy
  - Twelve-step sexual addiction or compulsion recovery program

Key treatment options for paraphiliacs who are sex offenders

- Specialized sex offender program
- Group therapy
- Twelve-step sexual addiction or compulsion recovery program
- Structured sexual disorder process group
- Educational sessions focusing on psychological factors, victim impact, and human sexuality
- Alcohol and drug awareness programs
- Values clarification
- Independent living skills training

Pharmacologic options for treating paraphilias

- Drugs to reduce compulsive thinking associated with paraphilias
- Possibly hormones if patient experiences intrusive sexual thoughts or urges, or demonstrates frequent abnormal sexual behaviors

– Rational thinking group
– Structured sexual disorder process group
– Educational sessions focusing on psychological factors, victim impact, and human sexuality
– Therapeutically structured recreational activities, adventure-based programming, arts and crafts, and team sports
– Patient and parent participation in treatment reviews
– Alcohol and drug awareness programs
– Values clarification
– Independent living skills training

Nursing interventions for patients with sexual disorders

These general interventions are useful when caring for a patient with any sexual disorder.

ENSURE A THERAPEUTIC RELATIONSHIP

- Arrange to spend uninterrupted time with the patient; encourage him to express his feelings, and accept what he says.
- Assess the patient's sexual history to provide a baseline.
- Assess the patient's perception of the problem.
- Explain all treatments and procedures, and answer the patient's questions to allay his fears and help him regain a sense of control.
- Never say anything that would make the patient feel ashamed; his needs and feelings – not your opinions – are what matter.
- Realize that treating the patient with empathy doesn't threaten your sexuality.

PROMOTE SELF-KNOWLEDGE

- Initiate a discussion about how the need for self-esteem, respect, love, and intimacy influences a person's sexual expression; this helps the patient understand his disorder.
- Encourage the patient to identify feelings – such as pleasure, reduced anxiety, increased control, or shame – associated with his sexual behavior and fantasies.
- Help the patient distinguish between practices that are distressing because they don't conform to social norms or personal values, and those that may place him or others in emotional, medical, or legal jeopardy; doing this reinforces the need to stop behaviors that could harm himself or others.
- Encourage him to express his sexual preferences as well as his feelings about them.

INCREASE THE LEVEL OF INTERACTION

- Spend specific, non-care-related time with the patient during each shift to encourage social interaction.
- Start with one-on-one interaction and increase to group interaction when his social skills indicate he's ready; increasing social interaction gradually eases his feeling of being overwhelmed and minimizes sensory input that may renew cognitive or perceptual disturbances.
- Give positive reinforcement for appropriate and effective interactions.

– Vocational exploration
- Certain drugs may be used to reduce the compulsive thinking associated with paraphilias; occasionally, hormones are prescribed if the patient experiences intrusive sexual thoughts or urges, or demonstrates frequent abnormal sexual behaviors

● **Nursing interventions**
- Assess the patient for signs and symptoms of paraphilia
- Assist with treatments as needed (see *Nursing interventions for patients with sexual disorders*)

Key nursing interventions for a patient with a paraphilia

- Assess patient for signs and symptoms of paraphilia.
- Assist with treatments as needed.

PROMOTE PARTICIPATION IN CARE
- Encourage the patient to make decisions about his care; this helps enhance his self-esteem and increase his sense of mastery over the current situation.
- Assist the patient and his family or close friends in progressive participation in care and therapies.
- Have the patient increase his self-care performance levels gradually so he can progress at his own pace.
- Initiate or participate in multidisciplinary, patient-centered conferences to evaluate progress and plan discharge; these conferences should involve the patient and his family in a cooperative effort to individualize his care plan.

IMPROVE COPING SKILLS
- Encourage the patient to use support systems to assist with coping, thereby helping to restore psychological equilibrium and prevent crises.
- Try to identify factors that cause or exacerbate poor coping ability, such as a fear of being fired from a job.
- Help the patient look at his current situation and evaluate various coping behaviors to encourage a realistic view of the crisis.
- Urge the patient to try new coping behaviors; a patient in crisis tends to accept interventions and develop new coping behaviors more readily than at other times.

- Request feedback from the patient about behaviors that seem to work; this encourages him to evaluate the effect of these behaviors.
- Praise the patient for making decisions and performing activities (to reinforce coping behaviors).

PROVIDE REFERRALS
- Refer the patient for professional psychological counseling; if his maladaptive behavior has high crisis potential, formal counseling can help ease your frustration, increase your objectivity, and foster a collaborative approach to patient care. (As appropriate, refer the patient to a physician, nurse, psychologist, social worker, or counselor trained in sex therapy.)

OTHER ACTIONS
- Be aware that, whenever possible, a primary nurse should be assigned to the patient to ensure continuity of care and promote a therapeutic relationship.
- Initially, allow the patient to partially depend on you for self-care because he may regress to a lower developmental level during the initial crisis phase.
- If the patient poses a threat to himself and others, institute safety precautions according to facility protocol.
- Identify and reduce unnecessary environmental stimuli.

General nursing interventions for patients with sexual disorders

- Ensure therapeutic relationship.
- Promote patient's self-knowledge.
- Increase patient's level of interaction.
- Promote patient's participation in care.
- Improve patient's coping skills.
- Provide referrals.
- Be aware that a primary nurse should be assigned to patient to ensure continuity of care and therapeutic relationship.
- Initially, allow patient to partially depend on you for self-care.
- If patient is threat to self or others, institute safety precautions according to facility protocol.
- Identify and reduce unnecessary environment stimuli.

Characteristics of female sexual arousal disorder and orgasmic disorder

- Female sexual arousal disorder: inability to achieve or maintain an adequate lubrication-swelling response of sexual excitement
- Primary disorders: person has never experienced sexual arousal or orgasm
- Secondary disorders: physical, mental, or environmental condition inhibits or prevents previously normal sexual functioning

Common causes of female sexual arousal disorder and orgasmic disorder

- Depression
- Drug use
- Discordant relationships
- Gynecological factors
- Lifestyle disruptions
- Psychological factors
- Pregnancy

Key signs and symptoms of female sexual arousal disorder

- Report of limited or absent sexual desire and little or no pleasure from sexual stimulation
- Pattern of dysfunctional sexual response
- Conceptual problems during childhood and adolescence about sex, masturbation, incest, rape, sexual fantasies, and homosexual or heterosexual practices
- Poor self-esteem and body image
- Lack of vaginal lubrication
- Absence of signs of genital vasoconstriction

FEMALE SEXUAL AROUSAL DISORDER AND FEMALE ORGASMIC DISORDER

● Defining characteristics
- Female sexual arousal disorder is defined as the inability to achieve or maintain an adequate lubrication-swelling response of sexual excitement
- Female orgasmic disorder (inability to achieve orgasm) is the most common sexual dysfunction in women and one of the most severe
  - May desire sexual activity and become aroused but feels inhibited as approaches orgasm
- These disorders can be primary or secondary
  - Primary disorders: person has never experienced sexual arousal or orgasm
  - Secondary disorders: physical, mental, or environmental condition inhibits or prevents previously normal sexual functioning

● Causes
- Depression
- Drug use (such as CNS depressants, antidepressants, hormonal contraceptives, alcohol, or street drugs)
- Discordant relationships (poor communication, hostility or ambivalence toward the partner, or fear of abandonment or of asserting independence)
- Diseases (general systemic illness, endocrine or nervous system disorders, or diseases that impair muscle tone or contractility)
- Fatigue
- Gynecologic factors (chronic vaginal or pelvic infection or pain, congenital anomalies, or genital cancer, trauma, or surgery)
- Inadequate or ineffective sexual stimulation
- Lifestyle disruptions
- Psychological factors (such as stress, anxiety, anger, hostility, boredom with sex, guilt, depression, unconscious conflicts about sexuality, or fear of losing control of one's feelings or behavior)
- Pregnancy
- Religious or cultural taboos that reinforce guilt feelings about sex

● Signs and symptoms
- Female sexual arousal disorder
  - Report of limited or absent sexual desire and little or no pleasure from sexual stimulation
  - Decreased sexual desire
  - Individual or family stress or fatigue (common in many working mothers with children younger than age 5, who are too exhausted to care about sex)
  - Misinformation about sex and sexuality
  - Pattern of dysfunctional sexual response
  - Conceptual problems during childhood and adolescence about sex in general and, specifically, about masturbation, incest, rape, sexual fantasies, and homosexual or heterosexual practices
  - Concerns about contraception and reproductive ability
  - Problems in the current sexual relationship
  - Poor self-esteem and body image
  - Lack of vaginal lubrication
  - Absence of signs of genital vasoconstriction

- Female orgasmic disorder
  - Inability to achieve orgasm (either totally or under certain circumstances)

Diagnosis
- Thorough physical examination, laboratory tests, and medical history (to rule out physical causes)
- Sexual dysfunction diagnosed if *DSM-IV-TR* criteria met

Treatment
- Sexual arousal disorder
  - Can be challenging, especially if the patient has never experienced sexual pleasure
  - Patient's goal: relaxation, becoming aware of sexual feelings, and eliminating guilt and fear of rejection
  - Providing reassurance about patient's activities or offering suggestions or more intensive therapy
  - Psychotherapy or behavioral therapy
    - Psychotherapy: may consist of free association, dream analysis, and discussion of life patterns to achieve greater sexual awareness
    - Behavioral approach: attempts to correct maladaptive patterns through systematic desensitization to situations that provoke anxiety (for example, by encouraging patient to fantasize about these situations)
  - Sensate focus exercises
    - Minimize importance of intercourse and orgasm while emphasizing touching and awareness of sensual feelings over entire body (not just genital sensations)
    - Done with a partner; each takes turns giving and then receiving touch and massage
    - At first, partners instructed to give pleasure without touching the breasts or genitals
    - Person receiving pleasure places his or her hand over the giver's to show where the touch should be and what it should feel like (improves communication and teaches the couple what they can achieve rather than what they can't)
    - Later, ban against genital touching and orgasm is reduced as the couple realizes that mutual pleasure can be derived from simple touching
    - Program may also include masturbation, either alone or together
- Female orgasmic disorder
  - Patient's goal: decrease or eliminate involuntary inhibition of the orgasmic reflex
  - Experiential therapy, psychoanalysis, or behavior modification; individual therapy, marital or couples therapy, or sex therapy
  - Treating underlying disorder
  - For primary orgasmic disorder: teaching the patient self-stimulation and distraction techniques, such as focusing on fantasies, breathing patterns, and muscle contractions to relieve anxiety
    - Patient learns new behavior through exercises she does at home between sessions
    - Eventually, therapist involves patient's sexual partner in treatment sessions (although some therapists treat the couple as a unit from the beginning)

Key signs and symptoms of female orgasmic disorder
- Inability to achieve orgasm (either totally or under certain circumstances)

Diagnosing female sexual arousal disorder and orgasmic disorder
- Thorough physical examination, laboratory tests, and medical history to rule out physical causes
- Confirmed if *DSM-IV-TR* criteria met

Key treatment options for female sexual arousal disorder and orgasmic disorder

Female sexual arousal disorder
- Psychotherapy or behavioral therapy
- Sensate focus exercises

Female orgasmic disorder
- Experiential therapy, psychoanalysis, or behavior modification
- Individual therapy, marital or couples therapy, or sex therapy
- For primary orgasmic disorder: teaching patient self-stimulation and distraction techniques
- For secondary orgasmic disorder: decreasing anxiety and promoting factors necessary for patient to achieve orgasm

Key nursing interventions for a female with sexual arousal disorder or orgasmic disorder

- Assess for signs and symptoms of female sexual dysfunction.
- Assist with necessary treatment.

Characteristics of gender identity

- Gender identity: the intimate, personal feeling one has about being male or female
- Three components: self-concept, perception of an ideal partner, and external presentation of masculinity or femininity through behavior, dress, and mannerisms

Common causes of gender identity disorder

- Chromosomal anomalies
- Hormonal imbalances (particularly in utero during brain formation)
- Pathologic deficiencies in early parent-child bonding and child-rearing practices

– For secondary orgasmic disorder: decreasing anxiety and promoting the factors necessary for the patient to achieve orgasm
- Therapist communicates accepting and permissive attitude
- Therapist helps patient understand that satisfactory sexual experiences don't always require coital orgasm

● **Nursing interventions**
- Assess for signs and symptoms of female sexual dysfunction
- Assist with necessary treatment (see *Nursing interventions for patients with sexual disorders,* pages 336 and 337)

GENDER IDENTITY DISORDER

● **Defining characteristics**
- Disorder is marked by discomfort with one's apparent or assigned gender, and a strong, persistent identification with the opposite sex
- Diagnosed cases of gender identity disorder occur six times more frequently in males than in females
- Gender identity (the intimate, personal feeling one has about being male or female) includes three components: self-concept, perception of an ideal partner, and external presentation of masculinity or femininity through behavior, dress, and mannerisms
  - Patient may have a problem with one or all of these components
  - Typically behaves and presents himself as person of the opposite sex
  - Person (sometimes called a *transsexual*) wants to be like or to become the opposite sex
- Disorder shouldn't be confused with the far more common phenomenon of feeling inadequate in meeting the expectations normally associated with a particular gender
- Children with gender identity disorder, particularly boys, are likely to be rejected by their peer group; girls may not experience social difficulties until early adolescence
- It may seriously impair social and occupational functioning (because of psychopathology and problems associated with trying to live as the opposite sex)
- Anxiety and depression are common among those with this disorder; may lead to suicide attempts
- With or without treatment, females with gender identity disorder have shown more stable adjustment patterns than males have
- It usually arises during childhood; onset after marriage may significantly disrupt the marital (and parental) relationship

● **Causes**
- Combination of predisposing factors
  - Chromosomal anomalies
  - Hormonal imbalances (particularly in utero during brain formation)
  - Pathologic deficiencies in early parent-child bonding and child-rearing practices
- Other contributing factors
  - Concurrent paraphilias, especially transvestic fetishism
  - Feelings of sexual inadequacy
  - Generalized anxiety disorder
  - Personality disorders

Signs and symptoms

- Adults and adolescents
  - Belief of being "born the wrong sex"
  - Preoccupation with eliminating primary and secondary sex characteristics
    - Attempts to mask or remove sex organs
    - Disturbed body image
    - Finding one's genitals "disgusting"
  - Lifelong history of feeling feminine and pursuing feminine activities (males); similar propensities for opposite-sex activities and discomfort with the female role (females)
    - Cross-dressing
    - Dreams of cross-gender identification
    - Preoccupation with appearance
    - Strong attraction to stereotypical activities of opposite sex
  - Anxiety
  - Depression
  - Fear of abandonment by family and friends
  - Ineffective coping strategies
  - Peer ostracism
  - Self-hatred
  - Self-medication (such as with hormonal therapy)
  - Suicide attempts or ideation
- Children
  - Expression of desire to be — or insisting that they are — the opposite sex
  - Disgust with their genitalia, along with an ardent hope to become the opposite sex when they grow up
  - Acute crisis during puberty
    - Development of secondary sex characteristics (breasts and pubic hair in the female, enlarged penis and testes in the male) possibly triggering intense distress
    - Possible intensification of feeling that one is a misfit

Diagnosis

- Karyotyping for sex chromosomes (may show abnormalities)
- Psychological tests (may reveal cross-gender identification or behavior patterns)
- Sex hormone assay (may reveal abnormality)
- Diagnosis of gender identity disorder confirmed if *DSM-IV-TR* criteria met

Treatment

- Individual and couples therapy to help an adult patient cope with the decision to live as the opposite sex or, depending on the circumstances, to cope with the knowledge that he or she won't be able to live as the opposite sex
- Psychiatric management (group or individual, depending on circumstances); may involve hospitalization if the patient has the potential for violence, such as suicidal ideation or self-mutilation fantasies
- For a child, individual and family therapy
  - Therapist of same sex helpful for role-modeling
  - Improved prognosis with earlier diagnosis and treatment
- Sex reassignment through hormonal therapy and sex-change surgery

---

Key signs and symptoms of gender identity disorder

Adults and adolescents
- Belief of being "born the wrong sex"
- Preoccupation with eliminating primary and secondary sex characteristics
- Lifelong history of feeling like the opposite sex and pursuing opposite sex activities
- Anxiety and depression
- Fear of abandonment
- Self-hatred
- Self-medication
- Suicide attempts or ideation

Children
- Acute crisis during puberty
- Development of secondary sex characteristics possibly triggering intense distress
- Possible intensification of feeling that one is a misfit

Diagnosing gender identity disorder

- Karyotyping for sex chromosomes
- Psychological tests
- Sex hormone assay
- Confirmed if *DSM-IV-TR* criteria met

Key treatment options for gender identity disorder

- Individual and couples therapy
- Psychiatric management
- For child, individual and family therapy
- Sex reassignment through hormonal therapy and sex-change surgery

Key nursing interventions for a patient with gender identity disorder

- Assess for signs and symptoms of gender identity disorder.
- Assist with necessary treatment.
- Demonstrate nonjudgmental approach with patient.

Characteristics of premature ejaculation

- A male's inability to control the ejaculatory reflex during sexual activity
- Causes ejaculation to occur before or immediately after penetration, or before the wishes of both partners
- Doesn't affect the ability to have or maintain an erection

Common causes of premature ejaculation

- Possible psychological factors
- Underlying degenerative neurologic disorder
- Other physical factors

Key signs and symptoms of premature ejaculation

- Excessively long foreplay or ejaculating immediately or soon after penile insertion
- Partner seeking treatment
- Anxiety
- Depression
- Disturbance in body image
- Frustration and feelings of being unattractive
- Poor self-concept

- – Sex reassignment not as beneficial as first hoped; severe psychological problems may persist afterward (sometimes even leading to suicide)
- – Seeking sex reassignment may be linked with larger pattern of depression and concomitant personality disorders such as borderline personality disorder

● **Nursing interventions**
- Assess for signs and symptoms of gender identity disorder
- Assist with necessary treatment (see *Nursing interventions for patients with sexual disorders,* pages 336 and 337)
- Demonstrate nonjudgmental approach with the patient

PREMATURE EJACULATION

● **Defining characteristics**
- Premature ejaculation refers to a male's inability to control the ejaculatory reflex during sexual activity
  - – Causes ejaculation to occur before or immediately after penetration or before the wishes of both partners
  - – Affects men of all ages
- Unlike male erectile disorder, premature ejaculation doesn't affect the ability to have or maintain an erection (see *Understanding male erectile disorder*)
- Premature ejaculation can seriously disrupt intimate relationships; it can lead to generalized anxiety disorder or pervasive feelings of inadequacy, guilt, and self-doubt

● **Causes**
- Possible psychological factors
  - – Stress
  - – Performance anxiety or limited sexual experiences
  - – Ambivalence toward or unconscious hatred of women
  - – Negative sexual relationships (patient unconsciously denies partner's sexual fulfillment)
  - – Guilt feelings about sex
- Underlying degenerative neurologic disorder (multiple sclerosis, or an inflammatory process, such as posterior urethritis or prostatitis)
- Other physical factors (drug or alcohol use, genital surgery, trauma)

● **Signs and symptoms**
- Excessively long foreplay or ejaculating immediately or soon after penile insertion
- Partner seeking treatment (may complain that patient is indifferent to her sexual needs)
- Anxiety
- Depression
- Disturbance in body image
- Frustration and feelings of being unattractive
- Ineffective coping
- Pain during sexual intercourse
- Poor self-concept
- Social isolation

Understanding male erectile disorder

Male erectile disorder (commonly called *impotence*) refers to the inability to attain or maintain penile erection long enough to complete sexual intercourse. The patient's history may reveal a longstanding inability to achieve erection, a sudden loss of erectile function, or a gradual decline in function. It may also include a medical condition, drug therapy, or psychological trauma that could contribute to erectile disorder.

When the cause of the disorder is psychogenic rather than organic, the patient may report that he can achieve erection through masturbation but not with a partner. He may show signs of anxiety when discussing his condition, such as sweating and palpitations — or he may appear disinterested. Depression, another common complaint, may be either a cause or an effect of erectile disorder.

TREATMENT

Sex therapy designed to reduce performance anxiety may effectively cure psychogenic impotence.

Treatment for organic impotence focuses on eliminating the underlying cause. If this isn't possible, counseling may help the couple deal with their situation realistically and explore alternatives for sexual expression. Some patients may benefit from a surgically inserted, inflatable or semirigid penile prosthesis. Others may benefit from such medications as sildenafil (Viagra), vardenafil (Levitra), or tadalafil (Cialis).

Diagnosing premature ejaculation

- Physical examination and diagnostic tests to rule out medical causes
- Confirmed if *DSM-IV-TR* criteria met

Key treatment options for premature ejaculation

- Masters' and Johnson's intensive treatment program
- Mutual physical exploration
- Sensate focus exercises
- Squeeze technique
- Stop-and-start technique

Key treatment options for male erectile disorder

- Sex therapy designed to reduce performance anxiety
- Elimination of underlying cause (organic impotence)
- Counseling
- Surgically inserted inflatable or semirigid penile prosthesis
- Medications (sildenafil, vardenafil, tadalafil)

Key nursing interventions for a patient with premature ejaculation

- Assess for signs and symptoms of male sexual dysfunction.
- Assist with necessary treatment.

● Diagnosis

- Physical examination and diagnostic tests to rule out medical causes
- Disorder diagnosed if *DSM-IV-TR* criteria met

● Treatment

- Masters' and Johnson's intensive treatment program for premature ejaculation: helps the patient focus on sensations of impending orgasm; combines insight therapy, behavioral techniques, and experiential sessions involving both partners; sessions last 2 weeks or longer and may involve variety of approaches
  - Mutual physical exploration to enhance the couple's awareness of anatomy and physiology while reducing shameful feelings about sexual body parts
  - Sensate focus exercises
  - Squeeze technique, which helps the patient gain control of ejaculatory tension (see *Squeeze technique for premature ejaculation,* page 344)
  - Stop-and-start technique (performed with the woman in the superior position), which also helps to delay ejaculation
    - Involves pelvic thrusting until orgasmic sensations begin; thrusting then stops and is restarted to promote control of ejaculation
    - Couple eventually allowed to achieve orgasm

● Nursing interventions

- Assess for signs and symptoms of male sexual dysfunction
- Assist with necessary treatment (see *Nursing interventions for patients with sexual disorders,* pages 336 and 337)

TIME-OUT FOR TEACHING

Squeeze technique for premature ejaculation

The squeeze technique, used to overcome premature ejaculation, may be practiced either with a partner or alone (during masturbation).

- Advise the patient or his partner to position the fingers correctly around the penis and apply the correct amount of pressure.
- When the patient feels the urge to ejaculate, tell him or his partner to place a thumb on the frenulum of the penis and place the index and middle fingers above and below the coronal ridge, as shown here.
- Instruct the patient or partner to squeeze the penis from front to back — more firmly for an erect penis and less firmly for a partially flaccid one.
- Advise the partner to apply and release pressure every few minutes during a touching exercise.

Explain that the goal of this technique is to delay ejaculation by keeping the man at an earlier phase of the sexual response cycle. Inform the patient that he should feel pressure but no pain. After several squeezes, he should have a more intense ejaculation than usual.

Patient instructions for the squeeze technique

- Position fingers correctly around the penis and apply correct amount of pressure.
- Place thumb on frenulum of penis and place index and middle fingers above and below coronal ridge.
- Squeeze penis from front to back.
- Apply and release pressure every few minutes during a touching exercise. Patient should feel pressure but no pain.
- Delay ejaculation by keeping the man at an early phase of sexual response cycle.
- After several squeezes, ejaculation should be more intense than usual.

ANATOMIC STRUCTURES

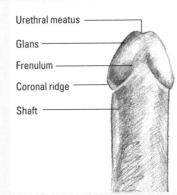

- Urethral meatus
- Glans
- Frenulum
- Coronal ridge
- Shaft

HAND POSITION

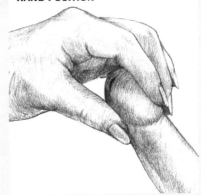

NCLEX CHECKS

It's never too soon to begin your NCLEX preparation. Now that you've reviewed this chapter, carefully read each of the following questions and choose the best answer. Then compare your responses to the correct answers.

1. A student is reviewing content for a test on the phases of the sexual response cycle. The student demonstrates understanding of the material by identifying which phase as the one involving fantasy and expectation?

☐ **1.** Desire phase
☐ **2.** Excitement phase
☐ **3.** Orgasm phase
☐ **4.** Resolution phase

2. Which behavior or disorder would the nurse identify as a possible cause of or contributing factor to sexual dysfunction?

☐ **1.** Drug use
☐ **2.** Dissociative disorders
☐ **3.** Supplemental vitamin use
☐ **4.** Exercise

3. The history of a patient reveals a persistent urge to show his genitalia to a stranger. The nurse identifies this as:

☐ **1.** fetishism.
☐ **2.** pedophilia.
☐ **3.** exhibitionism.
☐ **4.** transsexualism.

4. Which treatment would the nurse expect to include in the care plan for a woman with orgasmic disorder?

☐ **1.** Use of soothing bubble baths
☐ **2.** Exercises involving touching her partner
☐ **3.** More frequent sexual intercourse
☐ **4.** Increase in the degree of sexual arousal

5. A patient reports achieving orgasm only by caressing suede boots when he's alone. His history reveals no other human partner. The nurse suspects:

☐ **1.** fetishism.
☐ **2.** gender identity disorder.
☐ **3.** transsexualism.
☐ **4.** hypoactive sexual desire disorder.

6. The multidisciplinary care team would suspect gender identity disorder if a patient:

☐ **1.** has a strong desire to be of the same sex.
☐ **2.** insists that he or she is of the opposite sex.
☐ **3.** prefers the opposite sex.
☐ **4.** engages in sexual activities with the same sex.

7. During an interview, a patient reveals a sexual attraction to children. The nurse documents this as:

☐ **1.** sexual sadism.
☐ **2.** necrophilia.
☐ **3.** exhibitionism.
☐ **4.** pedophilia.

8. Which disorders are classified as paraphilias according to the *DSM-IV-TR?* Select all that apply:

☐ **1.** Sexual masochism
☐ **2.** Voyeurism
☐ **3.** Fetishism
☐ **4.** Protracted promiscuity
☐ **5.** Compulsive masturbation
☐ **6.** Severe sexual desire

TOP 10

Items to study for your next test on sexual disorders

1. Four components of sexual identity
2. Normal and abnormal sexual behaviors
3. Categories of sexual dysfunction
4. Stages of sexual development
5. Five phases of human sexual response cycle
6. Eight recognized paraphilias
7. Nursing interventions for patients with sexual disorders
8. Signs and symptoms of female sexual arousal disorder and female orgasmic disorder
9. Treatment for gender identity disorder
10. Treatment for premature ejaculation and male erectile disorder

9. When developing the care plan for a patient diagnosed with premature ejaculation, which intervention would the nurse expect to include?

- ☐ **1.** Administration of sildenafil (Viagra)
- ☐ **2.** Preparation for insertion of a penile prosthesis
- ☐ **3.** Instructions in the squeeze technique
- ☐ **4.** Sex therapy to reduce performance anxiety

10. During an initial assessment, a female patient states, "It hurts so much when my husband and I have sexual intercourse that sometimes I don't even want to think about having sex." The nurse interprets this statement as suggesting:

- ☐ **1.** vaginismus.
- ☐ **2.** dyspareunia.
- ☐ **3.** female orgasmic disorder.
- ☐ **4.** sexual aversion disorder.

ANSWERS AND RATIONALES

1. CORRECT ANSWER: 1
The desire phase of the sexual response cycle involves fantasy and expectation. The excitement phase is the arousal phase that prepares both partners for intercourse. The orgasm phase is the peak of sexual excitement. In the resolution phase, the body returns to its normal unexcited state.

2. CORRECT ANSWER: 1
Sexual dysfunctions sometimes stem from transient conditions such as drug or alcohol use. They aren't typically associated with dissociative disorders, supplemental vitamin use, or exercise.

3. CORRECT ANSWER: 3
An exhibitionist has sexual fantasies, urges, or behaviors involving exposing his genitals to strangers. Fetishism is characterized by sexual fantasies, urges, or behaviors that involve the use of an inanimate object or a nonsexual part of the body to produce or enhance sexual arousal. Pedophilia is characterized by sexual fantasies, urges, or activity involving a child. Transsexualism is a gender identity disorder marked by discomfort with one's apparent or assigned sex, and a strong, persistent identification with the opposite sex.

4. CORRECT ANSWER: 2
Sensate focus exercises are recommended for female orgasmic disorder. These exercises emphasize touching and awareness of sensual feelings throughout the entire body while minimizing the importance of intercourse and orgasm. The couple takes turns giving and receiving touch. Soothing bubble baths, increased frequency of intercourse, and increased degree of sexual arousal would be inappropriate.

5. CORRECT ANSWER: 1
In one form of fetishism, an inanimate object completely replaces a human partner. The object may be undergarments, shoes, or a fabric, such as velvet or silk. Gender identity disorder, or transsexualism, is marked by discomfort with one's apparent or assigned gender and a strong, persistent identification with the opposite sex. Hypoactive sexual desire disorder involves a deficiency or absence of sexual fantasies or desire for sexual activity.

6. CORRECT ANSWER: 2

Gender identity disorder is marked by a repeatedly stated desire to be the opposite sex or an insistence that one is the opposite sex. Heterosexual individuals prefer members of the opposite sex; homosexual individuals engage in sexual activities with members of the same sex.

7. CORRECT ANSWER: 4

In pedophilia, the patient has sexual fantasies, urges, or activity involving a child. Sadism involves the achievement of sexual gratification by inflicting cruelty or emotional abuse on another person. Necrophilia involves sexual attraction to corpses. Exhibitionism is marked by sexual fantasies, urges, or behaviors involving exposing the genitals to strangers.

8. CORRECT ANSWER: 1, 2, 3

Sexual masochism, voyeurism, and fetishism are paraphilias identified by the *DSM-IV-TR*. Protracted promiscuity, compulsive masturbation, and severe sexual desire are similar to paraphilias but don't fall into the main classifications of the *DSM-IV-TR*.

9. CORRECT ANSWER: 3

For the patient with premature ejaculation, treatment may include the squeeze technique to help the patient gain control of ejaculatory tension. Sildenafil, a penile prosthesis, and sex therapy for performance anxiety would be appropriate treatments for a patient with erectile dysfunction.

10. CORRECT ANSWER: 2

The woman is describing dyspareunia, a sexual pain disorder involving genital pain that occurs before, during, or after intercourse. Vaginismus, also a sexual pain disorder, involves involuntary spasmodic muscle contractions that occur at the vaginal entrance when the male attempts penile insertion. A patient with female orgasmic disorder typically experiences a persistent or recurrent delay in or absence of orgasm following a normal sexual excitement phase. Sexual aversion disorder is characterized by dislike and avoidance of genital sexual contact with a sexual partner.

NANDA nursing diagnoses
Glossary
Selected references
Index

NANDA nursing diagnoses

The following is a list of the current 2005-2006 nursing diagnosis classifications according to their domains.

DOMAIN
HEALTH PROMOTION

- Effective therapeutic regimen management
- Health-seeking behaviors (specify)
- Impaired home maintenance
- Ineffective community therapeutic regimen management
- Ineffective family therapeutic regimen management
- Ineffective health maintenance
- Ineffective therapeutic regimen management
- Readiness for enhanced management of therapeutic regimen
- Readiness for enhanced nutrition

DOMAIN
NUTRITION

- Deficient fluid volume
- Excess fluid volume
- Imbalanced nutrition: Less than body requirements
- Imbalanced nutrition: More than body requirements
- Impaired swallowing
- Ineffective infant feeding pattern
- Readiness for enhanced fluid balance
- Risk for deficient fluid volume
- Risk for imbalanced fluid volume
- Risk for imbalanced nutrition: More than body requirements

DOMAIN
ELIMINATION/EXCHANGE

- Bowel incontinence
- Constipation
- Diarrhea
- Functional urinary incontinence
- Impaired gas exchange
- Impaired urinary elimination
- Perceived constipation
- Readiness for enhanced urinary elimination
- Reflex urinary incontinence
- Risk for constipation
- Risk for urge urinary incontinence
- Stress urinary incontinence
- Total urinary incontinence
- Urge urinary incontinence
- Urinary retention

DOMAIN
ACTIVITY/REST

- Activity intolerance
- Bathing or hygiene self-care deficit
- Decreased cardiac output
- Deficient diversional activity
- Delayed surgical recovery
- Disturbed energy field
- Disturbed sleep pattern
- Dressing or grooming self-care deficit
- Dysfunctional ventilatory weaning response
- Fatigue
- Feeding self-care deficit
- Impaired bed mobility
- Impaired physical mobility
- Impaired spontaneous ventilation
- Impaired transfer ability
- Impaired walking
- Impaired wheelchair mobility
- Ineffective breathing pattern
- Ineffective tissue perfusion (specify type: renal, cerebral, cardiopulmonary, gastrointestinal, peripheral)
- Readiness for enhanced sleep
- Risk for activity intolerance
- Risk for disuse syndrome
- Sedentary lifestyle
- Sleep deprivation
- Toileting self-care deficit

DOMAIN
PERCEPTION/COGNITION

- Disturbed sensory perception (specify: visual, auditory, kinesthetic, gustatory, tactile, olfactory)
- Impaired environmental interpretation syndrome
- Impaired verbal communication
- Readiness for enhanced communication
- Unilateral neglect
- Wandering

DOMAIN
SELF-PERCEPTION

- Chronic low self-esteem
- Disturbed body image
- Disturbed personal identity
- Hopelessness
- Powerlessness
- Readiness for enhanced self-concept
- Risk for loneliness
- Risk for powerlessness
- Risk for situational low self-esteem
- Situational low self-esteem

DOMAIN
ROLE RELATIONSHIPS

- Caregiver role strain
- Dysfunctional family processes: Alcoholism
- Effective breast-feeding
- Impaired parenting
- Impaired social interaction
- Ineffective breast-feeding
- Ineffective role performance
- Interrupted breast-feeding
- Interrupted family processes
- Parental role conflict
- Readiness for enhanced family processes
- Readiness for enhanced parenting
- Risk for caregiver role strain
- Risk for impaired parent/infant/child attachment
- Risk for impaired parenting

DOMAIN
SEXUALITY

- Ineffective sexuality patterns
- Sexual dysfunction

DOMAIN
COPING/STRESS TOLERANCE

- Anticipatory grieving
- Anxiety
- Autonomic dysreflexia
- Chronic sorrow
- Compromised family coping
- Death anxiety
- Decreased intracranial adaptive capacity
- Defensive coping
- Disabled family coping
- Disorganized infant behavior
- Dysfunctional grieving
- Fear
- Impaired adjustment
- Ineffective community coping
- Ineffective coping
- Ineffective denial
- Posttrauma syndrome
- Rape-trauma syndrome
- Rape-trauma syndrome: Compound reaction
- Rape-trauma syndrome: Silent reaction
- Readiness for enhanced community coping
- Readiness for enhanced coping
- Readiness for enhanced family coping
- Readiness for enhanced organized infant behavior
- Relocation stress syndrome
- Risk for autonomic dysreflexia
- Risk for disorganized infant behavior
- Risk for dysfunctional grieving
- Risk for posttrauma syndrome
- Risk for relocation stress syndrome

DOMAIN
LIFE PRINCIPLES

- Decisional conflict (specify)
- Impaired religiosity
- Noncompliance (specify)
- Readiness for enhanced religiosity
- Readiness for enhanced spiritual well-being
- Risk for impaired religiosity
- Risk for spiritual distress
- Spiritual distress

DOMAIN
SAFETY/PROTECTION

- Hyperthermia
- Hypothermia
- Impaired dentition
- Impaired oral mucous membrane
- Impaired skin integrity
- Impaired tissue integrity
- Ineffective airway clearance
- Ineffective protection
- Ineffective thermoregulation
- Latex allergy response
- Risk for aspiration
- Risk for falls
- Risk for imbalanced body temperature
- Risk for impaired skin integrity
- Risk for infection
- Risk for injury
- Risk for latex allergy response
- Risk for other-directed violence
- Risk for perioperative-positioning injury
- Risk for peripheral neurovascular dysfunction
- Risk for poisoning
- Risk for self-directed violence
- Risk for self-mutilation
- Risk for sudden infant death syndrome
- Risk for suffocation
- Risk for suicide
- Risk for trauma
- Self-mutilation

DOMAIN
COMFORT

- Acute pain
- Chronic pain
- Nausea
- Social isolation

DOMAIN
GROWTH/DEVELOPMENT

- Adult failure to thrive
- Delayed growth and development
- Risk for delayed development
- Risk for disproportionate growth

Glossary

acetylcholine: neurotransmitter

acting out: repeatedly performing actions without weighing the possible results of those actions

agnosia: loss of sensory ability to recognize objects

ambivalence: coexisting, strong, positive and negative feelings, leading to emotional conflict

amphetamines: stimulant drugs used to increase alertness, relieve fatigue, and feel stronger and more decisive; used for euphoric effects or to counteract the "down" feeling of tranquilizers or alcohol

anhedonia: diminished capacity to experience pleasure; may be reflected by a lack of interest in activities with substantial time spent in purposeless activity

antisocial personality disorder: pervasive lack of remorse or lack of exhibiting feelings that leads to a total disregard for the rights of others

aphasia: loss of language ability

apraxia: loss of purpose without loss of muscle power leads to difficulty carrying out complex tasks

asociality: lack of interest in relationships

attention level: ability to concentrate on a task for an appropriate length of time

avoidant personality disorder: negativity, poor self-esteem, and issues surrounding social interaction; difficulty looking at situations and interactions in an objective manner

Beck Depression Inventory: helps diagnose depression and determine its severity

bipolar disorder: mood disorder characterized by severe, frequent pathologic mood swings

blunted affect: flattening of emotions in which the person's face may appear immobile with poor eye contact and lack of expressiveness

body dysmorphic disorder: preoccupation with an imagined or an actual slight defect in physical appearance; perceived thoughts are typically distorted, making the problem, or perceived problem, bigger than it actually is; in many cases, the flaw doesn't exist

borderline personality disorder: pattern of instability or impulsiveness in a person's mood, interpersonal relationships, self-esteem, self-identity, behavior, and cognition; originates in early childhood

clang association: words that rhyme or sound alike used in an illogical, nonsensical manner — for example: "It's the rain, train, pain."

clanging: choice of a word based on the sound rather than the meaning

cocaine: narcotic and stimulant, which may be ingested, injected, sniffed, or smoked to obtain its effects; street names include coke, flake, snow, nose candy, hits, crack (hardened form), rock, and crank

Cognitive Assessment Scale: measures orientation, general knowledge, mental ability, and psychomotor function

Cognitive Capacity Screening Examination: measures orientation, memory, calculation, and language

comorbidity: coexistence of two disorders, such as mental and somatic disorders, occurring together in a person

compensation: hiding a weakness by stressing too strongly the desirable strength

comprehension: ability to understand, retain, and repeat material

compulsion: preoccupation that's acted out such as constantly washing one's hands

concept formation: testing the patient's ability to think abstractly

concrete thinking: inability to form or understand abstract thoughts

confabulation: unconscious filling of gaps in memory with fabricated facts and experiences

conversion disorder: (previously called *hysterical neurosis, conversion type*) disorder in which patients resolve psychological conflicts through the loss of a specific physical function; examples include paralysis, blindness, or the inability to swallow; patients exhibit symptoms that suggest a physical disorder, but evaluation and observation can't determine a physiological cause

cyclothymia: short periods of mild depression alternating with short periods of hypomania

delusions: false ideas or beliefs accepted as real by the patient; somatic illness, depersonalization, and delusions of grandeur, persecution, and reference are common in schizophrenia

denial: protecting oneself from unpleasant aspects of life by refusing to perceive, acknowledge, or deal with them

dependent personality disorder: an extreme need to be taken care of that leads to submissive, clinging behavior and fear of separation; pattern begins by early adulthood, when behaviors designed to elicit caring from others become predominant

depersonalization: feeling that one has become detached from one's mind or body or has lost one's identity

depression: persistent sad mood lasting 2 weeks or longer

derailment: speech that vacillates from one subject to another; the subjects are unrelated; ideas slip off the track between clauses

displacement: misdirecting pent-up feelings toward something or someone that's less threatening than that which triggered the response

dissociation: separating objects from their emotional significance

dysthymia: mild depression that lasts at least 2 years in adults or 1 year in a child

Eating Attitudes Test: detects patterns that suggest an eating disorder

echolalia: meaningless repetition of words or phrases

echopraxia: involuntary repetition of movements observed in others

electroconvulsive therapy: treatment that involves inducing a seizure to improve depression

extinction: technique that simply ignores undesirable behavior, provided that the behavior isn't dangerous or illegal

fantasy: creation of unrealistic or improbable images to escape from daily pressures and responsibilities

flat affect: unresponsive range of emotion, possibly an indication of schizophrenia or Parkinson's disease

flight of ideas: rapid succession of incomplete and poorly connected ideas

flooding: frequent full-intensity exposure, possibly through the use of imagination, to an object that triggers a symptom; produces extreme discomfort

fluid intelligence: form of intelligence defined as the ability to solve novel problems

focusing: technique in which the nurse assists the patient in redirecting attention toward something specific, especially if the patient is vague or rambling

Functional Dementia Scale: measures orientation, affect, and the ability to perform activities of daily living

Global Deterioration Scale: assesses and stages primary degenerative dementia based on orientation, memory, and neurologic function

grandiosity: exaggerated sense of self-importance, power, and status

hallucinations: false sensory perceptions with no basis in reality; usually visual or auditory, hallucinations also may be olfactory (smell), gustatory (taste), or tactile (touch)

hallucinogens: drugs with no known medical use that produce behavioral changes that are commonly multiple and dramatic; however, some block sensation to pain and use may result in self-inflicted injuries

histrionic personality disorder: pervasive pattern of excessive emotionality and attention-seeking; usually begins in early adulthood and may be present in a variety of contexts

hypochondriasis: misinterpretation of the severity and significance of physical signs or sensations or the fear of contracting a disease; leads to the preoccupation with having a serious disease, which persists despite medical reassurance to the contrary; significant distress or impairment in functioning occurs

ideas of reference: misinterpreting acts of others in a highly personal way

identification: unconscious adoption of the personality characteristics, attitudes, values, and behavior of another person

illusions: false sensory perceptions with some basis in reality; for example, a car backfiring mistaken for a gunshot

implicit memory: information that can't be brought to mind but can be seen to affect behavior

implosion therapy: form of desensitization; requires repeated exposure (that increases in graduated levels) to a highly feared object, requires strong interpersonal support or anxiolytic medication

inappropriate affect: inconsistency between expression (affect) and mood; for example, a patient who smiles when discussing an anger-provoking situation

incoherence: incomprehensible speech

intellectualization: hiding feelings about something painful behind thoughts; keeping opposing attitudes apart by using logic-tight comparisons

introjection: adopting someone else's values and standards without exploring whether they actually fit; often responds to "should" or "ought to"

lability of affect: rapid, dramatic fluctuation in the range of emotion

loose associations: not connected or related by logic or rationality

magical thinking: belief that thoughts or wishes can control other people or events

magnetoencephalography: measures the brain's magnetic field

Mini–Mental Status Examination: structured interview that measures orientation, registration, recall, calculation, language, and graphomotor function

Minnesota Multiphasic Personality Inventory: helps assess personality traits and ego function in adolescents and adults

modeling: provides a reward when the patient imitates the desired behavior

monoamine oxidase inhibitors: atypical antidepressants used cautiously due to food and drug interactions

mood stabilizers: medications used to treat bipolar disorder

narcissistic personality disorder: projecting an image of perfection and personal invincibility because of a fear of personal weakness and imperfection; commonly projecting an inflated sense of self to hide low self-esteem

negative reinforcement: involves the removal of a negative stimulus only after the patient provides a desirable response

neologisms: distorted or invented words that have meaning only for the patient

nonverbal communication: eye contact, posture, facial expression, gestures, clothing, affect, silence, and other body movements that can convey a powerful message

obsessions: intense preoccupations that interfere with daily living

obsessive-compulsive personality disorder: lack of openness and flexibility in daily routines as well as in interpersonal relationships and expectations; a preoccupation with orderliness and perfectionism; treatment options that don't fit in with the patient's cognitive schema will be rejected quickly

opiates: narcotics and depressants used medicinally to relieve pain, but have a high potential for abuse; cause relaxation with an immediate "rush," but also have initial unpleasant effects, such as restlessness and nausea; includes codeine, heroin, meperidine, and opium; street names include junk, horse, H, and smack

paranoid personality disorder: extreme distrust of others and an avoidance of relationships in which the person isn't in control or has the potential of losing control

perseveration: repeating the same words or movements despite efforts to make a new response

pharmacodynamics: drug's effect on its target organ

phencyclidine: hallucinogen that produces behavioral changes that are usually multiple and dramatic; flashbacks may occur long after use; street names include hog, angel dust, peace pill, crystal superjoint, elephant tranquilizer, and rocket fuel

phobia: irrational and disproportionate fear of objects or situations

positive reinforcement: increase of the likelihood of a desirable behavior being repeated by promptly praising or rewarding the patient when performing it

poverty of speech: diminution of thought reflected in decreased speech and terse replies to questions, creating the impression of inner emptiness

processing capacity: understanding text, making inferences, and paying attention, which all depend on working memory capability

projection: displacement of negative feelings onto another person

prospective memory: remembering things that one needs

punishment: discouraging of problem behavior by inflicting a penalty such as temporary removal of a privilege

rationalization: substitution of acceptable reasons for the real or actual reasons motivating behavior

reaction formation: conduct in a manner opposite from the way the person feels

recent memory: event experienced in the past few hours or days

regression: return to an earlier developmental stage

remote memory: ability to remember events in the more distant past, such as birthplace or high school days

repression: unconsciously blocking out painful thoughts

response prevention: form of behavior therapy that may require hospitalization as well as family involvement to be effective

schizoid personality: pervasive pattern of detachment from social relationships and restricted range of expression of emotions in interpersonal settings

schizotypal personality disorder: pervasive pattern of social and interpersonal deficits marked by acute discomfort with, and reduced capacity for, close relationships as well as by cognitive or perceptual distortions and eccentricities of behavior; begins in early adulthood and is present in various contexts

selective serotonin reuptake inhibitors: class of antidepressants used to treat depression that works on serotonin receptor sites

self-efficacy: personality measure defined by the ability to organize and execute actions required to deal with situations likely to happen in the future

serotonin norepinephrine reuptake inhibitors: class of antidepressants used to treat depression that works on serotonin and norepinephrine receptor sites

shaping: initially rewards any behavior that resembles the desirable one; then, step by step, the behavior required to gain a reward becomes progressively closer to the desired behavior

sharing impressions: describing the patients feelings to him and then seeking corrective feedback from the patient

somatization disorder: experiencing multiple signs and symptoms that suggest a physical disorder, but no verifiable disease or pathophysiologic condition exists to account for them; unexplained symptoms appear to represent an unconscious somatized plea for attention and care; commonly familial with unknown etiology

sublimation: transforming unacceptable needs into acceptable ambitions and actions; for instance, a person can funnel anger and resentment into an obsession to excel in a lucrative career

substance abuse: maladaptive pattern of substance use coupled with recurrent and significant adverse consequences

substance dependence: physical, behavioral, and cognitive changes resulting from persistent substance use; persistent drug use results in tolerance and withdrawal

substance intoxication: development of a reversible substance-specific syndrome due to the ingestion of or exposure to a substance; the clinically significant maladaptive behavior or psychological changes vary from substance to substance

suicide ideation: thoughts of self-harm, doing away with or taking one's life

sundowning: confused behavior late in the day or at night when environmental stimulation is low

Thematic Apperception Test: test in which, after seeing a series of pictures that depict ambiguous situations, the patient tells a story describing each picture

thought blocking: sudden interruption in the patient's train of thought

thought replacement or switching: replacement of fear-inducing self-instructions with competent self-instructions, which teaches the patient to replace negative thoughts with positive ones until the positive thoughts become strong enough to overcome the anxiety-provoking ones

thought stopping: method that breaks the habit of fear-inducing anticipatory thoughts; to stop unwanted thoughts by saying the word "stop" and then focus attention on achieving calmness and muscle relaxation

tolerance: increased need for a substance or need for an increased amount of the substance to achieve an effect

tricyclic antidepressants: class of antidepressants used to treat depression that works on serotonin, dopamine, and norepinephrine receptor sites

undoing: trying to superficially repair or make up for an action without dealing with the complex effects of that deed; also called *magical thinking*

withdrawal: becoming emotionally uninvolved by pulling back and being passive

word salad: illogical word groupings; the extreme form of loose associations; for example, "She had a star, barn, plant."

working memory: part of the brain that enables not paying attention to irrelevancies

Selected references

Averill, P.M., et al. "Is Schizoaffective Disorder a Stable Diagnostic Category: A Retrospective Examination," *Psychiatric Quarterly* 75(3):215-27, Fall 2004.

Boyd, M.A. *Psychiatric Nursing Contemporary Practice,* 3rd ed. Philadelphia: Lippincott Williams & Wilkins, 2004.

Cutcliffe, J.R., and Barker, P. "The Nurses' Global Assessment of Suicide Risk (NGASR): Developing a Tool for Clinical Practice," *Journal of Psychiatric Mental Health Nursing* 11(4):393-400, August 2004.

Dearing, K.S. "Getting It Together: How the Nurse-Patient Relationship Influences Treatment Compliance for Patients with Schizophrenia," *Archives of Psychiatric Nursing* 18(5):155-63, October 2004.

Diagnostic and Statistical Manual of Mental Disorders, Fourth Edition, Text Revision. Washington, D.C.: American Psychiatric Association, 2000.

Fortinash, K., and Worret, P.H. *Psychiatric Mental Health Nursing,* 3rd ed. St. Louis: Mosby–Year Book, Inc., 2004.

Gallop, R., and O'Brien, L. "Re-establishing Psychodynamic Theory as Foundational Knowledge for Psychiatric/Mental Health Nursing," *Issues in Mental Health Nursing* 24(2):213-27, March 2003.

Haverkamp, R., et al. "Problem Solving Treatment for Complicated Depression in Later Life: A Case Study in Primary Care," *Perspectives in Psychiatric Care* 40(2):45-52, April-June 2004.

Holmes, D., et al. "The Mentally Ill & Social Exclusion: A Critical Examination of the Use of Seclusion from the Patient's Perspectives," *Issues in Mental Health Nursing* 25(6):559-78, September 2004.

Keltner, N.L., et al. *Psychiatric Nursing,* 4th ed. St. Louis: Mosby–Year Book, Inc., 2003.

Kemppainen, J.K., et al. "Psychiatric Nursing and Medication Adherence," *Journal of Psychosocial Nursing and Mental Health Services* 41(2):38-49, February 2003.

Killeen, M. "Private Matters, "*Journal of Child and Adolescent Psychiatric Nursing* 15(4):41-42, October-December 2002.

Kools, S., and Spiers J. "Caregiver Understanding of Adolescent Development in Residential Treatment," *Journal of Child and Adolescent Psychiatric Nursing* 15(4):151-62, October-December 2002.

Latvala, E., et al. "Developing and Testing Instruments for Improving Cooperation and Patient's Participation in Mental Health Care," *Journal of Psychiatric and Mental Health Nursing* 11(5):614-19, October 2004.

McAllister, M., and Walsh, K. "CARE: A Framework for Mental Health Practice," *Journal of Psychiatric and Mental Health Nursing* 10(1):39-48, February 2003.

Piaget, J. "The Stages of the Intellectual Development of the Child," *Bulletin of the Menninger Clinic* 26:120-28, 1962.

Raue, P.J., et al. "Assessing Behavioral Health Using OASIS: Part 1: Depression and Suicidality," *Home Healthcare Nurse* 20(3):154-61, March 2002.

Raue, P.J., et al. "Assessing Behavioral Health Using OASIS: Part 2: Cognitive Impairment, Problematic Behaviors, and Anxiety," *Home Healthcare Nurse* 20(4):230-35, April 2002.

Scott, S.R., et al. "A Staff Perspective of Early Warning Signs Intervention for Individuals with Psychosis: Clinical and Service Implications," *Journal of Psychiatric and Mental Health Nursing* 11(4):469-75, August 2004.

Shives, L.R. *Basic Concepts of Psychiatric-Mental Health Nursing,* 6th ed. Philadelphia: Lippincott Williams & Wilkins, 2004.

Stuart, G., and Laraia, M. *Principles and Practice of Psychiatric Nursing,* 8th ed. St. Louis: Mosby–Year Book, Inc., 2005.

Szczesny, S., and Miller, M. "PRN Medication Use in Inpatient Psychiatry," *Journal of Psychosocial Nursing and Mental Health Services* 41(1):16-21, January 2003.

SELECTED REFERENCES

Townsend, M.C. *Psychiatric Mental Health Nursing: Concepts of Care,* 4th ed. Philadelphia: F.A. Davis Co., 2003.

Van Meijel, B., et al. "Recognition of Early Warning Signs in Patients with Schizophrenia: A Review of the Literature," *International Journal of Mental Health Nursing* 13(2):107-16, June 2004.

Varcarolis, E. *Foundation of Psychiatric Mental Health Nursing: A Clinical Approach.* Philadelphia: W.B. Saunders Co., 2002.

Videbeck, S.L. *Psychiatric Mental Health Nursing,* 2nd ed. Philadelphia: Lippincott Williams & Wilkins, 2003.

Wright, M. "Violence Against Psychiatric Nurses: Team Approach is Needed," *Journal of Psychosocial Nursing and Mental Health Services* 41(1):8, January 2003.

Index

A

Abandonment, fear of, 231
Abilify, 105
Ace, 287
Acid, 294
Acting out, as defense mechanism, 21
Activated charcoal, for benzodiazepine abuse, 316
Acupressure, 190
Acupuncture, 190
  for nicotine dependence, 305
  for opioid abuse, 311
Acute distress disorder, 144-146, 170, 171
Adam, 295
Addiction, 274
Admission, involuntary, 34
Adolescence, disorders of, 39-64
Adolescents
  communicating with, 42
  depression in, 2, 53-57
  sexual development in, 329
  suicide rate in, 2
Adult day care, 74
Adults, sexual development in, 329
Advanced practice, 5
  in geropsychiatric nursing, 70
Advanced practice interventions, 7
Advocacy, 33
Aerosols, inhaling, 300
Affect
  blunted, in schizophrenia, 99, 114, 116
  in mood disorders, 118
Aging, neurobiological changes of, 66-67
Agoraphobia, 146-147, 170, 171
  panic disorder and, 154
Akathisia, antipsychotics and, 104
Al-Anon, 282
Alateen, 282
Alcohol, and cocaine, effects of, 291

Alcohol abuse, 2. *See also* Alcohol dependence.
Alcohol dependence, 276-282
  causes of, 276-277
  characteristics of, 276
  complications of, 277
  diagnosis of, 278
  nursing interventions for, 281-282
  signs and symptoms of, 277-278
  treatment of, 279-280
Alcohol use, excessive, signs and symptoms of, 277, 278
Alcohol withdrawal
  assessing for, 279t
  signs and symptoms of, 277, 278, 320, 321, 322
Alcoholics Anonymous, 280
Alfenta, 306
Alfentanil, 306
Alprazolam, for anxiety disorders, 164-165t
Alternative therapies
  common, 190
  for pain disorder, 189
Alzheimer's disease. *See* Dementia of Alzheimer's type.
Ambivalence, 98
Amenorrhea, anorexia nervosa and, 259
American Association on Mental Retardation's Adaptive Behavior Scale, 60
Americans with Disabilities Act of 1990, 31
American Nurses Association Standards, 5, 6-7
Amitriptyline, 132-133t
  for anxiety disorders, 166-167t
  patient teaching for, 140, 141
Amnesia, dissociative, 208-210, 216, 218
Amphetamine abuse, 282-285
  causes of, 283
  diagnosis of, 284

Amphetamine abuse *(continued)*
  and health hazards and impairments, 283
  nursing interventions for, 285
  signs and symptoms of, 283-284
  treatment of, 284
Amphetamines
  characteristics of, 282
  effects of, 282
Amyloid, 82
Analgesics
  opioids as, 307
  for pain disorder, 189
Anesthetic, cocaine as, 291
Angel dust, 312
Anorexia nervosa, 259-264
  causes of, 260-261
  characteristics of, 259
  complications of, 259-260, 268, 270
  diagnosis of, 262, 269, 270
  forms of, 259
  nursing interventions for, 263-264, 269, 271
  signs and symptoms of, 261-262, 269, 270
  treatment of, 262-263
Antabuse, 280
Antagonist therapy
  for alcohol dependence, 280
  for nicotine dependence, 305
Antianxiety agents
  for generalized anxiety disorder, 149
  for panic disorder, 157
Anticholinergic effects, antipsychotics and, 104
Anticonvulsants, for bipolar disorder, 134-135t
Antidepressants
  for anxiety disorders, 166-167t
  atypical, 131
  for bipolar disorders, 122
  for major depressive disorder, 131
  for mood disorders, 132-133t
Antiemetic, cannabis as, 287

i refers to an illustration; t refers to a table.

Antimanics, for mood disorders, 134-135t
Antipsychotics
  adverse effects of, 104
  atypical, 104-105
  patient teaching for, 103
  for schizophrenia, 102-103
Antisocial personality disorder, 222-227
  causes of, 223
  characteristics of, 222-223
  diagnosis of, 224
  nursing interventions for, 226-227
  risk factors for, 223
  setting limits in, 227
  signs and symptoms of, 223-224
  and somatization disorder, 196
  treatment of, 224-226
Antitussive, codeine as, 307
Anxiety, easing, patient teaching for, 150
Anxiety disorders, 142-172
  causes of, 143-144
  characteristics of, 143
  classifying, 143
  pharmacologic therapy for, 164-167t
  and somatoform disorders, 174
Anxiolytic abuse, 314-319
  causes of, 315
  characteristics of, 314
  diagnosis of, 316
  effects of, 314-315
  and health hazards and impairments, 315
  nursing interventions for, 319
  signs and symptoms of, 315-316
  treatment of, 316-319
Apartments, supervised, 106
Apolipoprotein E, 83
Appearance, assessing, 18
Appetite, in alcohol withdrawal, 279t
Aripiprazole, 105
Arnica, 190
Aromatherapy, 190
Arousal phase, of sexual response cycle, 330
Assertiveness training, 28
Assessment, 15-25
  of children and adolescents, 42-44
  of elderly people, 70-71
  interview during, 15-18
  mental status evaluation during, 18-22
  as standard of care, 6

Attention deficit hyperactivity disorder, 44-45, 61, 62, 63
  treatment of, 46-47t
Attention-seeking, in histrionic personality disorder, 238
Attentive listening, as communication tool, 12
Auriculotherapy, for opioid abuse, 311
Autism Screening Questionnaire, 49
Autistic disorder, 47-50, 62, 63
  patient teaching for, 50
  screening tools for, 49
Autocratic behavior, 238
Autonomic arousal, heightened, and somatization, 176
Aversion therapy, 28, 182, 199, 201
  for alcohol dependence, 279t
  for nicotine dependence, 305
  for paraphilias, 335
Avoidant personality disorder, 227-230
  causes of, 228
  characteristics of, 227-228
  diagnosis of, 229
  nursing interventions for, 229-230
  signs and symptoms of, 228-229
  treatment of, 229

B

"Bad trips," 297, 298
Bagging, 300
Bandler's model of behavior, 9
Bang, 300
Bayley Scale of Infant Development, 60
Beck Depression Inventory, 22, 23, 24, 224
Bed-wetting, 178
Behavior modification, for hypochondriasis, 186
Behavior, assessing, 19
Behavior, autocratic, 236
Behavior, theoretical models of, 8-9
Behavioral disturbances, in schizotypal personality disorder, 252
Behavioral model of behavior, 9
Behavioral theory
  of anorexia nervosa, 260
  of mood disorders, 119
  of obsessive-compulsive disorder, 152
  of pain disorder, 188
  of paraphilias, 334
  of somatoform disorders, 175
  of substance abuse, 275

Behavioral therapy, 26, 28-29
  for acute distress disorder, 146
  for amphetamine abuse, 284
  for body dysmorphic disorder, 182
  for cocaine abuse, 294
  dialectical, 232, 233
  for female sexual arousal disorder, 339
  for nicotine dependence, 305
  for opioid abuse, 311
  for panic disorder, 156
  for somatoform disorders, 178
  types of, 182
Bennies, 282
Benzodiazepine abuse, 314-319
  causes of, 315
  characteristics of, 314
  diagnosis of, 316
  effects of, 314-315
  and health hazards and impairments, 315
  nursing interventions for, 319
  signs and symptoms of, 315-316
  treatment of, 316-319
Benzodiazepines
  for anxiety disorders, 164-165t
  for generalized anxiety disorder, 149
  for panic disorder, 157
Bereavement, 67, 68, 88, 90
Berne's model of behavior, 9
Beta amyloid, 82, 83
Beta-adrenergic blockers
  for anxiety disorders, 164-165t
  for social phobia, 159
Big D, 294
Bill of rights for mental health patients, 31
Binge eating, 259, 264
Biofeedback, for generalized anxiety disorder, 149
Biological theory
  of anorexia nervosa, 260
  of antisocial personality disorder, 223
  of avoidant personality disorder, 228
  of borderline personality disorder, 231
  of bulimia nervosa, 265
  of dissociative disorders, 204
  of eating disorders, 258
  of gender identity, 324
  of paraphilias, 334
  of personality disorders, 221

---

i refers to an illustration; t refers to a table.

Bipolar disorders, 119-125
    causes of, 121, 139, 140
    characteristics of, 119-120
    classifying, 120-121
    diagnosis of, 122
    nursing interventions for, 122-125
    signs and symptoms of, 121-122,
        138, 140
    treatment of, 122
Bisexual identity, 324
Bisexuality, 324
Black pepper oil, 190
Blackouts, 205
Blood pressure, in alcohol
        withdrawal, 279t
Blotter acid, 295
Blow, 290
Blunt, 287
Boarding homes, 106
Body dysmorphic disorder, 179-180,
        200, 202
    causes of, 180
    characteristics of, 179-180
    diagnosis of, 181
    nursing interventions for, 182-183
    signs and symptoms of, 180-181,
        199, 201
    treatment of, 181-182
Body language, 11
Body sensations, heightened, and
        somatization, 175
Bolt, 300
Boo, 287
Boppers, 300
Borderline personality disorder,
        230-235
    causes of, 231
    characteristics of, 230-231
    diagnosis of, 232
    nursing interventions for, 234-235
    signs and symptoms of, 231-232,
        253, 255
    treatment of, 232-234
Bowel changes
    in anorexia nervosa, 259
    in bulimia nervosa, 265
Brain abnormalities, and
        schizophrenia, 96, 114, 116
Brain scans, in schizophrenia, 101
Brief respite homes, 106
Broccoli, 287
Bromelain, 190
Bulimia nervosa, 264-268
    causes of, 265
    characteristics of, 264

Bulimia nervosa (continued)
    complications of, 264-265
    diagnosis of, 266
    medication guidelines for, 268
    nursing interventions for, 267-268,
        270, 271
    signs and symptoms of, 265-266
    treatment of, 266-267, 269, 270
Bullet, 300
Bupropion, 131
    for nicotine dependence, 305
BuSpar
    for anxiety disorders, 166-167t
    for generalized anxiety disorder, 149
Buspirone
    for anxiety disorders, 166-167t,
        171, 172
    for generalized anxiety disorder, 149

C
C, 290
Caffeine, common sources of, 287,
        320, 322
Caffeine intoxication, 285-286
Caffeine withdrawal, 286
CAGE questionnaire, 24
Cannabis
    characteristics of, 287-288
    effects of, 288
Cannabis abuse, 287-290
    causes of, 288
    diagnosis of, 289
    and health hazards and
        impairments, 288
    nursing interventions for, 290
    risk factors for, 288-289
    signs and symptoms of, 289
    treatment of, 289-290
Caplan's model of behavior, 8
Capsaicin, 190
Carbamazepine, for bipolar
        disorders, 122
Cardiopulmonary complications
    alcohol dependence and, 277
    anorexia nervosa and, 259
Cardiovascular disease, smoking
        and, 304
Care plan, 25
Care settings, for elderly people, 72-74
Cartwheels, 282
Case management, as standard of
        care, 7
Catapres, for nicotine dependence, 305
Catatonic schizophrenia, 107-110,
        115, 116

Certification, 5
Chamomile, 190
Checklist for Autism in Toddlers, 49
Child abuse, and dissociative identity
        disorder, 212
Childhood, disorders of, 39-64
Childhood Autism Rating Scale, 49
Childhood development, 40-41
Children
    communicating with, 42, 61, 63
    depression in, 53-57, 62, 63
    mental illness in, 40-42
    sexual development in, 328, 329
    stress-related disorders in, 177-178
Chlorpromazine, 102
Cigarette smoking, 302
Cinnamon, 190
Clang associations, 98, 114, 115
Clarify, 295
Clarifying, as communication tool, 13
Climax, 300
Clonidine, for nicotine
        dependence, 305
Clozapine, 102, 103-104
Clozaril, 102
Cocaethylene, 291
Cocaine
    characteristics of, 290-291
    effects of, 291
Cocaine abuse, 290-294
    causes of, 292
    diagnosis of, 293
    nursing interventions for, 294
    physiologic effects of, 291-292
    signs and symptoms of, 292
    treatment of, 293-294
Cocaine addiction severity test, 24
Cocaine assessment profile, 24
Cocaine binge, 291
Codeine overdose, 320, 321
Codeine, 306
Cognitive assessment scale, 24
Cognitive capacity screening
        examination, 24
Cognitive decline, age-related, 80-82,
        88, 89, 90
Cognitive development, 41
Cognitive performance, in elderly
        people, 67
Cognitive theory
    of gender identity, 324
    of mood disorders, 119
    of schizotypal personality
        disorder, 252

i refers to an illustration; t refers to a table.

Cognitive therapy, 27
    for acute distress disorder, 146
    for amphetamine abuse, 284
    for body dysmorphic disorder, 182
    for cocaine abuse, 294
    for dissociative fugue, 211
    for generalized anxiety disorder, 149
    for obsessive-compulsive personality
        disorder, 245
    for opioid abuse, 311
    for panic disorder, 156
    for schizoid personality disorder, 250
    for somatoform disorders, 178
Coke, 290
Colombian, 287
Communication
    with children and adolescents, 42
    nontherapeutic, 13, 14
    nonverbal, 11-12
    patient, 11-14
    therapeutic, 12-14
    verbal, 11
Communication barriers, reducing,
    11, 12-13
Communication models of behavior, 9
Community education programs, 74
Compensation, as defense
    mechanism, 21
Competence, 33-34
    assessing, 20
Compliance, 75, 109
Computed tomography, in schizo-
    phrenia, 101
Concrete thinking, excessive, 98
Conduct disorder, 51-53
Confidential information,
    disclosing, 33
Confidentiality, for older adults, 71
Conflict resolution therapy, for
        borderline personality
        disorder, 233
Confusion, in alcohol withdrawal, 279t
Consultation, as standard of care, 7
Contingency management, for cocaine
        abuse, 293
Conversion disorder, 191-195
    causes of, 193-194
    characteristics of, 191-193
    diagnosis of, 194-195
    nursing interventions for, 195
    risk factors for, 194
    signs and symptoms of, 194,
        200, 201
    treatment of, 195
Coping skills, improving, 306

Counseling
    for alcohol dependence, 280
    as standard of care, 7
Couples therapy, for gender identity
        disorder, 341
Crack, 290
Crank, 282, 290
Creative therapies
    for dissociative fugue, 211
    for obsessive-compulsive personality
        disorder, 245
Crisis homes, 106
Crisis intervention, 27
Crystal, 282, 319, 321
Crystal supergrass, 312
Cultural considerations, 16
    in somatoform disorders, 174-175
Cyclothymic disorder, 125-127
Cylert, for attention deficit
        hyperactivity disorder, 46-47t

D

Darvocet, 306
Date rape drug, 295
Day care, adult, 74
Daydreams, 203
Deep breathing, 187
Defense mechanisms, assessing, 20, 21
Deinstitutionalization, 30
Delirium, as communication
        barrier, 13
Delirium tremens, 319
Delta-1-tetrahydrocannabinol, 288
Delusions, 98, 115, 116
    in bipolar disorders, 120
    as communication barrier, 13
    in schizophrenia, 98, 99
Dementia
    as communication barrier, 13
    multi-infarct, 86
    vascular, 86-88
Dementia of Alzheimer's type, 82-86
    causes of, 82-84
    characteristics of, 82
    diagnosis of, 84-85
    nursing interventions for, 85-86
    signs and symptoms of, 84, 89, 90
    treatment of, 85
Demerol, 306
Denial, as defense mechanism, 21
Denver Developmental Screening
        test, 60
Depakote
    for bipolar disorders, 122
    for mood disorders, 134-135t

Dependent personality disorder,
        235-238
    causes of, 236
    characteristics of, 235-236
    diagnosis of, 237
    nursing interventions for, 238,
        254, 255
    signs and symptoms of, 236-237
    treatment of, 237
Depersonalization disorder, 206-207,
        215, 216, 217
Depression
    in adolescents, 2
    in adults versus children, 54
    in bipolar disorders, 119, 120,
        121, 124
    in cyclothymic disorder, 126
    major. *See* Major depression.
    in older adults, 67-69
    secondary, 129
    unipolar, 53
Desensitization, 28
    for agoraphobia, 147
    for social phobia, 159
    for specific phobia, 163
Desire phase, of sexual response cycle,
        330, 344, 346
Desyrel, 131
Detoxification programs, 26, 317
Development, childhood, 40-41
Developmental abnormalities, and
        schizophrenia, 96
Dexamethasone depression test, for
        major depressive disorder, 131
Dexedrine, for attention deficit
        hyperactivity disorder, 46-47t
Dexies, 282
Dextroamphetamine, 283
    for attention deficit hyperactivity
        disorder, 46-47t
Dextromethorphan, 295
Dextromethorphan use, assessing
        for, 299
Diagnosis, 6, 25
*Diagnostic and Statistical Manual of
        Mental Disorders*, 3, 4
Diagnostic Drawing Series, 205
Dialectical behavior therapy, 232, 233
Diazepam, for anxiety disorders,
        164-165t
Disorganized schizophrenia, 110-111
Displacement, as defense
        mechanism, 21
Dissociation, in acute distress dis-
        order, 145

i refers to an illustration; t refers to a table.

Dissociative amnesia, 208-210, 216, 218
Dissociative Disorders Interview Schedule, 205
Dissociative disorders, 203-218
  causes of, 204-205
  characteristics of, 204
  classifying, 204
  evaluation and diagnosis of, 205
Dissociative Experiences Scale, 205, 216, 217
Dissociative fugue, 210-212, 215, 217
Dissociative identity disorder, 212-214
  promoting recovery from, 214
Disulfiram, 280
Disulfiram reaction, 280, 319, 321
Diuresis, forced, for cocaine abuse, 293
Documentation, in evaluation, 30
Dolls, 314
Dolophine, 306
Dopamine, and schizophrenia, 95
Dosage calculations, 171, 172, 254, 255, 270, 271
Dosages, for older adults, 75
Draw-a-Person Test, 22, 24, 224
Drug abuse. See also Substance abuse.
  assessing for, 308
  consequences of, 273
  and mental illness, 30, 31
  neurobiologic theories of, 275
Drug administration, in older adults, 75
Drug detoxification programs, 317
Drug intoxication, nursing interventions for, 281
Drug overdose, nursing interventions for, 318
Drug rape, 295
Drug therapy
  for elderly people, 74-75
  in schizophrenia, 102-105
Dry-bed therapy, 178
DSM-IV-TR, 3, 4
Duramorph, 306
Duty to inform, 33
DXM, 295
Dynamic psychotherapy, for opioid abuse, 311
Dyskinesia Identification System, 75, 76-79i
Dyspareunia, 326, 327, 346, 347
Dysthymia, 127
Dysthymic disorder, 127-128
Dystonia, antipsychotics and, 104, 115, 116

E
Eating aptitudes test, 24
Eating disorders, 257-271. See also Anorexia nervosa; Bulimia nervosa.
  causes of, 258
  characteristics of, 257-258
  effects of, 258
Echolalia, 98
Echopraxia, 98
Ecstasy, 295
Ecstasy use, assessing for, 299
Ego, 8
Elavil
  for anxiety disorders, 166-167t
  for mood disorders, 132-133t
Elder abuse and neglect, 184
Elderly people
  assessment and treatment of, 70-71
  barriers to treatment of, 66
  care settings for, 72-74
  depression in, 2, 67-69
  disorders of, 65-91
  drug therapy for, 74-75
  and mental health, 66-67
  somatoform disorders in, 184
Electroconvulsive therapy, 27
  for major depressive disorder, 136, 139, 140, 141
  for schizophrenia, 107
Elephant tranquilizer, 312
Embalming fluid, 312
Emergency department, for elder care, 73
Emotional disorders, contributing factors to, 2
Encopresis, functional, 178
Enuresis, functional, 178
Environmental theory
  of anorexia nervosa, 260
  of avoidant personality disorder, 228
  of bulimia nervosa, 265
Erikson's theory of growth and development, 41
Eserine, for phencyclidine abuse, 313, 320, 322
Eskalith
  for bipolar disorders, 122
  for mood disorders, 134-135t
Essence, 295
Ethical issues, 31-35
Ethnicity, and somatoform disorders, 174-175
Eucalyptus oil, 190

Evaluation, 29-30
  as standard of care, 7
Excitement phase, of sexual response cycle, 330
Exhibitionism, 332, 345, 346
Existential model of behavior, 8
Exploration phase, of nurse-patient relationship, 10
Exposure and response technique, for obsessive-compulsive disorder, 152
Exposure therapy, for specific phobia, 163
Extrapyramidal effects, antipsychotics and, 104
Eysenck's model of behavior, 9

F
Factitious disorders, 192-193, 200, 202
Family, impact of schizophrenia on, 94
Family dynamics, and anorexia nervosa, 261
Family history, 17
Family living, for schizophrenics, 106
Family stress, and somatoform disorders, 175, 176
Family therapy, 27
  for antisocial personality disorder, 226
  for conversion disorder, 195
  for dissociative fugue, 211
  for gender identity disorder 341
  for hypochondriasis, 186
  for somatoform disorders, 178
Fantasy, as defense mechanism, 21
Female orgasmic disorder, 326, 338-340, 345, 346
Female sexual arousal disorder, 326, 338-340
Fennel, 190
Fentanyl, 306
Fetishism, 332, 334, 345, 346
  transvestic, 333
Flake, 290
Flashbacks, 297
Flight of ideas, 98
Flooding, 28, 182
Flumazenil, for benzodiazepine abuse, 316
Fluoxetine
  for anxiety disorders, 164-165t
  for major depression, 56-57t, 62, 63
  for mood disorders, 132-133t
Fluphenazine, 103
Flush, sexual, 330

i refers to an illustration; t refers to a table.

Focusing, as communication tool, 14
Formication, 283
Foster homes, 106
François, Donatien Alphonse, 333
Frankl's model of behavior, 8
Freebase, 290
Freud's model of behavior, 8
Freud's theory of growth and
        development, 41
Frotteurism, 333
Fugue, 205
    dissociative, 210-212, 215, 217
Functional dementia scale, 24
Functional encopresis, 178
Functional enuresis, 178
Funding cuts, 30

G

Gamma-aminobutyric acid
    and generalized anxiety
        disorder, 148
    in phencyclidine abuse, 312
Gases, inhaling, 300
Gastrointestinal complications, alcohol
        dependence and, 277, 279t
Gender, and personality disorders, 220
Gender identity, 324, 340
Gender identity disorder, 340-342,
        345, 347
Gender role, 324
General adaptation syndrome, 3
Generalized anxiety disorder, 147-150,
        171, 172
    causes of, 148
    characteristics of, 147-148
    diagnosis of, 149
    nursing interventions for, 150
    risk factors for, 148
    signs and symptoms of, 148-149
    treatment of, 149-150
Genetic theory
    of alcohol dependence, 276
    of anorexia nervosa, 260
    of antisocial personality
        disorder, 223
    of avoidant personality disorder, 228
    of borderline personality
        disorder, 231
    of bulimia nervosa, 265
    of eating disorders, 258
    of personality disorders, 221
    of schizotypal personality
        disorder, 251
    of substance abuse, 275
Geodon, 105

Geropsychiatric nursing, 70
Geropsychiatric units, inpatient, 73
Ginger, 190
Glading, 300
Global deterioration scale, 24
Gluey, 300
Glutamate, and schizophrenia, 96
Goals, evaluation and, 29
Goal setting, 25
Grannies, 282
Grass, 287
Green and whites, 314
Green dragon, 294
Grief, 68, 69
Grindler's model of behavior, 9
Group homes, transitional, 106
Group therapy, 27, 242
    for antisocial personality
        disorder, 226
    for body dysmorphic disorder, 181
    for borderline personality
        disorder, 232
    for dependent personality
        disorder 237
    for dissociative fugue, 211
    for hypochondriasis, 186
    for obsessive-compulsive personality
        disorder, 245
    for opioid abuse, 311
    for posttraumatic stress disorder, 169
    for schizoid personality disorder,
        249, 250
    for schizotypal personality
        disorder, 253
Growth and development, theories of,
        40, 41
Guardianship, 33

H

H, 307
Haldol, 103
Hallucinations
    in alcohol withdrawal, 279t
    bereavement and, 68
    in bipolar disorders, 120
    as communication barrier, 13
    nursing interventions for,
        108-109, 110
    in schizophrenia, 98
Hallucinogen abuse, 294-299
    assessing for, 299
    causes of, 297-298
    diagnosis of, 298
    and health hazards and
        impairments, 296-297

Hallucinogen abuse (continued)
    nursing interventions for, 298-299
    and psychological impairments, 297
    signs and symptoms of, 298
    treatment of, 298
Hallucinogens
    characteristics of, 294
    classifying, 294-296
    effects of, 296
Haloperidol, 103
Hardware, 300
Hashish. See Cannabis.
Head cleaner, 300
Health promotion and maintenance,
        as standards of care, 7
Health teaching, as standard of care, 7
Hearing, impaired, as communication
        barrier, 12
Hearts, 282
Hemodialysis, for cocaine abuse, 293
Hemoperfusion, for cocaine abuse, 293
Hepatic complications, alcohol
        dependence and, 277
Herb, 287
Herbal therapy, 190
Heroin, 306
Heterosexuality, 324
High, amphetamine, 282
Highway hypnosis, 203
Hippie crack, 300
Histrionic personality disorder, 238-241
    causes of, 239
    characteristics of, 238-239
    and conversion disorder, 194
    diagnosis of, 240
    nursing interventions for, 241
    signs and symptoms of, 239-240
    treatment of, 240-241
Hits, 290
Hog, 312
Home care, for elderly people, 72
Homeopathic remedies, 190
Homosexuality, 324, 325
Horse, 307
Hospitalization
    for anorexia nervosa, 263, 269, 270
    for antisocial personality
        disorder, 226
    for benzodiazepine abuse, 319
    for borderline personality disorder,
        233, 234
    for bulimia nervosa, 267
    for narcissistic personality
        disorder, 242
    partial, 74

i refers to an illustration; t refers to a table.

Huffing, 300
Humanistic model of behavior, 9
Hydrocodone, 306
Hydrotherapy, 190
Hypericum, 190
Hypnosis
  for conversion disorder, 195
  for dissociative amnesia, 209
  for dissociative fugue, 211
  for dissociative identity disorder, 214
  highway, 203
Hypnotic abuse, 314-319
  causes of, 315
  diagnosis of, 316
  and health hazards and
    impairments, 315
  nursing interventions for, 319
  signs and symptoms of, 315-316
  treatment of, 316-319
Hypnotics
  characteristics of, 314
  effects of, 314-315
Hypoactive sexual desire disorder, 326
Hypochondriasis, 183-187
  causes of, 184
  characteristics of, 183-184
  diagnosis of, 185-186
  nursing interventions for, 186-187,
    200, 202
  signs and symptoms of, 185,
    200, 202
  and somatization disorder, 175
  treatment of, 186
Hypomania
  in bipolar disorders, 119, 120
  in cyclothymic disorder, 125, 126
Hypothyroidism, and bipolar disorder,
  139, 140
Hypoxyphilia, sexual, 333

I

Id, 8
Identification, as defense
    mechanism, 21
Identity
  during dissociative fugue, 210
  gender, 324, 340
Imipramine
  for anxiety disorders, 166-167t
  for functional enuresis, 178
  for mood disorders, 132-133t
Implementation, 6-7, 26-29
Implosion therapy, 28, 182
Impotence, 342, 343

Impressions, sharing, as
    communication tool, 14
Independent living, for
    schizophrenics, 106
Inderal, for anxiety disorders, 164-165t
Individual therapy, 27
  for antisocial personality
    disorder, 224-225
  for avoidant personality
    disorder, 229
  for borderline personality
    disorder, 232
  for dependent personality
    disorder, 237
  for gender identity disorder, 341
  for histrionic personality
    disorder, 240
  for hypochondriasis, 186
  for obsessive-compulsive personality
    disorder, 245
  for paranoid personality
    disorder, 247
  for posttraumatic stress disorder, 169
  for schizoid personality disorder,
    249, 250
  for schizotypal personality
    disorder, 252
Infantilism, 333
Infants, sexual development in, 328
Information, offering, as
    communication tool, 14
Informed consent, right to, 32
Inhalant abuse, 300-302
Intellectualization, as defense mecha-
    nism, 21
Interpersonal model of behavior, 8
Interventions, American Nurses
    Association standards and, 6-7
Interview, 15-18, 16, 248
Interview do's and don'ts, 16
Intoxication, 274
Introductory phase, of nurse-patient
    relationship, 10
Introjection, as defense mechanism, 21
Inversine, for nicotine
    dependence, 305
Involuntary admission, 34
IQ, and mental retardation, 58
Isocarboxazid, for mood disorders,
    132-133t
Isolation, as defense mechanism, 21

J

Joints, 287
Junk, 307

K

K, 295
Ket, 295
Ketamine, 295
Ketamine use, assessing for, 299
Kick, 300
Killer joint, 312
Kit, 295

L

La belle indifference, 194
Language difficulties, as
    communication barrier, 12
Lavender oil, 190
Learning theory
  of dissociative disorders, 204
  of panic disorder, 155
Legal and ethical issues, 31-35
Lemon balm, 190
Level of consciousness, assessing, 18
Levomethadyl acetate, for opioid
    abuse, 311
Limits, setting, in personality
    disorders, 227
Lithium
  for autistic disorder, 49
  for bipolar disorders, 122
  for mood disorders, 134-135t
  patient teaching for, 123, 139, 140
Lithium toxicity, 123, 140, 141
Locker room, 300
Long-term care, 72-73
Loose association, 98
"Lost" time, 205, 208
Love boat, 312
LSD. *See* Lysergic acid diethylamide.
Lysergic acid diethylamide, 294, 320
Lysergic acid diethylamide use,
    assessing for, 299
Lung cancer, smoking and, 304

M

Magical thinking, 98
  in schizotypal personality
    disorder, 252
Magnetic resonance imaging, in
    schizophrenia, 101
Major depression
  characteristics of, 53
  in children and adolescents, 53-57
  diagnosis of, 55
  nursing interventions in, 56-57
  possible causes of, 53-54
  risk factors for, 54

i refers to an illustration; t refers to a table.

Major depression (continued)
  signs and symptoms of, 54
  treatment of, 55-56, 56-57t
Major depressive disorder, 128-138
  body dysmorphic disorder and, 180
  causes of, 129-130
  characteristics of, 128-129
  diagnosis of, 131
  nursing interventions for, 136-138
  signs and symptoms of, 130
  treatment of, 131-136
Male erectile disorder, 326, 342, 343
Male orgasmic disorder, 326
Malingering, 192, 211
Mania, in bipolar disorders, 119, 120,
    121, 122, 139, 141
Manic-depressive disorders. See
    Bipolar disorders.
Manipulation, in histrionic personality
    disorder, 240
Marijuana. See Cannabis.
Marjoram oil, 190
Marplan, for mood disorders, 132-133t
Mary Jane, 287
Maslow's model of behavior, 9
Masochism, sexual, 333
Massage, 190
Masturbation, 325
  compulsive, 331
May's model of behavior, 8
MDMA, 295
Meadowsweet, 190
Mecamylamine, for nicotine
    dependence, 305
Medical model of behavior, 9
Medical record, 30
Medical research, consent to, 32-33
Medication history, 18
Meditation, 187, 206
Mellaril, 103
Memory, assessing, 19
Mental disorders
  in children, 40-42
  classification of, 3-4
  contributing factors to, 2
Mental health field, changes in, 2-4
Mental health programs, community, 2
Mental Health Systems Act, 31
Mental retardation
  causes of, 59
  characteristics of, 57-59
  in children and adolescents, 57-61
  classifying, 58, 61, 62, 63, 64
  diagnosis of, 59-60
  nursing interventions for, 60-61

Mental retardation (continued)
  signs and symptoms of, 59
  treatment of, 60
Mental status evaluation, 18-22, 43
Meperidine, 306
Mescaline, 295
Mescaline use, assessing for, 299
Meth, 282
Methadone, 306, 310
Methamphetamine, 282
Methamphetamine abuse, 283
N-methyl-D-aspartate receptors, 312
3,4-methylenedioxymethampheta-
    mine, 295
Methylphenidate
  for attention deficit hyperactivity
      disorder, 46-47t, 61, 63
  for autistic disorder, 49
Michigan alcoholism screening test, 24
Microdot, 294
Milieu therapy, 7, 26, 234
Mini-Mental Status Examination, 24
Minnesota Multiphasic Personality
    Inventory, 22, 24
Minnesota Multiphasic Personality
    Inventory-2, 224
Minors, rights of, 32
Mirtazapine, 131
MJ, 287
Moban, 103
Modeling behavior, for social
    phobia, 159
Molindone, 103
Monoamine oxidase inhibitors
  for anxiety disorders, 164-165t
  food interactions and, 138
  for major depressive disorder, 131
  for mood disorders, 132-133t
Mood, assessing, 19
Mood disorders, 117-141
  causes of, 118-119
  challenges in caring for patients
      with, 118
  characteristics of, 118
  classifying, 118
  pharmacologic therapy for, 132-135t
Mood swings, in borderline
    personality disorder, 232
Morphine, 306
Motor impairment, in alcohol
    withdrawal, 279t
Multidisciplinary care, 30
Multi-infarct dementia, 86
Multiple personality disorder, 212,
    215, 217

Munchausen syndrome, 192-193
Munchausen syndrome by proxy, 193

N
NA, 311
Naloxone, for opioid overdose,
    320, 321
Naltrexone
  for alcohol dependence, 280
  for nicotine dependence, 305
  for opioid abuse, 311
Narcan
  for nicotine dependence, 305
  for opioid overdose, 320, 321
Narcissistic personality disorder,
    241-243
Narcoanalysis, for conversion
    disorder, 195
Narcotics. See Opioid abuse; Opioids.
Nardil, for anxiety disorders, 164-165t
National Association for Children of
    Alcoholics, 282
Naturopathic manipulative
    therapy, 190
Navane, 103
Nefazodone, 131
Negative thought stopping, for social
    phobia, 159
Neologisms, 98
Neurobiologic theories, of substance
    abuse, 275
Neurofibrillary tangles, 82
Neuroleptic malignant syndrome,
    antipsychotics and, 104
Neurologic complications, alcohol
    dependence and, 277
Nicotine, effects of, 303
Nicotine dependence, 302-306
  adverse effects of, 304
  causes of, 303
  characteristics of, 302-303
  diagnosis of, 304
  and health hazards and
      impairments, 303
  nursing interventions for, 306
  risk factors for, 303-304
  treatment of, 305-306
Nicotine-mimicking agents, 305
Nicotine replacement, 305
Nicotine withdrawal, 304
Nitrites, inhaling, 300
Norepinephrine
  and panic disorder, 155
  and schizophrenia, 96
Nose candy, 290

i refers to an illustration; t refers to a table.

Numorphan, 306
Nurse practice acts, 5
Nurse-patient relationship, 10-11
Nursing diagnoses, developing, 25
Nursing model of behavior, 9
Nutritional therapy, 190

O

O, 307
Obsessive-compulsive disorder,
    150-153
Obsessive-compulsive personality
    disorder, 243-246
  causes of, 244
  characteristics of, 243-244
  diagnosis of, 244
  nursing interventions for, 245-246
  signs and symptoms of, 244
  treatment of, 245
Offering information, as
    communication tool, 14
Olanzapine, 105
Omnibus Budget Reconciliation Act of
    1987, 72, 73, 89, 91
OP, 307
Ope, 307
Opioid abuse, 306-311
  assessing for, 308
  causes of, 307
  diagnosis of, 309
  and health hazards and
      impairments, 307
  nursing interventions for, 311
  signs and symptoms of, 307-309
  treatment of, 309-311
Opioid agonists, 310, 311
Opioid detoxification, 310
Opioid intoxication or overdose, 309
Opioid replacement therapy, 310
Opioids
  characteristics of, 306-307
  effects of, 307
Opioid withdrawal, 310
Opium, 307
Oranges, 282
Orem's model of behavior, 9
Orgasmic disorders, 326
Orgasm phase, of sexual response
    cycle, 330
Orientation phase, of nurse-patient
    relationship, 10
ORLAAM, for opioid abuse, 311
Orthostatic hypotension,
    antipsychotics and, 104

Outcome identification, as standard of
    care, 6
Outpatient therapy
  for dependent personality
      disorder, 237
  for older adults, 71
Overdose, nursing interventions
    for, 318
Oxycodone, 306
OxyContin, 306
Oxymorphone, 306
Ozone, 312

P

Pain disorder, 188-191
  causes of, 188
  characteristics of, 188
  diagnosis of, 189
  nursing interventions for, 191
  signs and symptoms of, 189
  treatment of, 189-190
Panic attacks, 154, 171, 172
  and agoraphobia, 146, 147
  narcissistic personality disorder
      and, 241
Panic disorder, 154-157
Paranoid personality disorder,
    246-248, 253, 255
Paranoid schizophrenia, 111-112,
    114, 115
Paranoid thinking, as communication
    barrier, 13
Paraphilias, 331-338. *See also specific*
    type.
  causes of, 334
  characteristics of, 331-332
  diagnosis of, 335
  nursing interventions for, 336-337
  risk factors for, 335
  treatment of, 335-336
  types of, 331, 333, 345, 347
Parkinsonism, antipsychotics and, 104
Parnate, for anxiety disorders, 164-165t
Paroxetine
  for anxiety disorders, 164-165t
  for major depression, 56-57t
Passive smoking, 304
Patient requests, responding to, 34
Paxil
  for anxiety disorders, 164-165t
  for major depression, 56-57t
PCP. *See* Phencyclidine abuse.
Peace pill, 312

Pediatric autoimmune neuropsychi-
    atric disorders associated with
    streptococcal infections
    (PANDAS), 151
Pedophilia, 334, 345, 347
Pemoline, for attention deficit
    hyperactivity disorder, 46-47t
Peplau's model of behavior, 8, 9
Peppermint, 190
Percocet, 306
Perls' model of behavior, 8
Perphenazine, 103
Personality and projective tests,
    224-225
Personality disorder clusters, 220, 221,
    222, 254, 255
Personality disorders, 219-258
  causes of, 221
  characteristics of, 220, 254, 256
  evaluation in, 221-222
  incidence and course of, 220-221
  interviewing patients with,
      guidelines for, 248
  and somatoform disorders, 174
  treatment of, 222, 253, 255
Personality profile, 17
Personality tests, 22-25
Phencyclidine abuse, 312-314
  treatment of, 320, 322
Phenelzine sulfate, for anxiety dis-
    orders, 164-165t
Phobia, specific. *See* Specific phobia.
Phobias, common, 161-163. *See also*
    specific type.
Physical dependence, 274
Physical examination, in personality
    disorders, 221
Physostigmine, for phencyclidine
    abuse, 313, 320, 322
Piaget's theory of growth and
    development, 41, 62, 64
Planning, 6, 25
Plateau phase, of sexual response
    cycle, 330
Polypharmacy, 75, 197
Poor man's pot, 300
Poppers, 300
Pornography dependency, 331
Positive conditioning, 29
Possession trance, 206
Posttraumatic stress disorder, 166-170
  causes of, 168
  characteristics of, 166-168
  diagnosis of, 168-169
  nursing interventions for, 169-170

i refers to an illustration; t refers to a table.

Posttraumatic stress disorder
    (*continued*)
  risk factors for, 168
  signs and symptoms of, 168, 170, 172
  treatment of, 169
Pot, 287
Preinteraction phase, of nurse-patient relationship, 10
Premature ejaculation, 326, 342-344, 346, 347
Prescriptions, writing, 5, 7
Primary gain, 175, 176
Privacy, right to, 33
Professional practice standards, 5
Projection, as defense mechanism, 21
Projective tests, 22-25, 224-225
Prolixin, 103, 114, 116
Promiscuity, protracted, 331
Propoxyphene, 306
Propranolol, for anxiety disorders, 164-165t
Prozac
  for anxiety disorders, 164-165t
  for major depression, 56-57t
  for mood disorders, 132-133t
Pseudoseizures, 194
Psilocybin use, assessing for, 299
Psilocybin, 295
Psychedelic drugs. *See* Hallucinogen abuse.
Psychiatric assessment tests, 22-25
Psychiatric care, trends and concerns in, 30-31
Psychiatric complications, alcohol dependence and, 277
Psychiatric disorders, classifying, 3-4
Psychiatric nurse
  clients of, 5
  level of performance of, 5, 10
  role of, 4-10
  scope of practice for, 5-10
  skills of, 5
Psychiatric nursing, theoretical frameworks of, 8-9, 10
Psychoanalysis, for somatoform disorders, 178
Psychoanalytic model of behavior, 8
Psychoanalytic theory
  of mood disorders, 119
  of obsessive-compulsive disorder, 152
  of schizotypal personality disorder, 252

Psychobiologic theory
  of somatization, 175-176
  of substance abuse, 275
Psychodynamic theory
  of conversion disorder, 194
  of gender identity, 324
  of narcissistic personality disorder, 242
  of obsessive-compulsive personality disorder, 244
  of personality disorders, 221
  of somatoform disorders, 175
Psychological examination, in personality disorders 222
Psychological theory
  of anorexia nervosa, 260
  of dissociative disorders, 204
  of pain disorder, 188
  of schizotypal personality disorder, 252
  of substance abuse, 276
Psychosexual development, 41
Psychosocial development, 41
Psychosocial history, 17
Psychosocial treatment, for schizophrenia, 105
Psychosomatic disorders. *See* Somatoform disorders.
Psychotherapy, 26, 27
  for acute distress disorder, 145
  for alcohol dependence, 280
  for anorexia nervosa, 262
  for antisocial personality disorder, 225, 226
  for borderline personality disorder, 232
  for bulimia nervosa, 267
  for dependent personality disorder, 237
  for depersonalization disorder, 207
  for dissociative fugue, 211
  for female sexual arousal disorder, 339
  for gender identity disorder, 341
  for generalized anxiety disorder, 149
  for histrionic personality disorder, 240
  for hypochondriasis, 186
  for mood disorders, 135
  for narcissistic personality disorder, 242
  for obsessive-compulsive personality disorder, 245
  for opioid abuse, 311
  for pain disorder, 189

Psychotherapy (*continued*)
  for paranoid personality disorder, 247
  for personality disorders, 222
  for posttraumatic stress disorder, 169
  for schizoid personality disorder, 249
  for schizophrenia, 106-107
  for schizotypal personality disorder, 252
  as standard of care, 7
Psychotropic drugs, in older adults, 75
Puberty, 329, 341
Pulse rate, in alcohol withdrawal, 279t
Purging, 259, 269, 270

Q

Questions, 13
Quetiapine, 105

R

Rationalization, as defense mechanism, 22
Reaction formation, as defense mechanism, 22
Recall, assessing, 19, 20
Red dragon, 294
Reefer, 287
Regression, 22, 98
Rehabilitation
  for alcohol dependence, 280
  for amphetamine abuse, 284
  for benzodiazepine abuse, 319
  for cocaine abuse, 293
  for inhalant abuse, 302
  for schizophrenia, 105, 107
Relationship, nurse-patient, 10-11
Relaxation response, 187
Relaxation techniques, 187
  for panic disorder, 156
Remeron, 131
Repression, as defense mechanism, 22
Reproductive and sexual rights, 33
Residual schizophrenia, 113
Resolution phase
  of nurse-patient relationship, 10
  of sexual response cycle, 331
Response prevention, 29, 182
Responses, inappropriate, as communication barrier, 12
Restating, as communication tool, 14
Restraints, 34-35
ReVia, for alcohol dependence, 280
Reward pathways, 303
Rhabdomyolysis, phencyclidine abuse and, 312

i refers to an illustration; t refers to a table.

Risperdal, 105
Risperidone, 105
Ritalin, for attention deficit
    hyperactivity disorder, 46-47t
Roach, 287
Roaches, 314
Robo, 295
Rock, 290
Rocket fuel, 312
Rogers' model of behavior, 9
Rolling, 295
Romazicon, for benzodiazepine
    abuse, 316
Rose oil, 190
Rosemary oil, 190
Roy, Sister, 9
Rush, 300
    amphetamine, 282

S

Sad syndrome, 151
Sade, Marquis de, 333
Sadism, sexual, 333
Sarapin, 190
Schizoid personality disorder, 248-251,
    254, 256
    causes of, 249
    characteristics of, 248-249
    diagnosis of, 249
    nursing interventions for, 250-251
    signs and symptoms of, 249
    treatment of, 249-250
Schizophrenia
    catatonic, 107-110, 115, 116
    causes of, 95-97
    classifying, 93
    course of, 100-101
    diagnosis of, 101
    disorganized, 110-111
    effects of, 93
    nursing interventions for, 108-109,
        110, 115, 116
    onset and course of, 93-94
    paranoid, 111-113
    phases of, 99-100
    prognosis in, 93, 94
    psychophysiologic markers of, 97
    psychosocial and economic issues
        of, 94
    residential options in, 106
    residual, 113
    versus schizotypal personality
        disorder, 251
    signs and symptoms of, 98

Schizophrenia (continued)
    symptom categories for, 97-99,
        114, 116
    treatment of, 102-107
    undifferentiated, 113-114
Schizophrenic disorders, 92-116
Schizotypal personality disorder,
    251-253, 255
Screening Test for Autism in 2-Year-
    Olds, 49
Seclusion, 34-35
Secondary gain, 175, 176
Secondhand smoke, 304
Sedative abuse, 314-319
    causes of, 315
    diagnosis of, 316
    and health hazards and
        impairments, 315
    nursing interventions for, 319
    signs and symptoms of, 315-316
    treatment of, 316-319
Sedative effects, antipsychotics
    and, 104
Sedatives
    characteristics of, 314
    effects of, 314-315
Seizures, in alcohol withdrawal, 279t
Selective serotonin reuptake inhibitors
    for anxiety disorders, 164-165t
    for autistic disorder, 49
    for major depressive disorder, 131
    for mood disorders, 132-133t
    patient teaching for, 269
Self-care activities, promoting, 7
Self-destructive behavior, assessing,
    20, 22
Self-injury, 22
Selye, Hans, 3
Sensate focus exercises, for female
    sexual arousal disorder, 339
Sensory replacement agents, for
    nicotine dependence, 305
Sentence Completion Test, 22, 25, 225
Seroquel, 105
Serotonin, and generalized anxiety
    disorder, 148
Serotonin/norepinephrine reuptake
    inhibitors, for major depressive
    disorder, 131
Sertraline, for major depression,
    56-57t
Serzone, 131
Sex drive, assessing, 20
Sex offenders, 335
Sexual accessories, 332

Sexual aversion disorder, 326
Sexual behavior, abnormal, 324-325
Sexual desire, 330, 332
Sexual development, stages of,
    328-329
Sexual disorders, 323-347
    nursing interventions for, 336-337
    types of, 325
Sexual dysfunctions, 325-328
    categories of, 325
    types of, 326
Sexual flush, 330
Sexual hypoxyphilia, 333
Sexual identity, 324
Sexuality, 324
Sexual masochism, 333
Sexual orientation or preference, 324
Sexual pain disorders, 327-328
Sexual response cycle, 329-331
Sexual sadism, 333
Sharing impressions, as
    communication tool, 14
Silence, as communication tool, 12
Silver acetate, for nicotine
    dependence, 305
Sinsemilla, 287
Skinner's model of behavior, 9
Sleep disturbance, in alcohol
    withdrawal, 279t
Sleep terrors, 177, 200, 202
Sleepwalking, 177
Smoke, 287
    secondhand, 304
Smoking
    cigarette, 302
    passive, 304
Smooth pursuit, 97
Snappers, 300
Snow, 290
Snowball, 290
Social anxiety, schizotypal personality
    disorder and, 251
Social anxiety disorder, 157-159
Social interactions, in
    schizophrenia, 98
Social learning theory, of gender
    identity, 324
Social model of behavior, 8
Social phobia, 157-159, 170, 171, 172
Social skills training, for
    paraphilias, 335
Social theories
    of personality disorders, 221
    of substance abuse, 276
Solvents, volatile, inhaling, 300

i refers to an illustration; t refers to a table.

Somatization, 174
Somatization disorder, 196-199, 200
    common assessment finds in, 198
    hypochondriasis and, 175
Somatoform disorders, 173-202
    alternative therapies for, 190
    causes of, 175-176
    characteristics of, 174
    classifying, 174
    coexisting disorders and, 174
    cultural and ethnic factors and,
        174-175
    diagnosis of, 176
    in elderly people, 184
    treatment of, 176-178
Special K, 295
Specific phobia, 160-166
    causes of, 160, 162
    characteristics of, 160
    diagnosis of, 162
    nursing interventions for, 166
    signs and symptoms of, 162
    treatment of, 163
Speech
    assessing, 19
    in histrionic personality
        disorder, 238
    in schizophrenia, 98, 99
    in schizotypal personality
        disorder, 252
Speed, 282
Speedball, 290
Splitting, 230, 254, 256
Standards
    American Nurses Association, 5, 6-7
    professional practice, 5
Starvation, self-imposed, 259, 261
Stelazine, 103
Stimulants, for autistic disorder, 49
Streptococcal infection, and obsessive-
        compulsive disorder, 151
Stress
    and childhood disorders, 177-178
    and disease, 3
    and dissociative amnesia, 209
    and pain disorder, 188
    and somatoform disorders, 175, 176
Structural Clinical Interview for
        Dissociative Disorders, 205
Stuttering, 177
Sublimation, as defense
        mechanism, 22
Sublimaze, 306
Submissiveness, 236
Subpersonalities, 212

Substance abuse, 2. *See also* Drug
        abuse.
    causes of, 275-276
    characteristics of, 273
    consequences of, 273
    schizophrenia and, 94
    scope of, 274
    and somatization disorder, 196
    terminology of, 273-274
Substance abuse disorders, 272-323
Substance dependence, 274
Substance screening, in personality
        disorders, 222
Substitution, as defense
        mechanism, 21
Sugar, 294
Suggestive collaboration, as
        communication tool, 14
Suicidal tendencies
    assessing, 20, 22
    dissociative identity disorder
        and, 213
    recognizing, 137
Suicidal threat, responding to, 23
Suicide
    major depressive disorder and,
        128, 130
    schizophrenia and, 93
Suicide attempts, in adolescents, 53
Suicide rate, in adolescents, 2
Sullivan's model of behavior, 8
Superego, 8
Superweed, 312
Support groups
    for alcohol dependence, 280
    for avoidant personality
        disorder, 229
    for borderline personality
        disorder, 234
    for bulimia nervosa, 267
    for dependent personality
        disorder, 237
    for older adults, 71
    for schizoid personality disorder, 250
Sweating, in alcohol withdrawal, 279t
Szasz's model of behavior, 8

T

Tardive dyskinesia
    antipsychotics and, 104
    diagnoses for, 78-79
Teenagers. *See* Adolescents.
Tegretol, for bipolar disorders, 122
Telephone sex, 331

Termination phase, of nurse-patient
        relationship, 10
THC, 287
Thematic Apperception test, 22,
        25, 225
Therapeutic communication, 12-14
Therapeutic communities, for cocaine
        abuse, 294
Therapeutic relationship,
        establishing, 10
Thinking, disturbed, in schizotypal
        personality disorder, 252
Thioridazine, 103
Thiothixene, 103
Thorazine, 102
Thought blocking, 98
Thought content and pattern,
        assessing, 20
Thought disorders, as communication
        barrier, 12-13
Thought distortions, in schizophrenia,
        98, 99
Thought replacement, 182
Thought stopping, 29, 182
Thought switching, 29, 182
Tobacco use, 302, 303, 304
Tofranil
    for anxiety disorders, 166-167t
    for functional enuresis, 178
    for mood disorders, 132-133t
Token economy, 29
Tolerance, 274
Tornado, 290
Tourette syndrome, and obsessive-
        compulsive disorder, 151
Trancelike states, 206
Transvestic fetishism, 333
Tranylcypromine sulfate, for anxiety
        disorders, 164-165t
Trauma
    and acute distress disorder, 144, 145
    and dissociative amnesia, 209
    and pain disorder, 188
    and posttraumatic stress
        disorder, 166
Trazodone, 131
Treatment
    criteria for, 31
    right to, 31
    right to refuse, 32
    types of, 26-29
Tricyclic antidepressants, patient
        teaching for, 268
Trifluoperazine, 103
Trilafon, 103

i refers to an illustration; t refers to a table.